The Health Physics SOLUTIONS MANUAL

Introduction to Health Physics
Problems Made Easy

Herman Cember, Ph.D.
Professor Emeritus, Northwestern University and
Visiting Professor, Purdue University

Thomas E. Johnson, Ph.D.
Assistant Professor, Department of Preventive Medicine and Biometrics
Uniformed Services University of the Health Sciences

PS&E Publications
Silver Spring, Maryland

Published by:

PS&E Publications
(an imprint of Bartleby Press)
P.O. Box 1516
Silver Spring, MD 20915

Library of Congress Catalog Card Number: 98-68614
ISBN 0-9625963-6-1

Review questions in this book are from *Introduction to Health Physics, Third Edition* by Herman Cember, published by McGraw Hill and are reprinted with permission.

The authors gratefully acknowledge the assistance of Professor W.P. Roach at the Uniformed Services University of the Health Sciences.

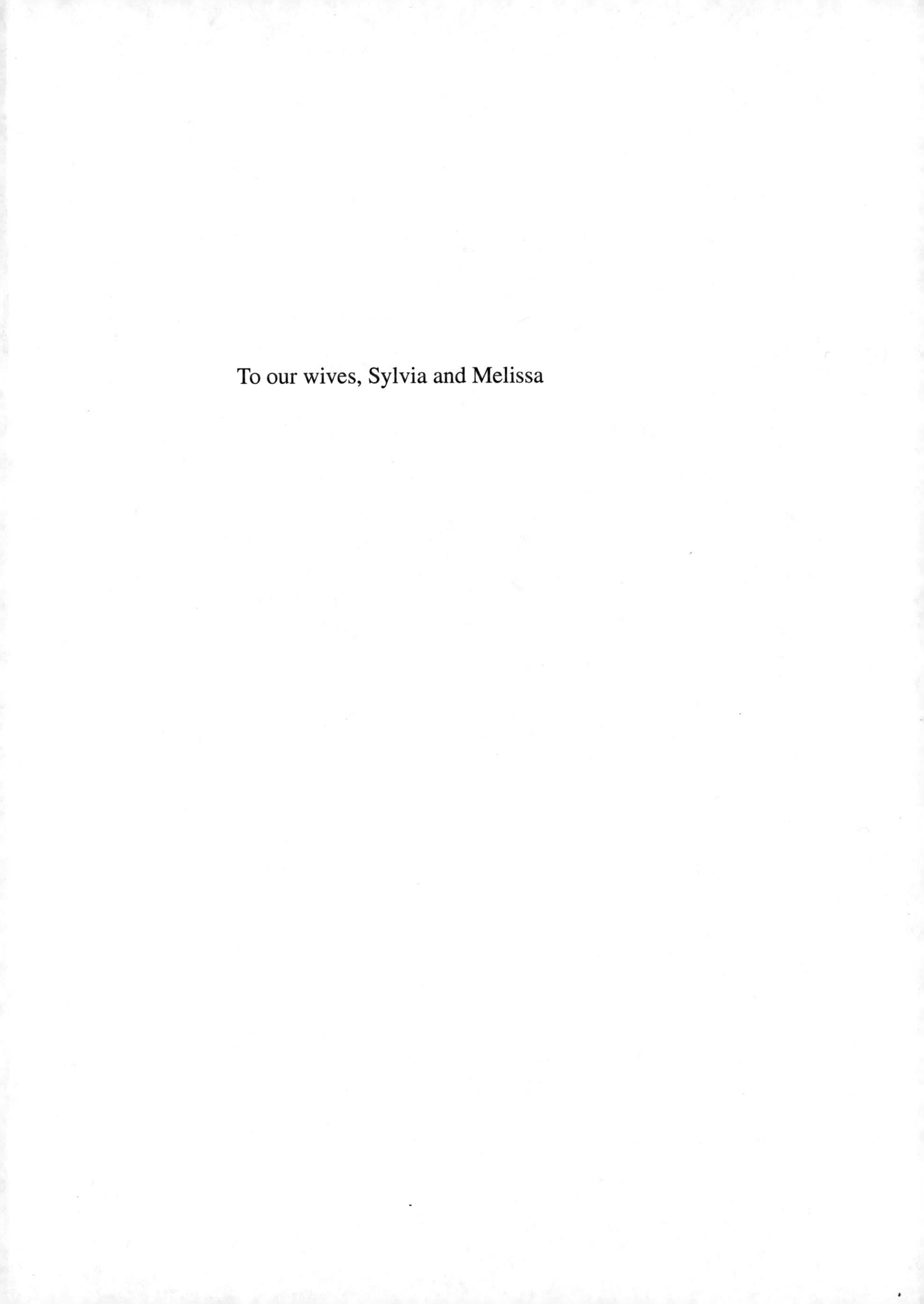

To our wives, Sylvia and Melissa

Contents

Introduction

The problems in the textbook *Introduction to Health Physics, 3rd edition*, are based mainly on Dr. Cember's experience as a practicing health physicist and teacher over a span of more than 40 years. They were formulated mainly to illustrate practical problems and the principles underlying the problem and its solution.

Although only one solution is shown for each problem, many of the problems have an answer that can be reached by more than one path.

As is true with all aspects of environmental and occupational health and safety, standards and calculational methods are continuously evolving and undergoing changes. Although the authors may attempt to do so, by practical necessity it is not possible for a textbook to keep current with the very latest recommendations, standards and computational methodology.

The purpose of a textbook, in contrast to a handbook or to a yearbook, is to present the basic ideas and principles on which standards an methodology are based. Thus, for example, in the field of ionizing radiation, the nomenclature, calculational methodology, the biological pharmaco-kinetic models (such as the successive lung models recommended by the NCRP and by the ICRP) and retention functions are undergoing continuous re-examination as more observational and scientific data become available. Even the basic radiation safety philosophy which forms the very basis for radiation safety standards has undergone a radical change from the concept of a "tolerance dose" to the zero threshold concept.

In the case of non-ionizing radiation too, we have changing methodologies. We recognize three radiation zones for the purpose of safety evaluation of RF and microwave radiation: the near, intermediate, and far fields. There are no sharp dividing lines that show where the near field ends and the far field begins. Rather, the transition from one to the other is very gradual. There is no definitive formulation, although there are several different formulas, for estimating the distance from an antenna to the end of the near field or to the beginning of the far field. Similarly, since there is no sharp boundary at the edge of a laser beam, and also because of the nonuniform (generally Gaussian) energy distribution across the beam, there are several different definitions of the beam diameter.

In the actual practice of health physics, the health physicist must be knowledgeable regarding the latest recommendations of the several non-governmental agencies, such as the American National Standards Institute (ANSI Standards), American Society for Testing Materials (ASTM), American Conference of Governmental Industrial Hygienists (ACGIH) These recommendations may be incorporated by reference directly into regulations, or may be applied in the interpretation of the regulations.

If the principles on which radiation safety is based are well understood, then the details of the continuing revisions may be easily applied to practical situations. The main purpose of these problems is to help to clarify these basic principles.

Solutions for Chapter 2
REVIEW OF PHYSICAL PRINCIPLES

2.1 Two blocks, of mass 0.1 kg and 0.2 kg, approach each other along a frictionless surface, at velocities 0.4 and 1 m/s, respectively. If the blocks collide, and remain together, calculate their joint velocity after the collision. **2.1**

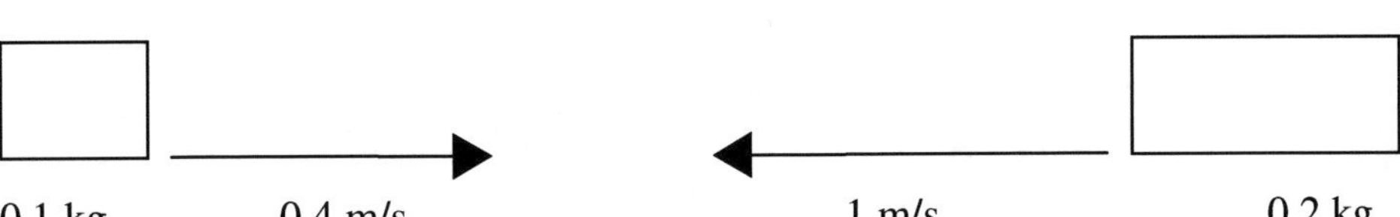

First, solve for the momentum of each block.

$p = mv$

0.1 kg × 0.4 m/s = 0.04 kg·m/s   0.2 kg × 1 m/s = 0.2 kg·m/s

Since the blocks are moving in opposite directions (remember that velocity has a direction associated with it), subtract the momentums:

0.04 kg·m/s – 0.2 kg·m/s = –0.16 kg·m/s

The negative sign indicates that after the blocks collide and join, they will have momentum to the left. Since the momentum of the 'combined' block is known, the velocity of the 'combined' block can be found.
The mass of the combined block is
0.1 kg + 0.2 kg = 0.3 kg

The momentum of the combined block is –0.16 kg·m/s

$$v = \frac{p}{m} = \frac{-0.16 \text{ kg} \cdot \text{m/s}}{0.3 \text{ kg}} = -0.53 \ \frac{\text{m}}{\text{s}}$$

So the 'combined' block would be moving at 0.53 m/s to the left.

2.2

2.2 A bullet whose mass is 50 g travels at a velocity of 500 m/s. It strikes a rigidly fixed wooden block, and penetrates a distance of 20 cm before coming to a stop.

(a) What is the deceleration of the bullet?

$$r = 20 \text{ cm} = 20 \text{ cm} \times \frac{1 \text{ meter}}{100 \text{ cm}} = 0.2 \text{ m}$$

$v = 500$ m/sec

$$m = 50 \text{ g} = 50 \text{ g} \times \frac{1 \text{ kg}}{1000 \text{ g}} = 0.05 \text{ kg}$$

Equation 2.5

$$W = \frac{1}{2} mv^2 = \frac{1}{2} \times 0.05 \text{ kg} \times \left(500 \frac{\text{m}}{\text{s}}\right)^2 = 6.25 \times 10^3 \ \frac{\text{kg} \cdot \text{m}^2}{\text{s}^2}$$

Equation 2.6A;

$$f = \frac{W}{r} = \frac{6.25 \times 10^3 \ \frac{\text{kg} \cdot \text{m}^2}{\text{sec}^2}}{0.2 \text{ m}} = 3.125 \times 10^4 \ \frac{\text{kg} \cdot \text{m}}{\text{sec}^2} = 3.125 \times 10^4 \text{ N}$$

Using equation 2.1,

$$a = \frac{f}{m} = \frac{3.125 \times 10^4 \ \frac{\text{kg} \cdot \text{m}}{\text{sec}^2}}{0.05 \text{ kg}} = 6.25 \times 10^5 \ \frac{\text{m}}{\text{sec}^2}$$ is the deceleration of the bullet.

(b) What was the decelerating force? 3.125×10^4 N as calculated in part (a).

(c) What was the initial momentum of the bullet?

Equation 2.77 is modified to use the initial velocity of the bullet, instead of the speed of light, so that

$$p = mv = 0.05 \text{ kg} \times 500 \text{ m/s} = 25 \ \frac{\text{kg} \cdot \text{m}}{\text{sec}}$$

(d) What was the impulse of the collision?

Equation 2.10A gives the impulse:

$f\,\Delta t = m\Delta v$

Since $m\Delta v$ is simply the change in momentum, and the final velocity is zero, the impulse is:

$25\ \frac{\text{kg}\cdot\text{m}}{\text{sec}}$ per second, which can be written as 25 N·sec

2.3 Compute the mass of the earth, assuming it to be a sphere of 25,000 miles circumference, if at its surface it attracts a mass of 1 g with a force of 980 dynes. **2.3**

$$f = 980\ \text{dynes} \times \frac{1\times 10^{-5}\,\text{N}}{1\text{dyne}} = 9.8 \times 10^{-3}\,\text{N} = 9.8 \times 10^{-3}\ \frac{\text{kg}\cdot\text{m}}{\text{sec}^2}$$

$$m_1 = 1\ \text{g} \times \frac{1\ \text{kg}}{1000\ \text{g}} = 1 \times 10^{-3}\ \text{kg}$$

Find the radius of the earth:

Circumference is 25,000 miles:

$$25000\ \text{miles} \times \frac{5280\ \text{ft}}{1\ \text{mile}} \times \frac{0.3048\ \text{m}}{1\ \text{ft}} = 4.02 \times 10^7\ \text{meters}$$

Circumference = $C = 2\pi\, r$

$r = \frac{C}{2\pi} = \frac{4.02\times 10^7\ \text{meters}}{2\pi} = 6.4 \times 10^6$ meters is the radius of the earth.

Solving equation 2.28 for m_2, the mass of the earth:

$$F = \frac{Gm_1m_2}{r^2}$$

$$G = 6.67 \times 10^{-11}\ \frac{\mathrm{N \cdot m^2}}{\mathrm{kg^2}}$$

$$m_2 = \frac{Fr^2}{Gm_1} = \frac{9.8 \times 10^{-3}\ \mathrm{N} \times \left(6.4 \times 10^{6}\ \mathrm{m}\right)^2}{6.67 \times 10^{-11}\ \frac{\mathrm{N \cdot m^2}}{\mathrm{kg^2}} \times \left(1 \times 10^{-3}\ \mathrm{kg}\right)} = 6.02 \times 10^{24}\ \mathrm{kg}$$

2.4

2.4 An automobile weighing 2000 kg, and going a speed of 60 km/hr, collides with a truck weighing 5 metric tons that was moving at right angles to the direction of the auto at a speed of 4 km/hr. If the two vehicles become joined in the collision, what is the magnitude and direction of their velocity after the collosion?

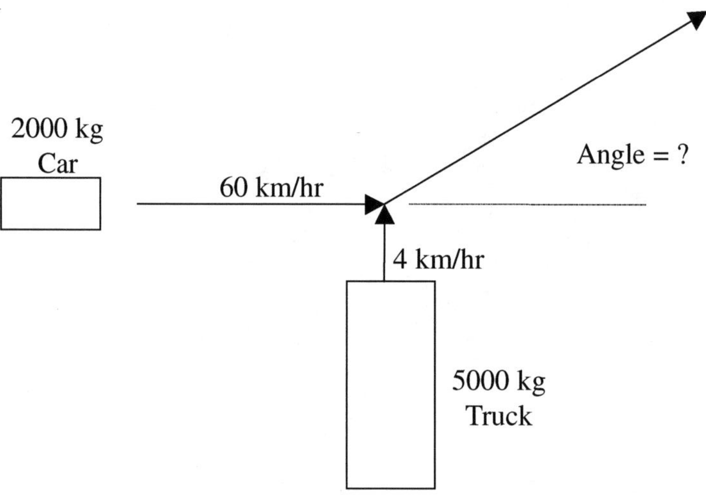

Calculate the initial momentum for each vehicle:

$p = mv$

$p_{car} = 2000\ \mathrm{kg} \times 60\ \mathrm{km/hr} = 120{,}000\ \mathrm{kg \cdot km/hr}$

$p_{truck} = 5000\ \mathrm{kg} \times 4\ \mathrm{km/hr} = 20{,}000\ \mathrm{kg \cdot kg/hr}$

Recalling that momentum is a vector, we can add the momentum for each vehicle as we would the sides of a triangle:

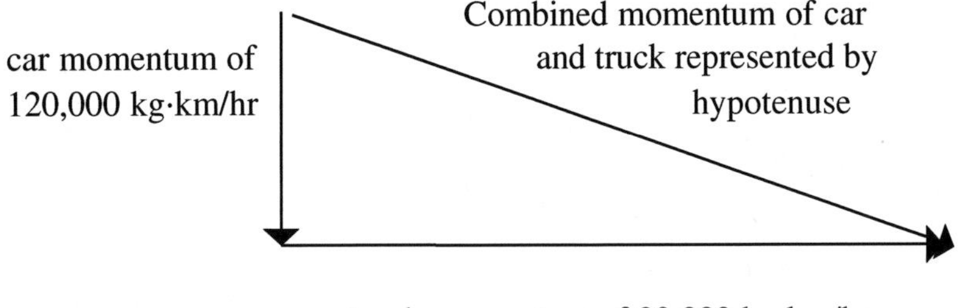

truck momentum of 20,000 kg·km/hr

Adding together the momenta, we obtain:

$$\sqrt{(120{,}000)^2 + (20{,}000)^2} = 121655\,\frac{\text{kg}\cdot\text{km}}{\text{hr}}$$

Because the car and truck 'stuck together', the combined mass of the truck and car must be used:

2000 kg + 5000 kg = 7,000 kg

Knowing the momentum, we can find the velocity of the 'combined' truck and car after the collision using the momentum equation in a rearranged form:

$v = \dfrac{p}{m} = \dfrac{121655\,\dfrac{\text{kg}\cdot\text{km}}{\text{hr}}}{7000\text{ kg}} = 17.38\dfrac{\text{km}}{\text{hr}}$ is the velocity of the combined truck and car after the collision.

The direction of the car and truck is determined through geometry, using the same momentum vectors. The angle corresponding to the tangent of the opposite over the adjacent sides would yield the angle θ:

$$\tan\theta = \frac{\text{opposite side}}{\text{adjacent side}} = \frac{20{,}000\dfrac{\text{kg}\cdot\text{km}}{\text{hr}}}{120{,}000\dfrac{\text{kg}\cdot\text{km}}{\text{hr}}} = 0.1667$$

Taking the inverse tangent, we obtain: $\tan^{-1}(0.1667) = 9.46°$

2.5

2.5 A small electrically charged sphere of mass 0.1 g hangs by a thread 100 cm long between two parallel vertical plates spaced 6 cm apart. If 100 volts are across the plates, and if the charge on the sphere is 10^{-9} coulombs, what angle does the thread make in the vertical direction?

$m = 1 \cdot 10^{-4}$ kg
$L = 1$ m
$d = 0.06$ m
$V = 100$ V
$q = 10^{-9}$ C
$\phi = ?$

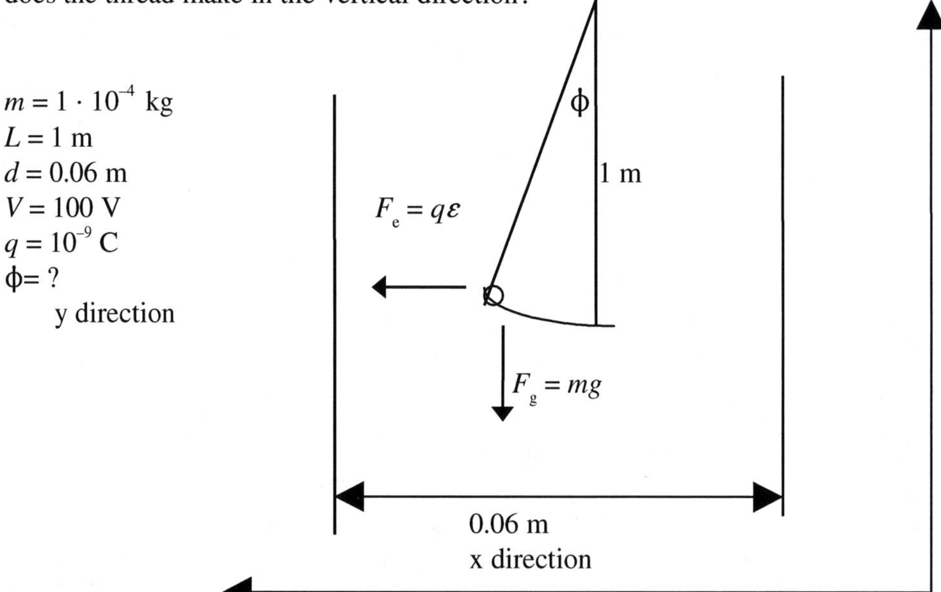

At static equilibrium, the sum of the horizontal forces, $F_H = 0$, and the sum of the vertical forces, $F_V = 0$. The only forces acting on the sphere are:
1. The force of gravity in the negative y direction ($F_g = -mg$)
2. The electrical force exerted by the plates ($F_e = q\varepsilon$)
3. The tension force on the string (T), which can be resolved into two components, one in the y direction $\{T(\cos\theta)\}$ and a second in the x direction $\{T(\sin\theta)\}$.

$$\Sigma F_H = F_e - T(\sin\theta) = 0$$
$$\Sigma F_V = -mg + T(\cos\theta) = 0$$

Dividing ΣF_H by ΣF_V, we have

$$\frac{q\varepsilon}{mg} = \frac{\sin\theta}{\cos\theta} = \tan\theta$$

According to equation 2.39

$$\varepsilon = \frac{V}{d}$$

Substituting into the equilibrium equation gives

$$\frac{q}{mg} \times \frac{V}{d} = \tan\theta$$

$$\tan\theta = \frac{1 \times 10^{-9}\ \text{C}}{1 \times 10^{-4}\,\text{kg} \times 9.8\ \frac{\text{m}}{\text{s}^2}} \times \frac{100\ \text{V}}{0.06\ \text{m}} = 1.7 \times 10^{-3}$$

$\theta = 0.00170$ radians = 0.092°
Note: for very small angles, the tangent of $\theta = \theta$ radian

2.6 A capacitor has a capacitance of 10 μF. How much charge must be removed to cause a decrease of 20 volts across the capacitor? **2.6**

$10\ \mu\text{F} = 10 \times 10^{-6}\,\text{F}$
Use equation 2.66 to solve for the charge:

$$Q = C \times V = 10 \times 10^{-6}\ \text{F} \times\ 20\ \text{volts} = 2 \times 10^{-4}\ \text{C}$$

2.7 A small charged particle whose mass is 0.01 g remains stationary in space when it is placed in an upward directed electric field of 10 V/cm. What is the charge on the particle? **2.7**

First, convert to SI units:
$\mathcal{E}$ = 10 V/cm = 1000 V/m
m = 0.01 g = 0.00001 kg
q = ? coulombs

The force acting in the downward direction is equal to the force acting in the upward direction. The electric force is 'pushing' the particle up, while the force of gravity is 'pulling' it down.

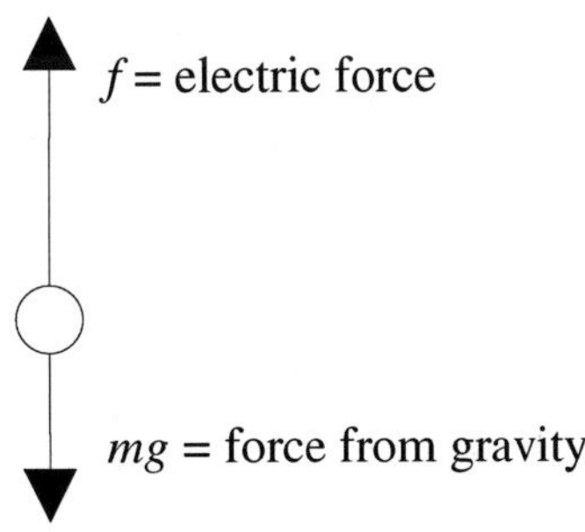

Since the particle is not moving, the forces are equal. Equation 2.36 gives the force from the electric field:

$$f = \varepsilon q$$

Equating the electric force and the gravitational force:

$$\varepsilon q = m g$$

Solving for q;

$$q = \frac{m \times g}{\varepsilon} = \frac{0.00001 \text{ kg} \times 9.8 \frac{\text{m}}{\text{sec}^2}}{1000 \frac{\text{V}}{\text{m}}} = 9.8 \times 10^{-8} \text{ C}$$

2.8

2.8 A 1 micron diameter droplet of oil, whose specific gravity is 0.9, is introduced into an electric field between two large parallel plates, separated by 5 mm, across which is placed a potential difference V volts. If the oil droplet carries a net charge of 100 electrons, how many volts must be placed across the plates if the droplet is to remain suspended between the plates?

To accomplish the desired outcome, the downward force of gravity, mg, acting on the drop must equal the upward electrical force, $q\varepsilon$, acting on the drop.

Find the volume of the droplet:

$$1 \text{ micron} = 1 \text{ micron} \times \frac{1 \times 10^{-6} \text{ m}}{1 \text{ micron}} = 1 \times 10^{-6} \text{ meter diameter}$$

$$\text{Volume of sphere} = \frac{4}{3}\pi r^3 = \frac{4}{3}\pi\left(\frac{1 \times 10^{-6}}{2}\right)^3 = 5.24 \times 10^{-19} \text{ m}^3$$

Find the mass of the droplet using the specific gravity:

mass = volume × density

$$\left[5.24 \times 10^{-19} \text{ m}^3 \times \frac{1 \times 10^6 \text{cm}^3}{1 \text{ m}^3}\right] \times \left[\frac{0.9 \text{ g}}{\text{cm}^3} \times \frac{\text{kg}}{1000 \text{ g}}\right] = 4.7 \times 10^{-16} \text{ kg}$$

The gravitational force can be found using equation 2.1;

$F_g = ma = mg$

$g = 9.8\ \text{m/s}^2$

The electrical force, F_e, is given by equation 2.36,

$F_e = q\varepsilon$

and the electric field intensity, ε, is related to the plate separation distance, d, and the voltage across the plates, V, by equation 2.39,

$$\varepsilon = \frac{V}{d}$$

Substituting the expression for ε, and equating the upward electrical force to the downward gravitational force, we have

$$q\frac{V}{d} = mg$$

$$V = \frac{dmg}{q} = \frac{5 \times 10^{-3}\,\text{m} \times 4.7 \times 10^{-16}\,\text{kg} \times 9.8\frac{\text{m}}{\text{sec}^2}}{100\ \text{electrons} \times 1.6 \times 10^{-19}\ \frac{\text{C}}{\text{electron}}}$$

$V = 1.44$ volts

2.9 A diode vacuum tube consists of a cathode and an anode spaced 5 mm apart. If 300 volts are placed across the electrodes, **2.9**
(a) What is the velocity of the electron midway between the electrodes, and at the instant of striking the plate, if the electrons are emitted by the cathode with zero velocity?

$$\text{KE} = \frac{1}{2}mv^2$$

$$v = \sqrt{\frac{2 \times \text{KE}}{m}}$$

The kinetic energy of an electron after having been accelerated to 300 V is 300 eV, or 300 eV × 1.6 × 10^{-19}J/eV = 4.8 × 10^{-17} J. Substituting the values for the kinetic energy and for the electron mass and solving for v gives the velocity at the instant of striking the plate:

$$v(300\ \text{eV}) = \sqrt{\frac{2 \times 4.8 \times 10^{-17}\ \text{J}}{9.11 \times 10^{-31}\ \text{kg}}} = 1.03 \times 10^{7}\ \frac{\text{m}}{\text{s}}$$

Since v is proportional to $(\text{KE})^{1/2}$, and since potential, and hence the electron's kinetic energy midway between the plates is ½ the total voltage drop, the electron's velocity at that point is

$$v(150\ \text{eV}) = \sqrt{\frac{1}{2}} \times 1.03 \times 10^{7}\ \frac{\text{m}}{\text{s}} = 0.73 \times 10^{7}\ \frac{\text{m}}{\text{s}}$$

(b) If the plate current is 20 mA, what is the average force exerted on the anode?

m = mass of each electron = 9.1 × 10^{-31} kg

Now calculate the number of electrons striking the plate in a one second time period;

$$20\ \text{mA} \times \frac{1\ \text{A}}{1000\ \text{mA}} \times \frac{1\frac{\text{C}}{\text{sec}}}{1\text{A}} \times \frac{6.2 \times 10^{18}\ \text{electrons}}{1\ \text{C}} = 1.24 \times 10^{17}\ \text{electrons per sec}$$

From part (a);

The electron's velocity is 1.03 × 10^{7} m/s and changes to zero after it impacts the plate.

Rearranging equation 2.10a;

$$f\Delta t = m\Delta v$$

$$f = \frac{m\Delta v}{\Delta t} = \frac{\left[9.1 \times 10^{-31}\ \frac{\text{kg}}{\text{electron}} \times \left(1.24 \times 10^{17}\ \text{electrons}\right)\right] \times \left(1.03 \times 10^{7}\ \frac{\text{m}}{\text{sec}}\right)}{\text{sec}}$$

f = 1.16 × 10^{-6} N

2.10

2.10 Calculate the ratios v/c and m/m_0 for a 1 MeV electron and for a 1 MeV proton.

Energy of the electron

$m_0 = 9.11 \times 10^{-31}$ kg
$c = 3 \times 10^8$ m/sec

$$E = 1 \text{ MeV} = 1 \text{ MeV} \times \frac{1.6 \times 10^{-13}\text{ J}}{\text{MeV}} = 1.6 \times 10^{-13} \text{ J}$$

Using equation 2.20

$$E = m_0 c^2 \left(\frac{1}{\sqrt{1 - \frac{v^2}{c^2}}} - 1 \right)$$

Using the respective values:

$$1.6 \times 10^{-13} \text{ J} = (9.11 \times 10^{-31} \text{ kg}) \times (3 \times 10^8 \text{ m/s})^2 \times \left(\frac{1}{\sqrt{1 - \frac{v^2}{c^2}}} - 1 \right)$$

$$v/c = 0.941$$

Find the electron mass ratios using equation 2.4;

$$\frac{m}{m_0} = \frac{1}{\sqrt{1 - \frac{v^2}{c^2}}} = \frac{1}{\sqrt{1 - 0.941^2}} = 2.96$$

For a 1 MeV proton

$m_0 = 1.67 \times 10^{-27}$ kg
$c = 3 \times 10^8$ m/sec

$$E = 1 \text{ MeV} = 1 \text{ MeV} \times \frac{1.6 \times 10^{-13}\text{ J}}{\text{MeV}} = 1.6 \times 10^{-13} \text{ J}$$

Using the relativistic expression for the kinetic energy, equation 2.20

$$E = m_0c^2\left(\frac{1}{\sqrt{1-\frac{v^2}{c^2}}}-1\right)$$

Substituting in the values:

$$1.6 \times 10^{-13}\text{ J} = 1.67 \times 10^{-27}\text{ kg} \times (3 \times 10^8\text{m/s})^2 \times \left(\frac{1}{\sqrt{1-\frac{v^2}{c^2}}}-1\right)$$

$$v/c = 0.046$$

Find the proton mass ratios using equation 2.4;

$$\frac{m}{m_0} = \frac{1}{\sqrt{1-\frac{v^2}{c^2}}} = \frac{1}{\sqrt{1-0.941^2}} = 1.001$$

2.11

2.11 Assuming an uncertainty in the momentum of an electron to be equal to one half its momentum, calculate the uncertainty in position of a 1 MeV electron.

$m_0 = 9.11 \times 10^{-31}$ kg
$c = 3 \times 10^8$ m/sec

$$E = 1\text{ MeV} = 1\text{ MeV} \times \frac{1.6 \times 10^{-13}\text{ J}}{\text{MeV}} = 1.6 \times 10^{-13}\text{ J}$$

Using equation 2.20

$$E = m_0c^2\left(\frac{1}{\sqrt{1-\frac{v^2}{c^2}}}-1\right)$$

Substituting align the values into the relativistic energy equation, we have

$$1.6 \times 10^{-13}\ \text{J} = 9.11 \times 10^{-31}\ \text{kg} \times (3 \times 10^{8}\text{m/s})^2 \times \left(\frac{1}{\sqrt{1-\frac{v^2}{c^2}}} - 1 \right)$$

$$v/c = 0.941$$

$v = 0.941 \times 3 \times 10^{8}$ m/sec $= 2.823 \times 10^{8}$ m/s

Find the electron mass using equation 2.4;

$$m = \frac{m_0}{\sqrt{1-\frac{v^2}{c^2}}} = \frac{9.11 \times 10^{-31}}{\sqrt{1-0.941^2}} = 2.7 \times 10^{-30}\,\text{kg}$$

The momentum of an electron is:

$m = 2.7 \times 10^{-30}$ kg

$v = 2.823 \times 10^{8}$ m/s

$p = mv = 2.7 \times 10^{-30}$ kg $\times\ 2.823 \times 10^{8}$ m/s $= 7.6 \times 10^{-22}$ kg · m/sec

Assuming the uncertainty associated with the momentum is one half the momentum:

$\Delta p = 1/2 \times 7.6 \times 10^{-22}$ kg · m/sec $= 3.8 \times 10^{-22}$ kg · m/sec

According to Heisenberg's Uncertainty Principle, equation 2.81,

$$\Delta x \times \Delta p \geq \frac{h}{2\pi}$$

Therefore, the minimum uncertainty $= \Delta x = \dfrac{h}{2\pi\Delta p}$

$$\Delta x = \frac{6.6 \times 10^{-34}\ \frac{\text{kg} \cdot \text{m}^2}{\text{sec}}}{2 \times \pi \times 3.8 \times 10^{-22}\ \frac{\text{kg} \cdot \text{m}}{\text{sec}}} = 2.77 \times 10^{-13}\ \text{m}$$

2.12

2.12 If light quanta have mass, they should be attracted by the earth's gravity. To test this hypothesis a parallel beam of light is directed horizontally at a receiver 10 miles away. How far would the photons have fallen during their flight to the receiver if their quanta have mass?

Calculate the time it takes for light to travel 10 miles:

$$10 \text{ miles} \times \frac{5280 \text{ ft}}{1 \text{ mile}} \times \frac{0.3048 \text{ m}}{1 \text{ ft}} = 1.61 \times 10^4 \text{ m}$$

Since light travels at 3×10^8 m/sec and 10 miles is 1.61×10^4 m

$$1.61 \times 10^4 \text{ m} \times \frac{\text{sec}}{3 \times 10^8 \text{ m}} = 5.36 \times 10^{-5} \text{ sec}$$ is the time it takes to travel 10 miles.

Velocity in the vertical direction at time zero is zero, so the distance fallen is given by:

$$y = \frac{1}{2} g t^2 = \frac{1}{2} \times 9.8 \frac{\text{m}}{\text{sec}^2} \times \left(5.36 \times 10^{-5} \text{sec}\right)^2 = 1.4 \times 10^{-8} \text{ meters}$$

2.13

2.13 The maximum wavelength of UV light observing the photoelectric effect in tungsten is 2730 angstroms. What will be the kinetic energy of photoelectrons produced by UV radiation of 1500 angstroms?

Use equation 2.76,
$h = 6.614 \times 10^{-34}$ J · sec
$c = 3 \times 10^8$ m/sec
λ = 1500 angstroms = 1.5×10^{-7} meters

$$E = h \frac{c}{\lambda}$$

$$E = 6.614 \times 10^{-34} \text{ J·s} \times \frac{3 \times 10^8 \frac{\text{m}}{\text{sec}}}{1.5 \times 10^{-7} \text{ m}} \times \frac{\text{eV}}{1.6 \times 10^{-19} \text{ J}} = 8.27 \text{ eV}$$

Thus 8.27 eV is the total energy carried by the incident photon. Since the energy carried by the 2730 angstrom UV photon is the energy, ϕ, that binds the electron to the atom,

$$\phi = h\frac{c}{\lambda} = 6.614 \times 10^{-34}\ \text{J} \cdot \text{sec} \times \frac{3 \times 10^{8}\ \frac{\text{m}}{\text{sec}}}{2.73 \times 10^{-7}\ \text{m}} \times \frac{\text{eV}}{1.6 \times 10^{-19}\ \text{J}} = 4.54\ \text{eV}$$

The kinetic energy of the photoelectron (E_{pe}) is equal to the difference between the photon energy $\left[h\frac{c}{\lambda}\right]$ and the energy required to remove the electron from the atom (the binding energy, ϕ).

$$E_{pe} = h\frac{c}{\lambda} - \phi$$

So the energy available to the photoelectron is the energy of the 1500 angstrom light less the energy of ionization:

$$E_{pe} = h\frac{c}{\lambda} - \phi = 8.27\ \text{eV} - 4.54\ \text{eV} = 3.73\ \text{eV}$$

2.14 Calculate the uncertainty in position of an electron that was accelerated across a potential difference of 100,000 ± 100 volts. **2.14**

Since the total energy is equal to the kinetic energy of the electron plus the rest mass energy;

$$E = E_k + E_0$$

To calculate the uncertainty in momentum (Δp), relativistic effects must be considered. The relationship among total energy, rest mass energy and momentum under relativistic conditions can be represented geometrically as a right triangle:

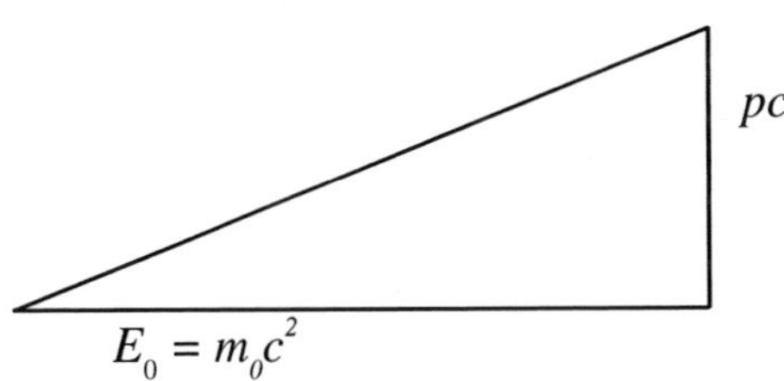

$$E = E_k + E_0 = mc^2$$
$$E^2 = E_0^2 + p^2c^2$$

Replacing E obtain:

$$(E_k + E_0)^2 = E_0^2 + p^2 c^2$$

Expanding the expression:

$$\left(E_k^2 + 2E_k E_0 + E_0^2\right) = E_0^2 + p^2 c^2$$

Collecting terms and solving for p;

$$\left(E_k^2 + 2E_k E_0\right) = p^2 c^2$$

$$p = \frac{1}{c}\sqrt{\left(E_k^2 + 2E_k E_0\right)}$$

From equation 2.32, the kinetic energy of the electron is equal to the charge times the applied voltage ($E_k = Vq$), so replacing E_k;

$$p = \frac{1}{c}\sqrt{\left(V^2 q^2 + 2(Vq)E_0\right)}$$

Differentiate momentum (p) with respect to voltage,

$$p = \frac{1}{c}\left(V^2 q^2 + 2(Vq)E_0\right)^{\frac{1}{2}}$$

$$dp = \frac{1}{c} \times \frac{1}{2}\left(V^2 q^2 + 2(Vq)E_0\right)^{-\frac{1}{2}} (q^2 2V dV + 2qE_0 dV)$$

$$dp = \frac{1}{c} \times \frac{1}{2}\left(V^2 q^2 + 2(Vq)E_0\right)^{-\frac{1}{2}} (q^2 2V + 2qE_0)dV$$

Where:

$c = 3 \times 10^8$ m/sec
$V = 1 \times 10^5$ volts
$dV = 100 \times 2 = 200$ V (accounts for the ±100 volts)
$q = 1.6 \times 10^{-19}$ C (charge on electron)
$m_0 = 9.11 \times 10^{-31}$ kg (Appendix A)
$c = 3 \times 10^8$ m/sec (Appendix A)

$$E_0 = m_0c^2 = 9.11 \times 10^{-31}\ \text{kg} \times \left(3\times10^{8}\ \frac{\text{m}}{\text{sec}}\right)^2 = 8.2\times10^{-14}\ \frac{\text{kg}\cdot\text{m}^2}{\text{sec}^2}$$

Placing values into the equation to find the change in momentum:

$$dp = \frac{1}{c}\times\frac{1}{2}\left(V^2q^2 + 2(Vq)E_0\right)^{-\frac{1}{2}}(q^2 2V + 2qE_0)dV$$

Please note that the following equation is in three lines:

$$dp = \frac{1}{3\times10^{8}\ \frac{\text{m}}{\text{sec}}}\times\frac{1}{2}\times$$

$$\left(\left(1\times10^{5}\,\text{V}\right)^2\times\left(1.6\times10^{-19}\,\text{C}\right)^2 + 2\times\left(\left(1\times10^{5}\,\text{V}\right)\times1.6\times10^{-19}\,\text{C}\right)\times8.2\times10^{-14}\ \frac{\text{kg}\cdot\text{m}^2}{\text{sec}^2}\right)^{-\frac{1}{2}}\times$$

$$\times\left(\left(1.6\times10^{-19}\,\text{C}\right)^2\times2\times\left(1\times10^{5}\,\text{V}\right) + 2\times\left(1.6\times10^{-19}\,\text{C}\right)\times8.2\times10^{-14}\ \frac{\text{kg}\cdot\text{m}^2}{\text{sec}^2}\right)\times200\text{V}$$

$$dp = 1.94\times10^{-25}\ \frac{\text{kg}\cdot\text{m}}{\text{sec}}$$

According to equation 2.81 where:

$$\Delta x\times\Delta p \geq \frac{h}{2\pi}$$

$$\Delta x \geq \frac{h}{2\pi\Delta p} = \frac{6.6\times10^{-34}\ \frac{\text{kg}\cdot\text{m}^2}{\text{sec}}}{2\times\pi\times1.94\times10^{-25}\ \frac{\text{kg}\cdot\text{m}}{\text{sec}}} = 5.4\times10^{-10}\ \text{m}$$

2.15(a) What voltage is required to accelerate a proton from zero velocity to a velocity corresponding to a de Broglie wavelength of 0.01 angstroms? **2.15**

First, find the momentum associated with this wavelength with equation 2.79:

$$\lambda = 0.01 \text{ Å} = 0.01 \text{ Å} \times \frac{1 \times 10^{-10} \text{ m}}{1 \text{ Å}} = 1 \times 10^{-12} \text{ meters}$$

$$mv = \frac{h}{\lambda} = \frac{6.63 \times 10^{-34} \text{ J} \cdot \text{sec}}{1 \times 10^{-12} \text{ m}} = 6.63 \times 10^{-22} \frac{\text{kg} \cdot \text{m}}{\text{sec}}$$

The equation from example 2.19 must be used to allow for relativistic effects. To determine whether relativistic effects are important, substitute the reset mass of the proton, $m_0 = 1.673 \times 10^{-27}$ kg into the equation for momentum in example 2.19 and solve for β:

$$p = mv = \frac{m_0}{\sqrt{1-\beta^2}} \beta c$$

Replacing values:

$$6.63 \times 10^{-22} \frac{\text{kg} \cdot \text{m}}{\text{sec}} = \frac{1.672 \times 10^{-27} \text{ kg}}{\sqrt{1-\beta^2}} \times \beta \times (\, 3 \times 10^{8} \frac{\text{m}}{\text{sec}})$$

$$\beta = \frac{v}{c} = 1.32 \times 10^{-3}$$

$$v = 1.32 \times 10^{-3} \times (3 \times 10^{8} \text{ m/sec}) = 3.95 \times 10^{5} \text{ m/sec}$$

Since $\beta < 0.1$, relativistic effects are negligible, and

$$\text{KE} = \frac{1}{2} mv^2$$

$$\text{KE} = \frac{1}{2} \times 1.673 \times 10^{-27} \text{ kg} \times \left(3.95 \times 10^{5} \frac{\text{m}}{\text{s}}\right)^2 \times \frac{1 \text{ eV}}{1.6 \times 10^{-19} \text{ J}} = 816 \text{ eV}$$

Since q(proton) = q(electron), accelerating voltage = 816 V

(b) What would be the kinetic energy of an electron with this wavelength?

The momentum associated with this wavelength would be the same as for the proton, the mass and velocity would be different, however:

$$mv = 6.63 \times 10^{-22}\ \frac{\text{kg}\cdot\text{m}}{\text{sec}}$$

The equation from example 2.19 must be used to allow for relativistic effects;
$c = 3 \times 10^8$ m/sec
$m_0 = 9.11 \times 10^{-31}$ kg

$$\beta = \frac{v}{c}$$

$$p = mv = \frac{m_0}{\sqrt{1-\beta^2}}\beta c$$

Replacing values:

$$6.63 \times 10^{-22}\ \frac{\text{kg}\cdot\text{m}}{\text{sec}} = \frac{9.11\times10^{-31}\,\text{kg}}{\sqrt{1-\beta^2}} \times \beta \times (\,3 \times 10^8\ \frac{\text{m}}{\text{sec}}\,)$$

$$\beta = \frac{v}{c} = 0.92$$

Since $\beta > 0.1$, relativistic effects must be considered
Substitute β into equation 2.20 and solve for the kinetic energy of the electron, using

$m_0c^2 = 0.511$ MeV (electron)

$$E = m_0c^2\left(\frac{1}{\sqrt{1-\beta^2}} - 1\right) = 0.511\ \text{MeV} \times \left(\frac{1}{\sqrt{1-0.85}} - 1\right) = 0.83\ \text{MeV}$$

(c) What is the energy of an X–ray photon whose wavelength is 0.01 angstrom?

$$E = \frac{hc}{\lambda} = \frac{6.614\times10^{-34}\,\text{J}\cdot\text{sec}\times\left(3\times10^8\ \frac{\text{m}}{\text{sec}}\right)}{1\times10^{-12}\,\text{m}} = 1.98 \times 10^{-13}\ \text{J}$$

$$1.98 \times 10^{-13}\ \text{J} \times \frac{\text{eV}}{1.6 \times 10^{-19}\ \text{J}} = 1.24 \times 10^{6}\ \text{eV} = 1.24\ \text{MeV}$$

2.16

2.16 A current of 25 mA flows through 25 gage wire, 0.0179 in. (17.9 mils) in diameter. If there are 5×10^{22} free electrons per cm^3 in copper, calculate the average speed with which electrons flow in the wire.

Find the number of electrons per cm:

$$d = 17.9\ \text{mils} = 17.9\ \text{mils} \times \frac{2.54 \times 10^{-3}\ \text{cm}}{1\ \text{mil}} = 0.0455\ \text{cm}$$

$$\text{Area of circle} = \pi r^2 = \pi \times \{0.5 \times 0.0455\ \text{cm}\}^2 = 1.62 \times 10^{-3}\ \text{cm}^2$$

$$\frac{5 \times 10^{22}\ \text{electrons}}{\text{cm}^3} \times 1.62 \times 10^{-3}\ \text{cm}^2 = 8.12 \times 10^{19}\ \frac{\text{electrons}}{\text{cm}}$$

Find the number of electrons traveling per second:

$$25\ \text{mA} \times \frac{1\ \text{A}}{1000\ \text{mA}} \times \frac{1\frac{\text{C}}{\text{sec}}}{1\ \text{A}} \times \frac{1\ \text{electron}}{1.6 \times 10^{-19}\ \text{C}} = 1.5625 \times 10^{17}\ \frac{\text{electrons}}{\text{sec}}$$

Combine the two above results:

$$\frac{1\ \text{cm}}{8.12 \times 10^{19}\ \text{electrons}} \times \frac{1.5625 \times 10^{17}\ \text{electrons}}{\text{sec}} \times \frac{1\ \text{m}}{100\ \text{cm}} = 1.92 \times 10^{-5}\ \text{m/sec}$$

2.17

2.17 An electron starts at rest on the negative plate of a parallel plate capacitor, and is accelerated by a potential of 1000 volts across a gap of 1 cm.

a. With what velocity does the electron strike the positive plate?

$V = 1000$ V
$d = 0.01$ m
$m = 9.109 \times 10^{-31}$ kg
$q = 1.602 \times 10^{-19}$ C

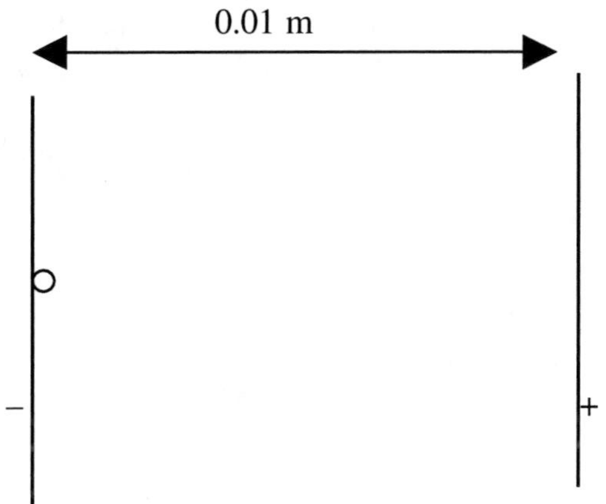

In this problem, the electron moves from a position of high potential energy, to a place of zero potential energy, converting the potential energy into kinetic energy.

The kinetic energy can be expressed as:

$$KE = \tfrac{1}{2} m v^2$$

The potential energy of a charged particle at an electrical potential is given by equation 2.38:

$$W = Vq$$

Now we have 2 expressions, one for the kinetic energy and another for potential energy. Setting them equal to each other:

$$\tfrac{1}{2} m v^2 = V q$$

Substituting in values to find velocity:

$$v = \sqrt{\frac{2 \times 1000 \text{ V} \times 1.602 \times 10^{-19} \text{ C}}{9.109 \times 10^{-31} \text{ kg}}} = 1.88 \times 10^7 \ \frac{\text{m}}{\text{sec}}$$

Since the velocity is less than 10% of the speed of light, relativistic corrections are not required.

b. How long does it take the electron to travel the 1 cm distance?

We cannot use the end velocity to find the time since the electron is continuously accelerating. However, we can find the acceleration and, knowing the distance, compute the time.
First, find the force acting on the electron. Using equation 2.36:

$$f = \varepsilon\, q$$

and combining this with equation 2.38:

$$V = \varepsilon\, d$$

Now replace ε in equation 2.36 with *V*/*d*:

$$f = \frac{V}{d} q$$

We can compute the acceleration of the particle across the 1 cm gap with equation 2.1:

$$f = ma$$

Since we have an expression for force (*f* = *(V/d) q),* install that into the classic *f* = *ma* equation and solve for acceleration;

$$a = \frac{Vq}{md} = \frac{1000\ \text{V} \times 1.6 \times 10^{-19}\ \text{C}}{9.109 \times 10^{-31}\ \text{kg} \times 0.01\ \text{m}} = 1.76 \times 10^{16}\ \frac{\text{m}}{\text{s}^2}$$

Since velocity = acceleration × time, and knowing the final velocity is 1.88×10^7 m/s from part a:

$$t = \frac{v}{a} = \frac{1.88 \times 10^7\ \frac{\text{m}}{\text{s}}}{1.76 \times 10^{16}\ \frac{\text{m}}{\text{s}^2}} = 1.07 \times 10^{-9}\ \text{sec}$$

2.18

2.18 A cylindrical capacitor is made of two coaxial conductors – the outer one has a diameter of 20.2 mm and the diameter of the inner one is 0.2 mm. The inner conductor is 1000 volts positive with respect to the outer conductor. Repeat parts (a) and (b) of problem 17, and compare the results to those of problem 17.

(a) With what velocity does the electron strike the positive plate?

$V = 1000$ V
$q = 1.6 \times 10^{-19}$ C
$m = 9.11 \times 10^{-31}$ kg

The kinetic energy of the electron depends only on the potential difference across which it was accelerated. From equation 2.33:

$$Vq = \frac{1}{2}mv^2$$

$$v = \sqrt{\frac{2Vq}{m}} = \sqrt{\frac{2 \times (1000\ \text{V}) \times 1.6\ \times 10^{-19}\,\text{C}}{9.11 \times 10^{-31}\,\text{kg}}} = 1.9 \times 10^7\ \text{m/sec}$$

Since this is less than 10% of the speed of light, relativistic effects are ignored.

(b) How long does it take the electron to travel the 1 cm distance?

The travel time is calculated from

velocity = acceleration × time

Since we already know the velocity (from part a), we must calculate the acceleration. From equations 2.1 and 2.36, we have

$$f = ma = \varepsilon q$$

$$a = \frac{\varepsilon q}{m}$$

However, the electric field intensity, ε varies radially in the case of coaxial electrodes. According to equation 2.40, ε at a radial distance r, is

$$\varepsilon = \frac{1}{r}\frac{V}{\ln\left(\dfrac{r_b}{r_a}\right)}$$

Where r_b is the larger radius and r_a is the smaller radius. Substituting for ε in the equation for a, we have

$$a = \frac{\varepsilon q}{m} = \frac{q}{m} \times \frac{V}{r \times \ln\left(\frac{r_b}{r_a}\right)}$$

Thus, $v = at = \dfrac{dr}{dt} = \dfrac{q}{m} \times \dfrac{V}{r \times \ln\left(\frac{r_b}{r_a}\right)} \times t$

$$rdr = \frac{q}{m} \frac{V}{\ln\left(\frac{r_b}{r_a}\right)} t\,dt$$

$$\int_{r_a}^{r_b} rdr = \frac{q}{m} \frac{V}{\ln\left(\frac{r_b}{r_a}\right)} \int_0^t t\,dt$$

Integrating between these limits, we have

$$\frac{1}{2}\left(r_b^2 - r_a^2\right) = \frac{q}{m} \frac{V}{\ln\left(\frac{r_b}{r_a}\right)} \times \frac{t^2}{2}$$

$$t = \left(\frac{\left(r_b^2 - r_a^2\right)}{\frac{q}{m} \times \frac{V}{\ln\left(r_b/r_a\right)}} \right)^{\frac{1}{2}}$$

Substituting the numerical values

$q = 1.6 \times 10^{-19}$ C
$m = 9.11 \times 10^{-31}$ kg
$V = 1000$ V
$r = 1$ cm = 0.01 m

$$r_a = \frac{0.2\ \text{mm}}{2} = 0.1\ \text{mm} = 1 \times 10^{-4}\ \text{m}$$

$$r_b = \frac{20.2\ \text{mm}}{2} = 10.1\ \text{mm} = 1.01 \times 10^{-2}\ \text{m}$$

and solving for t, we have

$$t = \left(\frac{\left((1.01 \times 10^{-2}\ \text{m})^2 - (1 \times 10^{-4}\ \text{m})^2 \right)}{\dfrac{1.6 \times 10^{-19}\ \text{C}}{9.11 \times 10^{-31}\ \text{kg}} \times \dfrac{1000\ \text{V}}{\ln(1.01 \times 10^{-2}\ \text{m}/1 \times 10^{-4}\ \text{m})}} \right)^{\frac{1}{2}}$$

$$t = 1.65 \times 10^{-9}\ \text{sec}$$

2.19 Two electrons are initially at rest, separated by 0.1 nm. After both electrons are released, they repel each other. What is the kinetic energy of each electron when they are 1.0 nm apart? **2.19**

The change in the potential energy of a system of 2 electrons separated by an initial distance r_1 which increases to r_2 as they repel each other is given by equation 2.31:

$$\Delta W = kq_1q_2\left(\frac{-1}{r_2} - \frac{-1}{r_1} \right)$$

This decrease in potential energy of the system appears as kinetic energy of the two particles as they move apart. If we substitute the following values into the above equation, we find that

$k = 9 \times 10^9\ \dfrac{\text{N}\cdot\text{m}^2}{\text{C}^2}$ (equation 2.25)
$q = 1.6 \times 10^{-19}\ \text{C}$
$r_1 = 0.1\ \text{nm} = 0.1 \times 10^{-9}\ \text{m}$
$r_2 = 1.0\ \text{nm} = 1 \times 10^{-9}\ \text{m}$

Note that the equation is split into two lines

$$\Delta W = 9 \times 10^9\ \frac{\text{N}\cdot\text{m}^2}{\text{C}^2} \times 1.6 \times 10^{-19}\ \text{C} \times 1.6 \times 10^{-19}\ \text{C}$$

$$\times\left(\frac{-1}{1\times10^{-9}\,\text{m}}-\frac{-1}{0.1\times10^{-9}\,\text{m}}\right)$$

$$DW = 2.07 \times 10^{-18}\ \text{J}$$

Since this is the total kinetic energy in the system, for each electron

$$\text{KE} = \tfrac{1}{2} \times 2.07 \times 10^{-18}\ \text{J} = 1.04 \times 10^{-18}\ \text{J}$$

2.20

2.20 A cyclotron produces a 100 microamp beam of 15 MeV deuterons. If the cyclotron were 100% efficient in converting electrical energy into kinetic energy of the deuterons, what is the minimum required power input, in kilowatts?

$$100\ \mu\text{A} \times \frac{1\frac{\text{C}}{\text{sec}}}{1\times10^{6}\ \mu\text{A}} \times \frac{\text{deuteron}}{1.6\times10^{-19}\,\text{C}} \times \frac{15\ \text{MeV}}{\text{deuteron}} \times \frac{1.6\times10^{-13}\,\text{J}}{1\ \text{MeV}} \times \frac{1\ \text{W}}{1\frac{\text{J}}{\text{s}}} = 1500\ \text{W}$$

2.21

2.21 A 1 μF capacitor is fully charged to 100 V by connecting it across the terminals of a 100 volt battery. Then, a 2 μF capacitor is charged to 100 V in the same manner. The two charged capacitors are then removed from the batteries, and connected as shown below. What is the charge on each capacitor?

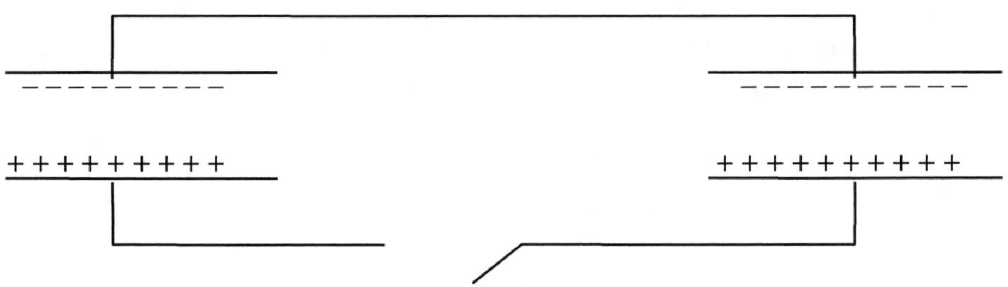

Use equation 2.66:

$C_1 = 1\ \mu\text{F} = 1 \times 10^{-6}\ \text{F}$
$V_1 = 100$ volts

$Q = CV$

$Q = 1 \times 10^{-6}\ \text{F} \times 100\ \text{V} = 1 \times 10^{-4}\ \text{C}$

$C_2 = 2\ \mu\text{F} = 2 \times 10^{-6}\ \text{F}$
$V_1 = 100\ \text{V}$

$Q = CV = 2 \times 10^{-6}\ \text{F} \times 100\ \text{V} = 2 \times 10^{-4}\ \text{C}$

2.22(a) What voltage must be applied across two oppositely charged parallel plates, 2 cm apart, in order to have an electron, starting from rest, strike the opposite plate in 10^{-8} second? **2.22**
(b) With what speed will the electron strike the plate?

Finding the velocity (speed) first, using classical physics since the electron is under constant acceleration:

$\Delta x = 2\ \text{cm} = 0.02\ \text{m}$

$t = 10^{-8}\ \text{sec}$

$v_0 = 0$

$$\Delta x = \bar{v} \times t = \frac{1}{2}(v_f + v_0)t$$

Solve for v_f:

$v_f = \dfrac{2\Delta x}{t} = \dfrac{2 \times (0.02\ \text{m})}{10^{-8}\ \text{sec}} = 4 \times 10^{6}$ m/sec is the speed the electron strikes the plate.

To find the required voltage, use equation 2.33:

$$Vq = \frac{1}{2}mv^2$$

$m = 9.11 \times 10^{-31}\ \text{kg}$
$q = 1.6 \times 10^{-19}\ \text{C}$
$v = 4 \times 10^{6}\ \text{m/sec}$

$$V = \frac{mv^2}{2q} = \frac{9.11\times10^{-31}\,\mathrm{kg}\times\left(4\times10^{6}\,\mathrm{m/sec}\right)^2}{2\times(1.6\times10^{-19}\,\mathrm{C})} = 45.55\ \mathrm{V}$$

2.23

2.23 When hydrogen "burns" it combines with oxygen according to

$$2H_2 + O_2 \rightarrow 2H_2O,$$

and emits about 2.3 x 10^5 Joules of heat energy in the production one mole of water. By what fraction is the mass of the reactants reduced in this reaction?

$E = 2.3 \times 10^5$ J
$c = 3 \times 10^8$ m/s

To find the mass reduction, calculate the mass lost:

$E = mc^2$

$$m = \frac{E}{c^2} = \frac{2.3\times10^5\,\mathrm{J}}{3\times10^8\,\frac{\mathrm{m}}{\mathrm{sec}}} = 2.56\times10^{-12}\ \mathrm{kg} = 2.56\times10^{-9}\ \mathrm{g}$$ is the total mass reduction

for one mole. The mass of one mole of water is:

2.016 g H_2 + 16 g O = 18.016 grams in one mole of water

To find the fraction of mass reduction, divide the mass reduction by the total mass:

$$\frac{2.56\times10^{-9}\,\mathrm{g}}{18.016\,\mathrm{g}} = 1.42\times10^{-10}$$ is the fraction mass reduced

2.24

2.24 (a) A 1000 MW(e) nuclear power plant operates at a thermal efficiency of 33% and at 75% capacity for 1 year. How many kilograms of nuclear fuel are consumed?

To solve this problem, the value "1000 MW(e)" must be understood. MW(e) means that this is how much electrical energy is produced from some thermal energy input into the plant. No power plant is 100% efficient, and the plant in this problem converts thermal energy to electrical energy with a 33% efficiency.

Therefore, the plant must make more thermal heat than it makes electrical energy. The energy input required to make 1000 MW in this plant is:

$$1000 \text{ MW(e)} \times \frac{100\%}{33\%} = 3030.3 \text{ MW(t)}$$

It is important to note that MW(t) stands for megawatts of thermal energy produced. Since the plant only operates at 75% capacity, the average MW(t) power would be:

3030.3 MW(t) × 75% = 2272.73 MW(t) during a year.

Converting into watts and subsequently, joules,

1 J/s = 1 W

$$2272.73 \text{ MW(t)} \times \frac{1\left(\text{J}/\text{sec}\right)}{\text{W}} \times \frac{3.1536 \times 10^{7}\text{ sec}}{\text{yr}} \times \frac{10^{6}\text{ W}}{1 \text{ MW}} = 7.17 \times 10^{16} \text{ J/yr}$$ produced by the power plant

The mass equivalent of this energy is

$$m = \frac{E}{c^2} = \frac{7.17 \times 10^{16}\text{ J}}{\left(3 \times 10^{8}\frac{\text{m}}{\text{sec}}\right)^2} = 0.8 \text{ kg nuclear fuel/yr.}$$

2.24(b) If a coal fired plant operates at the same efficiency and capacity factor, how many kilograms of coal must be burned during the year if the heat content of the coal is 27 MJ/kg (11,000 Btu/pound)?

Using the energy from part (a), the number of kilograms can be calculated.

7.17×10^{16} J are produced by the power plant burning coal (since the same amount of electricity was produced at the same efficiency and capacity).

Multiplying to obtain the kg of coal burned:

$$7.17 \times 10^{16}\text{ J} \times \frac{1 \text{ kg}}{27 \times 10^{6}\text{ J}} = 2.7 \times 10^{9} \text{ kg}$$

Since there are 1000 kg per metric tonne,

2.7×10^6 tonnes of coal are burned in a year.

2.25 **2.25** The solar constant is defined as the rate at which solar radiant energy falls on the earth's atmosphere on a surface normal to the incident radiation. The mean value for the solar constant is 1353 W/m^2, and the mean distance of the earth from the sun is 1.5×10^8 km.

(a) At what rate is energy being emitted from the sun?

The surface area of a sphere at the distance the earth is from the sun is the area throughout which the sun's energy is distributed. By taking the sun's power divided by the area over which it is distributed, the solar constant is found.

$r = 1.5 \times 10^8 \text{ km} = 1.5 \times 10^{11} \text{ m}$

$A_{sphere} = 4\pi r^2 = 4 \times \pi \times (1.5 \times 10^{11} \text{ m})^2 = 2.83 \times 10^{23} \text{ m}^2$

Sun power = surface area × power per unit area

Sun power = $2.83 \times 10^{23} \text{ m}^2 \times 1353 \text{ W/m}^2 = 3.83 \times 10^{26}$ W

(b) At what rate in tonnes per second, is the sun's mass being converted to energy?

$$3.83 \times 10^{26} \text{ W} \times \frac{1\frac{\text{J}}{\text{sec}}}{\text{W}} \times \frac{\text{MeV}}{1.6 \times 10^{-13}\text{J}} \times \frac{1 \text{ amu}}{931 \text{ MeV}} \times \frac{1.66 \times 10^{-27} \text{ kg}}{1 \text{amu}} \times \frac{1 \text{ tonne}}{1000 \text{ kg}}$$

$$= 4.3 \times 10^6 \frac{\text{tonnes}}{\text{sec}}$$

2.26 **2.26** What is the energy of a photon whose momentum is equal to that of a 10 MeV electron?

Since the electron has such high energy, relativistic equations must be used. To find the momentum associated with the electron, its mass and velocity must be determined.

The electron's total energy is

$mc^2 = \text{KE} + m_0c^2$

$$m = \frac{(10\ \text{MeV} + 0.51\ \text{MeV}) \times 1.6 \times 10^{-13}\ \frac{\text{J}}{\text{MeV}}}{\left(3 \times 10^8\ \text{m/s}\right)^2}$$

$m = 1.868 \times 10^{-29}$ kg

The electron's velocity at this energy is calculated by solving equation 2.4 for v:

$$m = \frac{m_0}{\sqrt{1 - \frac{v^2}{c^2}}}$$

Substituting

$m = 1.868 \times 10^{-29}$ kg
$m_0 = 9.109 \times 10^{-31}$ kg
$c = 3 \times 10^8$ m/sec

we find that

$$v = \left(c^2\left(1 - \frac{m_0}{m}\right)\right)^{\frac{1}{2}} = \left(\left(3 \times 10^8\ \frac{\text{m}}{\text{s}}\right)^2\left(1 - \frac{9.109 \times 10^{-31}\ \text{kg}}{1.868 \times 10^{-29}\ \text{kg}}\right)\right)^{\frac{1}{2}}$$

$v = 2.996 \times 10^8$ m/s

Using these values, we find that the electron's momentum

$p = mv = 1.868 \times 10^{-29}\ \text{kg} \times 2.996 \times 10^8\ \text{m/s}$

$$p = 5.597 \times 10^{-21}\ \frac{\text{kg} \cdot \text{m}}{\text{s}}$$

The energy of the photon that has this momentum is found by combining equations 2.76 and 2.78 to give

$E_\gamma = p_\gamma c$

$$E_\gamma = \frac{5.597 \times 10^{-21} \dfrac{\text{kg} \cdot \text{m}}{\text{s}} \times 3 \times 10^{8} \dfrac{\text{m}}{\text{s}}}{1.6 \times 10^{-13} \dfrac{\text{J}}{\text{MeV}}}$$

$$E_\gamma = 10.5 \text{ MeV}$$

2.27

2.27 What is the wavelength of
(a) an electron whose kinetic energy is 1000 eV?

Since the electron's KE << 15 keV, relativistic effects are negligible. Therefore

$$\text{KE} = \frac{1}{2} m v^2$$

$$v = \left(\frac{2 \times \text{KE}}{m} \right)^{\frac{1}{2}}$$

$$v = \left(\frac{2 \times 0.001 \text{ MeV} \times 1.6 \times 10^{-13} \dfrac{\text{J}}{\text{MeV}}}{9.11 \times 10^{-28} \text{ kg}} \right)^{\frac{1}{2}} = 1.87 \times 10^{7} \text{ m/s}$$

The de Broglie wavelength is found with equation 2.78:
$h = 6.614 \times 10^{-34}$ J · sec

$$\lambda = \frac{h}{mv} = \frac{6.614 \times 10^{-34} \text{ J} \cdot \text{s}}{9.11 \times 10^{-28} \text{ kg} \times 1.87 \times 10^{7} \dfrac{\text{m}}{\text{s}}} = 3.87 \times 10^{-11} \text{ m} \times \frac{1 \text{ Å}}{1 \times 10^{-10} \text{ m}} = 0.387 \text{ Å}$$

(b) a 10^{-8} kg oil droplet falling at a rate of 0.01 m/sec?

The de Broglie wavelength, equation 2.79, is:

$$\lambda = \frac{h}{mv} = \frac{6.614 \times 10^{-34} \text{ J} \cdot \text{sec}}{1 \times 10^{-8} \text{ kg} \times 0.01 \dfrac{\text{m}}{\text{sec}}} = 6.614 \times 10^{-24} \text{ m}$$

(c) a 1 MeV neutron?

Determine whether the 1 MeV neutron is relativistic. According to equation 2.20

$$\mathrm{KE} = m_0 c^2 \left(\left(1 - {v^2}/{c^2}\right)^{-1/2} - 1 \right)$$

The KE of the neutron is 4.7 MeV when $v = 0.1\ c$. Therefore, we have a non-relativistic situation in the case of a 1 MeV neutron. The neutron's KE = ½ mv^2 and it's momentum therefore is

$$p = mv = m\left(\frac{2 \times \mathrm{KE}}{m}\right)^{\frac{1}{2}}$$

The neutron's mass = 1.67×10^{-27} kg, and
its KE = 1 MeV × 1.6×10^{-13} J/MeV = 1.6×10^{-13} J

Substituting these values into the momentum equation above yields

$$p = 1.67 \times 10^{-27}\ \mathrm{kg}\left(\frac{2 \times 1.6 \times 10^{-13}\ \mathrm{J}}{1.67 \times 10^{-27}\ \mathrm{kg}}\right)^{\frac{1}{2}}$$

$$p = 2.31 \times 10^{-20}\ \frac{\mathrm{kg \cdot m}}{\mathrm{sec}}$$

The de Broglie wavelength is

$$\lambda = \frac{h}{p} = \frac{6.614 \times 10^{-34}\ \mathrm{J \cdot sec}}{2.31 \times 10^{-20}\ \frac{\mathrm{kg \cdot m}}{\mathrm{sec}}} = 2.86 \times 10^{-14}\ \text{meters}$$

2.28 (a) The specific heat of water in the English system of units is 1 Btu per pound degree F; in the cgs system, it is 1 calorie per gram degree C. Calculate the number of joules per Btu, if there are 4.186 joules per calorie. **2.28**

$$\frac{1\,\mathrm{Btu}}{\mathrm{lb \cdot ^\circ F}} \times \frac{1\ \mathrm{lb}}{454\ \mathrm{g}} \times \frac{9^\circ \mathrm{F}}{5^\circ \mathrm{C}} \times (X)\frac{\mathrm{J}}{\mathrm{Btu}} \times \frac{1\ \text{calorie}}{4.186\ \mathrm{J}} = 1\frac{\text{calorie}}{\mathrm{g \cdot ^\circ C}}$$

$X = 1.05 \times 10^3$ J in one Btu.

(b) What is the specific heat of water, in J/kg·°C

$$\frac{1 \text{ calorie}}{\text{gram}\cdot{}^\circ\text{C}} \times \frac{4.186 \text{ J}}{\text{calorie}} \times \frac{1000 \text{ g}}{\text{kg}} = 4186 \frac{\text{J}}{\text{kg}\cdot{}^\circ\text{C}}$$

2.29 **2.29** The maximum amplitude of the electric vector in a plane wave in free space is 275 V/m.

(a) What is the amplitude of the magnetic field vector?

In free space, the magnetic field vector is related to the electric field vector by equation 2.56

$$H_0\sqrt{\mu_0} = E_0\sqrt{\varepsilon_0}$$

$$E_0 = 275 \ \frac{\text{V}}{\text{m}}$$

$$\varepsilon_0 = 8.85 \times 10^{-12} \frac{\text{C}^2}{\text{N}\cdot\text{m}^2}$$

$$\mu_0 = 4 \times \pi \times 10^{-7} \frac{\text{C}^2}{\text{A}^2\cdot\text{m}^2}$$

Substituting these values into equation 2.56:

$$H_0 = \frac{E_0\sqrt{\varepsilon_0}}{\sqrt{\mu_0}} = \frac{275\frac{\text{V}}{\text{m}} \times \sqrt{8.85 \times 10^{-12} \frac{\text{C}^2}{\text{N}\cdot\text{m}^2}}}{\sqrt{4 \times \pi \times 10^{-7} \frac{\text{C}^2}{\text{A}^2\cdot\text{m}^2}}}$$

$$H_0 = 0.73 \ \frac{\text{A}}{\text{m}}$$

(b) What is the rms value of the electric vector?

$$\text{RMS value} = \frac{\text{Maximum amplitude}}{\sqrt{2}} = \frac{275\frac{\text{V}}{\text{m}}}{\sqrt{2}} = 194.5\ \frac{\text{V}}{\text{m}}$$

(c) What is the power density, in mW/cm^2, in this electromagnetic field?

Using the values from part (a) in equation 2.68:

$$H_0 = 0.73\ \frac{\text{A}}{\text{m}}$$

$$E_0 = 275\ \frac{\text{V}}{\text{m}}$$

$$Z = \frac{E_0}{H_0} = \frac{275\frac{\text{V}}{\text{m}}}{0.73\frac{\text{A}}{\text{m}}} = 377\ \text{ohms}$$

Solving with equation 2.71:

$$\overline{P} = \frac{\left(\frac{E_0}{\sqrt{2}}\right)^2}{Z} = \frac{\left(\frac{275\ \text{volts}}{\sqrt{2}}\right)^2}{377\ \text{ohms}} = 100\ \frac{\text{W}}{\text{m}^2} = 10\ \text{mW/cm}^2$$

2.30(a) What is the free space power density, in milliwatts per cm^2, of a 2450 MHz electromagnetic wave whose maximum electric intensity is 100 millivolts/m? 2.30

$$\overline{P} = \frac{\left(\frac{E_0}{\sqrt{2}}\right)^2}{Z} = \frac{\left(0.1\frac{\text{V}}{\text{m}}\Big/\sqrt{2}\right)^2}{377} = 1.33 \times 10^{-5}\ \frac{\text{W}}{\text{m}^2}$$

$$\overline{P} = 1.33 \times 10^{-5}\ \frac{\text{W}}{\text{m}^2} \times \frac{1\ \text{m}^2}{10^4\ \text{cm}^2} \times 10^3\ \frac{\text{mW}}{\text{m}^2} = 1.33 \times 10^{-6}\ \frac{\text{mW}}{\text{cm}^2}$$

(b) What is the maximum magnetic field intensity in this wave?

Equation 2.56:

$$H_0 \sqrt{\mu_0} = E_0 \sqrt{\varepsilon_0}$$

$$E_0 = 100 \frac{\text{mV}}{\text{m}} = 100 \times 10^{-3} \frac{\text{V}}{\text{m}}$$

$$\varepsilon_0 = 8.85 \times 10^{-12} \frac{\text{C}^2}{\text{N} \cdot \text{m}^2}$$

$$\mu_0 = 4 \times \pi \times 10^{-7} \frac{\text{C}^2}{\text{A}^2 \cdot \text{m}^2}$$

$$H_0 = \frac{E_0 \sqrt{\varepsilon_0}}{\sqrt{\mu_0}} = \frac{100 \times 10^{-3} \frac{\text{V}}{\text{m}} \times \sqrt{8.85 \times 10^{-12} \frac{\text{C}^2}{\text{N} \cdot \text{m}^2}}}{\sqrt{4 \times \pi \times 10^{-7} \frac{\text{C}^2}{\text{A}^2 \cdot \text{m}^2}}}$$

$$H_0 = 2.65 \times 10^{-4} \frac{\text{A}}{\text{m}}$$

2.31 **2.31** A radio station transmits at a power of 50,000 W. Assuming the electromagnetic energy to be isotropically radiated (in the case of a real radio transmitter, emission is not isotropic),

(a) What is the mean power density at a distance of 50 km?

50 km = 50,000 meters

$$A_{sphere} = 4\pi r^2 = 4\pi(50000 \text{ m})^2 = 3.14 \times 10^{10} \text{ m}^2$$

$$\frac{50000 \text{ W}}{3.14 \times 10^{10} \text{ m}^2} = 1.59 \times 10^{-6} \text{ W/m}^2 = 1.59 \times 10^{-7} \text{ mW/cm}^2$$

(b) What is the maximum electric field strength at this distance?

The mean power density and the maximum electric field strength are related by equation 2.71

$$\overline{P} = \frac{\left(\frac{E_0}{\sqrt{2}}\right)^2}{Z} = \frac{\left(E_0/\sqrt{2}\right)^2}{377} = 1.59 \times 10^{-6}\ \text{W/m}^2$$

$$E_0 = 0.035\frac{\text{V}}{\text{m}} = 3.5\times 10^{-2}\frac{\text{V}}{\text{m}}$$

(c) What is the maximum magnetic field strength at that distance?

Solving for H_0:

$$H_0 = \frac{2\overline{P}}{E_0} = \frac{2\times\left(1.59\times 10^{-6}\ \frac{\text{W}}{\text{m}^2}\right)}{0.035\frac{\text{V}}{\text{m}}} = 9.1\times 10^{-5}\frac{\text{A}}{\text{m}}$$

2.32 The mean value for the solar constant is 1.94 calories per cm^2. Calculate the electric and magnetic field strengths corresponding to the solar constant. **2.32**

$$\overline{P} = \frac{1.94\ \text{calories}}{\text{min}\cdot\text{cm}^2}\times\frac{4.186\ \text{J}}{\text{calorie}}\times\frac{1\ \text{min}}{60\ \text{sec}}\times\frac{10000\ \text{cm}^2}{1\ \text{m}^2}\times\frac{1\ \text{W}}{1\frac{\text{J}}{\text{sec}}} = 1353.5\ \frac{\text{W}}{\text{m}^2}$$

The maximum electric field strength is found by substituting equation 2.74

$$\overline{P} = \frac{\left(\frac{E_0}{\sqrt{2}}\right)^2}{Z} = \frac{\left(E_0/\sqrt{2}\right)^2}{377} = 1353.5\ \text{W/m}^2$$

$$\overline{E} = \frac{E_0}{\sqrt{2}} = 714\ \text{V/m}$$

The average power level, in terms of RMS values for E and H is, according to equation 2.73

$$\overline{P} = \overline{E}\times\overline{H}$$

$$\overline{H} = \frac{1353.5\,\frac{\text{W}}{\text{m}^2}}{714\,\frac{\text{V}}{\text{m}}} = 1.89\,\frac{\text{A}}{\text{m}}$$

2.33

2.33 What volume of water, m^3, must fall over a dam 10 m high to generate enough electricity to keep a 100 W electric bulb lit for 1 year, if the overall efficiency of the hydroelectric plant is 20%?

E = Power × time

$$E = 100\text{ W} \times \frac{1\,\text{J}/\text{sec}}{\text{W}} \times 1\text{ yr} \times \frac{365\text{ d}}{1\text{yr}} \times \frac{24\text{ hr}}{\text{d}} \times \frac{3600\text{ sec}}{\text{hr}} = 3.154 \times 10^9\text{ J}$$ is the

energy required over one year to light the light bulb. This energy required is equal to the amount of potential energy the water has due to its height behind the dam;

$PE = 3.154 \times 10^9$ J
$g = 9.8$ m/s^2 (gravitational acceleration)
$h = 10$ meters

Potential energy = $PE = mgh$
Solving for the mass of water required:

$$m = \frac{PE}{gh} = \frac{3.154 \times 10^9\text{ J}}{9.8\,\frac{\text{m}}{\text{sec}^2} \times 10\text{ m}} = 3.22 \times 10^7\text{ kg}$$ is the mass of water required to

produce 100 watts for 1 year.
However, since the plant is only 20% efficient,

$$\frac{3.22 \times 10^7\text{ kg}}{0.2} = 1.61 \times 10^8\text{ kg}$$ of water will be actually used.

The water density is 1000 kg/m^3:

$$1.61 \times 10^8\text{ kg} \times \frac{\text{m}^3}{1000\text{ kg}} = 1.61 \times 10^5\text{ m}^3$$ is the volume of water required.

Solutions for Chapter 3

ATOMIC AND NUCLEAR STRUCURE

3.1 What is the closest approach that a 5.3 MeV alpha particle can make to a gold nucleus? **3.1**

Gold has 79 protons, giving it a net charge on the nucleus of :

$$q_1 = 79 \text{ protons} \times \frac{1.6\times 10^{-19}\,\text{C}}{\text{proton}} = 1.264 \times 10^{-17}\ \text{C}$$

An alpha particle has 2 protons, giving it a net charge on the nucleus of :

$$q_2 = 2 \text{ protons} \times \frac{1.6\times 10^{-19}\,\text{C}}{\text{proton}} = 3.2 \times 10^{-19}\ \text{C}$$

$$k_0 = 9\ \times 10^9 \frac{\text{N}\cdot\text{m}^2}{\text{C}^2}$$

$$W = 5.3\ \text{MeV} = 5.3\ \text{MeV} \times \frac{1\times 10^6\,\text{eV}}{1\ \text{MeV}} \times \frac{1.6\times 10^{-19}\,\text{J}}{1\text{eV}} = 8.48 \times 10^{-13}\ \text{J}$$

Equation 2.24 is the equation for electrical force between two charged particles:

$$f = k_0 \frac{q_1 q_2}{r^2}$$

And equation 2.2 gives the equation for work:

$$W = fr$$

The work done by bringing these two widely separated charged particles to a separation r is given by combining equation 2.2 and 2.24;

$$\frac{W}{r} = k_0 \frac{q_1 q_2}{r^2}$$

Solving for *r*, the closest approach;

$$r = k_0 \frac{q_1 q_2}{W} = 9 \times 10^9 \frac{\text{N} \cdot \text{m}^2}{\text{C}^2} \times \frac{1.26 \times 10^{-17}\,\text{C} \times 3.2 \times 10^{-19}\,\text{C}}{8.48 \times 10^{-13}\,\text{J}} = 4.3 \times 10^{-14}\text{m}$$

3.2 **3.2** Calculate the number of atoms per cm^3 of lead, given the density of lead is 11.3 g/cm^3 and its atomic weight is 207.21.

$$\frac{11.3\ \text{g}}{\text{cm}^3} \times \frac{1\ \text{mole}}{207.21\ \text{g}} \times \frac{6.02 \times 10^{23}\ \text{atoms}}{\text{mole}} = 3.29 \times 10^{22}\ \frac{\text{atoms}}{\text{cm}^3}$$

3.3 **3.3** A μ^- meson has a charge of -4.8×10^{-10} sC and a mass 207 times that of a resting electron. If a proton should capture a μ^- to form a "mesic" atom, calculate
(a) the radius of the first Bohr orbit

find the ground state orbit radius using equation 3.6;

$n = 1$
$h = 6.625 \times 10^{-34}$ J·sec
$m_{meson} = 207 \times 9.11 \times 10^{-31}\ \text{kg} = 1.89 \times 10^{-28}\ \text{kg}$

$Z = 1$

$$k_0 = 9 \times 10^9\ \frac{\text{N} \cdot \text{m}^2}{\text{C}^2}$$

$$e = 4.8 \times 10^{-10}\ \text{sC} = 4.8 \times 10^{-10}\ \text{sC} \times \frac{1\ \text{C}}{3 \times 10^9\ \text{sC}} = 1.6 \times 10^{-19}\ \text{C}$$

$$r = \frac{n^2 h^2}{4\pi^2 m e^2 Z k_0}$$

$$r = \frac{1^2 \times \left(6.625 \times 10^{-34}\ \text{J} \cdot \text{sec}\right)^2}{4 \times \pi^2 \times (1.89 \times 10^{-28}\ \text{kg}) \times (1.62 \times 10^{-19}\ \text{C})^2 \times 1 \times \left(9 \times 10^9\ \dfrac{\text{N} \cdot \text{m}^2}{\text{C}^2}\right)}$$

$r = 2.49 \times 10^{-13}$ m $= 2.49 \times 10^{-11}$ cm

(b) the ionization potential equals the energy, eV, in orbit n_i, equation 3.10.

$$E = \frac{2\pi^2 k_0^{\,2} m Z^2 e^4}{h^2} \frac{1}{n^2}$$

$n = 1$
$h = 6.625 \times 10^{-34}$ J×sec
$m_{meson} = 207 \times 9.11 \times 10^{-31}$ kg $= 1.89 \times 10^{-28}$ kg
$Z = 1$

$$k_0 = 9 \times 10^9 \frac{\text{N} \cdot \text{m}^2}{\text{C}^2}$$

$$e = 4.8 \times 10^{-10} \text{ sC} = 4.8 \times 10^{-10} \text{sC} \times \frac{1\text{C}}{3 \times 10^9 \text{sC}} = 1.6 \times 10^{-19} \text{ C}$$

$$E = \frac{2 \times \pi^2 \times \left(9 \times 10^9 \frac{\text{N} \cdot \text{m}^2}{\text{C}^2}\right)^2 \times 1.89 \times 10^{-28} \text{kg} \times \left(1^2\right) \times \left(1.6 \times 10^{-19} \text{C}\right)^4}{\left(6.625 \times 10^{-34} \text{J} \cdot \text{sec}\right)^2} \times \frac{1}{1^2}$$

$$E = 4.5 \times 10^{-16}\text{J} = 4.5 \times 10^{-16}\text{J} \times \frac{\text{eV}}{1.6 \times 10^{-19} \text{J}} = 2.8 \times 10^3 \text{ eV}$$

3.4 Calculate the ionization potential of a singly ionized ^{4}He atom. **3.4**

The ionization potential represents the binding energy of an electron; it represents the work that must be done in order to remove the electron from the atom. For a one electron atom, such as a singly ionized helium atom, the energy level of an electron in orbit n_i, and hence the binding energy , is given by equation 3.10.

$$E = \frac{-2\pi^2 k_0^{\,2} m Z^2 e^4}{h^2} \frac{1}{n_i^2}$$

where,
$n = 1$ = ground state
$h = 6.625 \times 10^{-34}$ J·sec
$m_{electron} = 9.11 \times 10^{-31}$ kg

$Z = 2$

$k_0 = 9 \times 10^9 \ \dfrac{\mathrm{N \cdot m^2}}{\mathrm{C^2}}$

$e = 1.62 \times 10^{-19}$ C

Substituting these values into equation 3.10 we have:

$$E = \frac{2 \times \pi^2 \times \left(9 \times 10^9 \ \dfrac{\mathrm{N \cdot m^2}}{\mathrm{C^2}}\right)^2 \times 9.11 \times 10^{-31}\,\mathrm{kg} \times \left(2^2\right) \times \left(1.6 \times 10^{-19}\,\mathrm{C}\right)^4}{\left(6.625 \times 10^{-34}\,\mathrm{J \cdot sec}\right)^2} \times \frac{1}{1^2}$$

$E = 8.68 \times 10^{-18}$ J

In electron volts, we have

$$E = 8.68 \times 10^{-18}\,\mathrm{J} \times \frac{\mathrm{eV}}{1.6 \times 10^{-19}\,\mathrm{J}} = 54.4\ \mathrm{eV}$$

3.5 **3.5** Calculate the current due to the hydrogen electron in the ground state of hydrogen.

First, find the radius of the ground state orbit using equation 3.6;

$$r = \frac{n^2 h^2}{4\pi^2 m e^2 Z k_0}$$

where,

$n = 1$

$h = 6.625 \times 10^{-34}$ J·sec

$m_{electron} = 9.11 \times 10^{-31}$ kg

$Z = 1$

$k_0 = 9 \times 10^9 \ \dfrac{\mathrm{N \cdot m^2}}{\mathrm{C^2}}$

$e = 1.6 \times 10^{-19}$ C

$$r = \frac{n^2h^2}{4\pi^2 me^2 Zk_0}$$

$$r = \frac{1^2 \times \left(6.625 \times 10^{-34}\,\text{J}\cdot\text{sec}\right)^2}{4 \times \pi^2 \times (9.11 \times 10^{-31}\,\text{kg}) \times (1.62 \times 10^{-19}\,\text{C})^2 \times 1 \times \left(9 \times 10^9\,\dfrac{\text{N}\cdot\text{m}^2}{\text{C}^2}\right)}$$

$r = 5.17 \times 10^{-11}$ m

Use equation 3.3 to find the velocity of the electron:

$$v = \frac{nh}{2\pi rm} = \frac{(1) \times 6.625 \times 10^{-34}\,\text{J}\cdot\text{sec}}{2 \times \pi \times (5.17 \times 10^{-11}\,\text{m}) \times 9.11 \times 10^{-31}\,\text{kg}} = 2.24 \times 10^6\ \text{m/sec}$$

The distance that the orbital electron in hydrogen atom travels is the circumference of its orbit circumference = $2\pi r = 2 \times \pi \times (5.17 \times 10^{-11}$ m$) = 3.25 \times 10^{-10}$
Next, compute the time to make a revolution around the hydrogen atom.
$d = 3.25 \times 10^{-10}$ m
$v = 2.24 \times 10^6$ m/sec

$$t = \frac{d}{v} = \frac{3.25 \times 10^{-10}\,\text{m}}{2.24 \times 10^6\,\dfrac{\text{m}}{\text{sec}}} = 1.45 \times 10^{-16}\text{sec is the time for a complete revolution.}$$

Current is measured as the flow of electric charge per unit time:

$$\frac{1\ \text{electron}}{1.45 \times 10^{-16}\,\text{sec}} \times \frac{1.6 \times 10^{-19}\,\text{C}}{1\ \text{electron}} \times \frac{1\ \text{A}}{1\dfrac{\text{C}}{\text{sec}}} \times \frac{1000\ \text{mA}}{1\ \text{A}} = 1.1\ \text{mA}$$

3.6 Calculate the ratio of the velocity of a hydrogen electron in the ground state to the velocity of light. **3.6**
First, find the radius of the ground state orbit using equation 3.6;
$n = 1$
$h = 6.625 \times 10^{-34}$ J·sec
$m_{electron} = 9.11 \times 10^{-31}$ kg
$Z = 1$

$$k_0 = 9 \times 10^9\ \frac{\text{N}\cdot\text{m}^2}{\text{C}^2}$$

$e = 1.62 \times 10^{-19}$ C

$$r = \frac{n^2 h^2}{4\pi^2 m e^2 Z k_0}$$

$$r = \frac{1^2 \times \left(6.625 \times 10^{-34}\,\text{J}\cdot\text{sec}\right)^2}{4 \times \pi^2 \times (9.11 \times 10^{-31}\,\text{kg}) \times (1.62 \times 10^{-19}\,\text{C})^2 \times 1 \times \left(9 \times 10^9\,\frac{\text{N}\cdot\text{m}^2}{\text{C}^2}\right)}$$

$r = 5.17 \times 10^{-11}$ m

Use equation 3.3 to find the velocity of the electron:

$$v = \frac{nh}{2\pi r m} = \frac{(1) \times 6.625 \times 10^{-34}\,\text{J}\cdot\text{sec}}{2 \times \pi \times (5.17 \times 10^{-11}\,\text{m}) \times 9.11 \times 10^{-31}\,\text{kg}} = 2.24 \times 10^6 \text{ m/sec}$$

The speed of light is 3×10^8 m/sec

$$\frac{2.24 \times 10^6}{3 \times 10^8} = 0.0075$$

3.7

3.7 Calculate the Rydberg constant for deuterium.

Equation 3.12 is where the elements of the equation for Rydberg's constant for a single-electron atom is found:

$c = 3 \times 10^8$ m/sec

$n = 1$

$h = 6.625 \times 10^{-34}$ J·sec

$m_{electron} = 9.11 \times 10^{-31}$ kg

$Z = 1$

$k_0 = 9 \times 10^9\ \frac{\text{N}\cdot\text{m}^2}{\text{C}^2}$

$e = 1.6 \times 10^{-19}$ C

Substituting these values:

$$R = \frac{2\pi (k_0)^2 m Z^2 e^4}{ch^3}$$

$$R = \frac{2 \times \pi^2 \times \left(9 \times 10^9 \frac{N \cdot m^2}{C^2}\right)^2 \times 9.11 \times 10^{-31} kg \times (1)^2 \times \left(1.6 \times 10^{-19} C\right)^4}{(3 \times 10^8 \frac{m}{sec}) \times \left(6.625 \times 10^{-34} J \cdot sec\right)^3}$$

R= $1.093 \times 10^7 m^{-1}$= $1.1 \times 10^5 cm^{-1}$

3.8 What is the uncertainty in the momentum of a proton inside a nucleus of ^{27}Al? What is the kinetic energy of this proton? **3.8**

The maximum uncertainty in position of a proton inside the nucleus is the diameter of the nucleus. Find the radius of the ^{27}Al nucleus to determine its position with equation 3.1

$A = 27$

$r = 1.2 \times 10^{-15} A^{1/3} = 1.2 \times 10^{-15} \times (27)^{1/3} = 3.6 \times 10^{-15}$ meters

Since the furthest one can be away when determining the position is across the nucleus, the diameter is the maximum uncertainty:

3.6×10^{-15} meters $\times 2 = 7.2 \times 10^{-15}$ meters

From equation 2.81 find the momentum uncertainty:
$h = 6.625 \times 10^{-34}$ J·sec
$x = 7.2 \times 10^{-15}$ meters

$$\Delta p \geq \frac{h}{2\pi\, \Delta x} = \frac{6.625 \times 10^{-34} J \cdot sec}{2 \times \pi \times (7.2 \times 10^{-15} m)} = 1.46 \times 10^{-20} \frac{kg \cdot m}{sec}$$

$$\Delta p \geq 1.46 \times 10^{-15} \frac{g \cdot cm}{sec}$$

Since the mass of the proton is
$m_{proton} = 1.676 \times 10^{-27}$ kg, its velocity is

$$v = \frac{p}{m} = \frac{1.46 \times 10^{-20} \frac{\text{kg} \cdot \text{m}}{\text{sec}}}{1.676 \times 10^{-27} \text{ kg}} = 8.76 \times 10^{6} \text{ m/sec}$$

Now find the kinetic energy of the proton (equation 2.3)

$$E = \frac{1}{2} mv^2 = \frac{1}{2} \times 1.676 \times 10^{-27} \text{ kg} \times \left(8.76 \times 10^{6} \frac{\text{m}}{\text{sec}}\right)^2 = 6.42 \times 10^{-14} \text{ J}$$

$$6.42 \times 10^{-14} \text{ J} \times \frac{\text{MeV}}{1.6 \times 10^{-13} \text{ J}} = 0.4 \text{ MeV}$$

3.9

3.9 A sodium ion is neutralized by capturing a 1 eV electron. What is the wavelength of the emitted radiation if the ionization potential of Na is 5.41 volts?

Since it is an electron experiencing the 5.41V, the electron must lose not only the energy of ionization but also the 1 eV of kinetic energy. Thus, the energy lost in the ionization process is 6.41 eV. Equation 2.76 can be rearranged to find the wavelength:

$h = 6.625 \times 10^{-34}$ J·sec
$c = 3 \times 10^{8}$ m/sec

$$E = 6.41 \text{eV} \times \frac{1.6 \times 10^{-19} \text{ J}}{1 \text{ eV}} = 1.03 \times 10^{-18} \text{ J}$$

$$\lambda = \frac{hc}{E} = \frac{6.625 \times 10^{-34} \text{ J} \cdot \text{sec}\left(3 \times 10^{8} \frac{\text{m}}{\text{sec}}\right)}{1.03 \times 10^{-18} \text{ J}} = 1.93 \times 10^{-7} \text{ m} = 193 \text{ nm}$$

3.10

3.10(a) How much energy would be released if one gram deuterium were fused to form helium according to the equation $^{2}H + ^{2}H \longrightarrow ^{4}He + Q$?

Find the number of ^{2}H atoms present in 1 g ^{2}H:

$1 \text{ g } (^2\text{H}) \times \dfrac{\text{mole}}{2 \text{ g}} \times \dfrac{6.02 \times 10^{23} \text{ atoms}}{1 \text{ mole}} = 3.01 \times 10^{23}$ atoms, however it takes two atoms of ^{2}H to make one atom ^{4}He, so only 1.505×10^{23} atoms will be made from this reaction.

Sum the mass of the deuterium atoms and subtract that from the mass of the ^{4}He atom formed, to determine the mass deficit:
$^2\text{H} = 2.0140$ amu
$^4\text{He} = 4.0026$ amu
$2 \times (2.0140 \text{ amu}) - 4.0026 \text{ amu} = 0.0254$ amu per atom of ^{4}He formed
Since 1 amu= 931 MeV

$$1.505 \times 10^{23} \text{ atoms} \times \frac{0.0254 \text{ amu}}{\text{atom}} \times \frac{931 \text{ MeV}}{\text{amu}} \times \frac{1.6 \times 10^{-13} \text{ J}}{\text{MeV}} = 5.7 \times 10^{11} \text{J}$$

(b) How much energy is necessary to drive the two deuterium nuclei together?

The work done in overcoming the repulsive force when bringing the two nuclei together until they touch, at a center to center distance of the two nuclei radii, is given by equal 2.31:

$$W = k_0 q_1 q_2 \left(\frac{1}{r_1} - \frac{1}{r_2} \right)$$

where
$q_1 = q_2 = 1.6 \times 10^{-19}$ C

$$k_o = 9 \times 10^9 \, \frac{\text{N} \cdot \text{m}^2}{\text{C}^2}$$

The distance r_1 is calculated with equation 3.1
$r_1 = 2r = 2 \times 1.2 \times 10^{-15} A^{1/3} = 2 \times 1.2 \times 10^{-15} \times 2^{1/3} = 3 \times 10^{-15}$m

$$W = k_0 q_1 q_2 \left(\frac{1}{r_1} - \frac{1}{r_2} \right)$$

$$W = 9 \times 10^9 \, \frac{\text{N} \cdot \text{m}^2}{\text{C}^2} \times 1.6 \times 10^{-19} \text{C} \times 1.6 \times 10^{-19} \text{C} \times \left(\frac{1}{3 \times 10^{-15} \text{ m}} - \frac{1}{\infty} \right)$$

$$W = 7.68 \times 10^{-14} \text{ J} = 7.68 \times 10^{-14} \text{ J} \times \frac{1 \text{ MeV}}{1.6 \times 10^{-13} \text{J}} = 0.48 \text{ MeV}$$

3.11

3.11 The density of beryllium, atomic number 4, is 1.84 g/cm^3, and the density of lead, atomic number 82, is 11.3 g/cm^3. Calculate the density of a ^{9}Be and a ^{208}Pb nucleus.

$A(\text{Be}) = 9$
$r = 1.2 \times 10^{-15} A^{1/3} = 1.2 \times 10^{-15} \times 9^{1/3} = 2.5 \times 10^{-15}\text{m}$

Volume of the nucleus (assume sphere):

$$V = \frac{4}{3}\pi r^3 = \frac{4}{3} \times \pi \times (2.5 \times 10^{-15}\,\text{m})^3 = 6.545 \times 10^{-44}\,\text{m}^3$$

Now divide the atomic mass of beryllium by the volume of the nucleus:

$$\frac{9\text{ amu}}{6.545 \times 10^{-44}\,\text{m}^3} \times \frac{1.66 \times 10^{-27}\,\text{kg}}{1\text{ amu}} \times \frac{1000\text{ g}}{1\text{ kg}} \times \frac{1\text{ m}^3}{1 \times 10^6\,\text{cm}^3} = 2.3 \times 10^{14}\,\frac{\text{g}}{\text{cm}^3}$$

For lead:

$A(\text{Pb}) = 207$
$r = 1.2 \times 10^{-15} A^{1/3} = 1.2 \times 10^{-15} \times 207^{1/3} = 7.1 \times 10^{-15}\text{m}$

Volume of the nucleus (assume sphere):

$$V = \frac{4}{3}\pi r^3 = \frac{4}{3} \times \pi \times (7.1 \times 10^{-15}\,\text{m})^3 = 1.5 \times 10^{-42}\,\text{m}^3$$

Now divide the atomic mass of beryllium by the volume of the nucleus:

$$\frac{207\text{ amu}}{1.5 \times 10^{-42}\,\text{m}^3} \times \frac{1.66 \times 10^{-27}\,\text{kg}}{1\text{ amu}} \times \frac{1000\text{ g}}{1\text{ kg}} \times \frac{1\text{ m}^3}{1 \times 10^6\,\text{cm}^3} = 2.3 \times 10^{14}\,\frac{\text{g}}{\text{cm}^3}$$

Note that the nuclear density is generally independent of the atomic number.

3.12

3.12 Determine the electronic shell configuration for aluminum, atomic number 13.

From table 3.1

Shell number	Number of electrons in shell
K	2
L	8
M	3

3.13 What is the difference in mass between the hydrogen atom and the sum of the masses of a proton and an electron? Express the answer in energy equivalent (eV) of the mass difference. **3.13**

Masses
$^{1}H = 1.007825035423$ amu
$^{1}p = 1.00727647012$ amu
$e^{-} = 5.48579903 \times 10^{-4}$ amu

$(1.00727647012 \text{ amu} + 5.48579903 \times 10^{-4} \text{ amu}) - 1.007825035423 \text{ amu}$
$= 1.46 \times 10^{-8}$ amu

$1.07356 \times 10^{-9} \text{ amu} = 1 \text{ eV}$

$$1.46 \times 10^{-8} \text{ amu} \times \frac{\text{eV}}{1.07356 \times 10^{-9} \text{ amu}} = 13.6 \text{ eV}$$

3.14 If the heat of vaporization of water is 540 calories per gram at atmospheric pressure, what is the binding energy of a water molecule? **3.14**

$H_2O = 18$ g per mole

$$\frac{540 \text{ cal}}{\text{g}} \times \frac{4.186 \text{ J}}{\text{cal}} \times \frac{\text{eV}}{1.6 \times 10^{-19} \text{ J}} \times \frac{18 \text{ g } (H_2O)}{\text{mol}} \times \frac{1 \text{ mol}}{6.02 \times 10^{23} \text{ molecules}} = 0.42 \text{ eV}$$

3.15 The ionization potential of He is 24.5 eV. **3.15**
(a) What is the maximum velocity with which an electron is moving before it can ionize an unexcited He atom?

$m_e = 9.11 \times 10^{-31}$ kg

$$E = 24.5 \text{ eV} = 24.5 \text{ eV} \times \frac{1.6 \times 10^{-19} \text{ J}}{\text{eV}} = 3.92 \times 10^{-18} \text{ J}$$

Solve for velocity using equation 3.7:

$$v = \sqrt{\frac{2E}{m}} = \sqrt{\frac{2 \times 3.92 \times 10^{-18} \text{ J}}{9.11 \times 10^{-31} \text{ kg}}} = 2.93 \times 10^{6} \text{ m/sec}$$

(b) What is the minimum wavelength of a photon in order that it ionize the He atom?

Equation 2.76:
$h = 6.625 \times 10^{-34}$ J·sec
$c = 3 \times 10^{8}$ m/sec

$$E = 24.5 \text{ eV} = 24.5 \text{ eV} \times \frac{1.6 \times 10^{-19}\,\text{J}}{\text{eV}} = 3.92 \times 10^{-18}\,\text{J}$$

$$\lambda = \frac{hc}{E} = \frac{6.625 \times 10^{-34}\,\text{J} \cdot \text{sec} \times 3 \times 10^{8}\,\frac{\text{m}}{\text{sec}}}{3.92 \times 10^{-18}\,\text{J}} = 50.7 \times 10^{-9}\,\text{m} = 50.7\,\text{nm}$$

3.16

3.16 In a certain 25 watt mercury–vapor ultraviolet lamp, 0.1% of the electrical energy input appears as U.V. radiation of wavelength 2537 angstroms. What is the photon emission rate, per second, from this lamp?

Find the energy of each photon with equation 2.76:

$h = 6.625 \times 10^{-34}$ J·sec
$c = 3 \times 10^{8}$ m/sec

$$\lambda = 2537\ \text{Å} \times \frac{1 \times 10^{-10}\,\text{m}}{1\ \text{Å}} = 2.537 \times 10^{-9}\,\text{m}$$

$$E = \frac{hc}{\lambda} = \frac{6.625 \times 10^{-34}\,\text{J} \cdot \text{sec} \times 3 \times 10^{8}\,\frac{\text{m}}{\text{sec}}}{2.537 \times 10^{-9}\,\text{m}} = 7.834 \times 10^{-19}\,\text{J/photon}$$

Find the actual amount of energy given off in the UV range:

$$25\,\text{W} \times \frac{0.1}{100} \times \frac{1\frac{\text{J}}{\text{sec}}}{1\,\text{W}} = 0.025\,\frac{\text{J}}{\text{sec}}$$

Multiply the energy of the photons by the UV energy to find the photon emission rate:

$$\frac{0.025\text{ J}}{\text{sec}} \times \frac{\text{photon}}{7.834 \times 10^{-19}\text{ J}} = 3.19 \times 10^{16}\ \frac{\text{photons}}{\text{sec}}$$

3.17 The atomic mass of tritium is 3.017005 amu. How much energy in MeV is required to dissociate the tritium into its component parts? **3.17**

Sum the individual components which make up tritium and determine the mass deficit:

n = 1.008665 amu
p = 1.007276 amu
e = 5.485×10^{-4} amu

Tritium has 2 neutrons, 1 proton and 1 electron:

$(2) \times 1.008665\text{ amu} + (1) \times 1.007276\text{ amu} + (1) \times 5.485 \times 10^{-4}\text{ amu}$
$= 3.0251545\text{ amu}$

Subtract from this the mass of tritium to find the mass deficit:

$3.0251545\text{ amu} - 3.017005\text{ amu} = 8.1495 \times 10^{-3}\text{ amu}$

931 MeV = 1 amu

$$8.1495 \times 10^{-3}\text{ amu} \times \frac{931\text{ MeV}}{\text{amu}} = 7.587\text{ MeV}$$ is required to dissociate the tritium.

3.18 Compute the wave length frequency, and energy (electron volts) for the second and third lines in the Lyman series. **3.18**

Equation 3.2 to solve for the wavelength:
$R = 1.097 \times 10^{7}\text{ m}^{-1}$

$c = 3 \times 10^8$ m/sec

$n_1 = 1$
$n_2 = 3$ (since the first line would be formed between the 1st and 2nd orbits)

$$\frac{1}{\lambda} = R\left(\frac{1}{n_1^2} - \frac{1}{n_2^2}\right) = 1.097 \times 10^7 \left(\frac{1}{1_1^2} - \frac{1}{3_2^2}\right) = 9.76 \times 10^6\ \text{m}^{-1}$$

λ, the wavelength of the 2nd line, $= 1.023 \times 10^{-7}$ m

Equation 2.57 describes the frequency and wavelength relationship:

$$f = \frac{c}{\lambda} = \frac{3 \times 10^8\ \frac{\text{m}}{\text{sec}}}{1.023 \times 10^{-7}\ \text{m}} = 2.93 \times 10^{15}\ \text{sec}^{-1}$$ is the frequency of the 2nd line.

The energy of the 2nd line is found using equation 2.76A;

$h = 6.625 \times 10^{-34}$ J·sec

$$E = hf = 6.625 \times 10^{-34}\ \text{J·sec} \times 2.93 \times 10^{15}\ \frac{1}{\text{sec}} = 1.94 \times 10^{-18}\ \text{J}$$

$$1.94 \times 10^{-18}\ \text{J} \times \frac{1\ \text{eV}}{1.6 \times 10^{-19}\ \text{J}} = 12.11\ \text{eV}$$ is the energy of the 2nd line.

The third line is calculated using equation 3.2 to solve for the wavelength:

$R = 1.097 \times 10^7\ \text{m}^{-1}$

$c = 3 \times 10^8\ \frac{\text{m}}{\text{s}}$

$n_1 = 1$
$n_2 = 4$

$$\frac{1}{\lambda} = R\left(\frac{1}{n_1^2} - \frac{1}{n_2^2}\right) = 1.097 \times 10^7 \frac{1}{\text{m}} \times \left(\frac{1}{1_1^2} - \frac{1}{4_2^2}\right) = 10.28 \times 10^6\ \text{m}^{-1}$$

$\lambda = 9.7 \times 10^{-8}$ m is the wavelength of the 3rd line.

Equation 2.57 describes the frequency and wavelength relationship:

$$f = \frac{c}{\lambda} = \frac{3 \times 10^{8}\ \frac{\text{m}}{\text{sec}}}{9.7 \times 10^{-8}\ \text{m}} = 3.085 \times 10^{15}\ \text{sec}^{-1}$$ is the frequency of the 3rd line.

The energy of the 3rd line is found using equation 2.76A;

$h = 6.625 \times 10^{-34}$ J·sec

$$E = hf = 6.625 \times 10^{-34}\ \text{J·sec} \times 3.085 \times 10^{15} \frac{1}{\text{sec}} = 2.044 \times 10^{-18}\ \text{J}$$

$$2.044 \times 10^{-18}\ \text{J} \times \frac{\text{eV}}{1.6 \times 10^{-19}\ \text{J}} = 12.78\ \text{eV}$$ is the energy of the 3rd line.

3.19 Using the Bohr atomic model, calculate the velocity of the ground state electrons in hydrogen and in helium. **3.19**

First, find the ground state orbit radius for hydrogen using equation 3.6;
$n = 1$
$h = 6.625 \times 10^{-34}$ J·sec
$m_{electron} = 9.11 \times 10^{-31}$ kg

$Z = 1$

$k_0 = 9 \times 10^{9}\ \frac{\text{N} \cdot \text{m}^2}{\text{C}^2}$
$e = 1.62 \times 10^{-19}$ C

$$r = \frac{n^2 h^2}{4\pi^2 m e^2 Z k_0}$$

$$r = \frac{1^2 \times \left(6.625 \times 10^{-34}\ \text{J} \cdot \text{sec}\right)^2}{4 \times \pi^2 \times (9.11 \times 10^{-31}\ \text{kg}) \times (1.62 \times 10^{-19}\ \text{C})^2 \times 1 \times \left(9 \times 10^{9}\ \frac{\text{N} \cdot \text{m}^2}{\text{C}^2}\right)}$$

$r = 5.17 \times 10^{-11}$ m

Use equation 3.3 to find the velocity of the electron:

$$v = \frac{nh}{2\pi rm} = \frac{(1) \times 6.625 \times 10^{-34}\,\text{J} \cdot \text{sec}}{2 \times \pi \times (5.17 \times 10^{-11}\,\text{m}) \times 9.11 \times 10^{-31}\,\text{kg}} = 2.2 \times 10^{6}\ \text{m/sec is the}$$

velocity of the hydrogen electron.

For helium, find the ground state orbit radius using equation 3.6;

$n = 1$

$h = 6.625 \times 10^{-34}$ J·sec

$m_{electron} = 9.11 \times 10^{-31}$ kg

$Z = 2$

$$k_0 = 9 \times 10^9 \ \frac{\text{N} \cdot \text{m}^2}{\text{C}^2}$$

$e = 1.62 \times 10^{-19}$ C

$$r = \frac{n^2 h^2}{4\pi^2 m e^2 Z k_0}$$

$$r = \frac{1^2 \times \left(6.625 \times 10^{-34}\,\text{J} \cdot \text{sec}\right)^2}{4 \times \pi^2 \times (9.11 \times 10^{-31}\,\text{kg}) \times (1.62 \times 10^{-19}\,\text{C})^2 \times 1 \times \left(9 \times 10^9 \ \frac{\text{N} \cdot \text{m}^2}{\text{C}^2}\right)}$$

$r = 2.58 \times 10^{-11}$ m

Use equation 3.3 to find the velocity of the electron:

$$v = \frac{nh}{2\pi rm} = \frac{(1) \times 6.625 \times 10^{-34}\,\text{J} \cdot \text{sec}}{2 \times \pi \times (2.58 \times 10^{-11}\,\text{m}) \times 9.11 \times 10^{-31}\,\text{kg}} = 4.49 \times 10^{6}\ \text{m/sec is the}$$

velocity of the helium electron.

3.20 **3.20** The heat of combustion when H_2 combines with O_2 to form water is 60 kcal/mole water. How much energy (electron volts) is liberated per molecule of water produced?

$$\frac{60\ \text{kcal}}{\text{mole}} \times \frac{1\ \text{mole}}{6.02 \times 10^{23}\ \text{molecules}} \times \frac{1000\ \text{cal}}{\text{kcal}} \times \frac{4.186\ \text{J}}{\text{cal}} \times \frac{1\text{eV}}{1.6 \times 10^{-19}\ \text{J}} = 2.6 \frac{\text{eV}}{\text{molecule}}$$

3.21 The atomic weights of ^{16}O, ^{17}O and ^{18}O are 15.994915, 16.999131, and 17.999160 respectively. Calculate the atomic weight of oxygen. **3.21**

The abundance of each isotope can be found in the CRC handbook.

Type Oxygen	Weight	Abundance	Abundance × weight
16	15.994915	0.99759	15.956367
17	16.999131	0.00037	0.006289678
18	17.999160	0.00204	0.036718286
		Sum	15.999377522

3.22 Calculate the molecular weight of chlorine, Cl_2, using the exact atomic weights of the Cl isotopes given in the reference sources (CRC). **3.22**

Type Chlorine	Weight	Abundance	Abundance ×Weight
35	34.968852	0.7577	26.49589916
37	36.965903	0.2423	8.956838297
		Sum	35.45273746

3.23 If 9 grams of NaCl were dissolved in 1 liter of water, what would be the concentration, in atoms per mL, of each of the constituent elements in the solution? **3.23**

Na = 22.99 g/mole
Cl = 35.45 g/mole
NaCl = 22.99 g/mole + 35.45 g/mole = 58.43 g/mole

Calculate the number of atoms of Na added to the solution in the 9 grams:

$$\frac{9\text{ g NaCl}}{1\text{ L}} \times \frac{\text{mol NaCl}}{58.43\text{ g NaCl}} \times \frac{1\text{ mol Na}}{1\text{ mol NaCl}} \times \frac{6.02 \times 10^{23}\text{ atoms Na}}{1\text{ mol Na}} \times \frac{1\text{ L}}{1000\text{ mL}} =$$

$$9.27 \times 10^{19}\ \frac{\text{atoms Na}}{\text{mL}}$$

Calculate the number of atoms of Cl added to the solution in the 9 grams:

$$\frac{9\text{ g NaCl}}{1\text{ L}} \times \frac{\text{mol NaCl}}{58.43\text{ g NaCl}} \times \frac{1\text{ mol Cl}}{1\text{ mol NaCl}} \times \frac{6.02 \times 10^{23}\text{ atoms Cl}}{1\text{ mol Cl}} \times \frac{1\text{ L}}{1000\text{ mL}} =$$

$$9.27 \times 10^{19}\ \frac{\text{atoms Cl}}{\text{mL}}$$

H = 1 g/mole
O = 16 g/mole
H_2O = 2(1 g/mole) +16 g/mole = 18 g/mole

Calculate the number of atoms of H in 1 milliliter of water (assume 1 liter = 1000 g water):

$$\frac{1000\text{ g H}_2\text{O}}{1\text{ L}} \times \frac{\text{mol H}_2\text{O}}{18\text{ g H}_2\text{O}} \times \frac{2\text{ mol H}}{1\text{ mol H}_2\text{O}} \times \frac{6.02 \times 10^{23}\text{ atoms H}}{1\text{ mol H}} \times \frac{1\text{ L}}{1000\text{ mL}} =$$

$$6.69 \times 10^{22}\ \frac{\text{atoms H}}{\text{mL}}$$

Calculate the number of atoms of O in 1 milliliter of water (1 liter = 1000 g water):

$$\frac{1000\text{ g H}_2\text{O}}{1\text{ L}} \times \frac{\text{mol H}_2\text{O}}{18\text{ g H}_2\text{O}} \times \frac{1\text{ mol O}}{1\text{ mol H}_2\text{O}} \times \frac{6.02 \times 10^{23}\text{ atoms O}}{1\text{ mol O}} \times \frac{1\text{ L}}{1000\text{ mL}} =$$

$$3.34 \times 10^{22}\ \frac{\text{atoms O}}{\text{mL}}$$

3.24

3.24 The visual threshold of the normal human eye is about 7.3×10^{-15} W/cm^2 for light whose λ = 556 nm. What is the corresponding photon flux in photons/cm^2/sec?

$\lambda = 556\text{ nm} = 556 \times 10^{-9}\text{ m}$

Find the energy of the photons in joules using equation 2.76;

$$c = 3 \times 10^{8}\ \frac{\text{m}}{\text{sec}}$$

$h = 6.625 \times 10^{-34}$ J·sec

$$E = h\frac{c}{\lambda} = 6.625 \times 10^{-34}\text{ J·sec} \times \frac{3 \times 10^{8}\ \frac{\text{m}}{\text{sec}}}{556 \times 10^{-9}\text{ m}} = 3.57 \times 10^{-19}\text{ J is the energy per}$$

photon.

Multiplying the energy per unit area by the number of photons per joule (inverse of 3.57×10^{-19} J /photon):

$$\frac{7.3\times10^{-15}\,\text{W}}{\text{cm}^2}\times\frac{1\frac{\text{J}}{\text{sec}}}{1\text{W}}\times\frac{1\text{ photon}}{3.57\times10^{-19}\,\text{J}} = 2\times10^4\ \frac{\text{photon}}{\text{cm}^2\,\text{sec}}$$

3.25 What is the binding energy of the last neutron in ^{17}O? **3.25**

Find the mass deficit between ^{16}O plus 1 neutron, and ^{17}O, which is the energy of removing one neutron, to determine the binding energy:

From CRC:

^{17}O = 16.999131 amu
^{16}O = 15.994915 amu
^{1}n = 1.008665 amu

^{16}O + ^{1}n =15.994915 amu + 1.008665 amu = 17.00358 amu

The difference in masses is:
17.00358 amu – 16.999131 amu = 0.004449 amu

931 MeV = 1 amu

$$0.004449\text{ amu}\times\frac{931\text{ MeV}}{1\text{ amu}} = 4.14\text{ MeV}$$

Solutions for Chapter 4

RADIOACTIVITY

4.1 Carbon–14 is a pure beta emitter that decays to ^{14}N. If the exact atomic masses of the parent and daughter are 14.007687 and 14.007520 *atomic* mass units, respectively, calculate the kinetic energy of the most energetic beta particle? **4.1**

$14.007687 - 14.007520 = 1.67 \times 10^{-4}$ amu

931 MeV = 1 amu

$$1.67 \times 10^{-4} \text{ amu} \times \frac{931 \text{ MeV}}{1 \text{ amu}} = 0.156 \text{ MeV}$$

4.2 If 1.0 MBq (27 μCi) ^{131}I is needed for a diagnostic test, and if 3 days elapse between shipment of the radioiodine and its use in the test, how many Bq must be shipped? To how many μCi does this correspond? **4.2**

A = 1.0 MBq (Final quantity desired)
t = 3 days
T = 8.04 days (Half life of I–131)

Equation 4.21

$$\lambda = \frac{0.693}{T} = \frac{0.693}{8.04 \text{ d}} = 0.086 \text{ d}^{-1}$$

Using equation 4.18;

$$A_0 = \frac{A}{e^{-\lambda t}} = \frac{1 \text{ MBq}}{e^{-0.086 \times 3}} = 1.3 \text{ MBq is required to be shipped.}$$

To convert to curies:

$$1.3\ \text{MBq} \times \frac{1\ \text{Ci}}{3.7 \times 10^{10}\ \text{Bq}} \times \frac{10^6\ \text{Bq}}{\text{MBq}} \times \frac{10^6\ \mu\text{Ci}}{1\ \text{Ci}} = 35.135\ \mu\text{Ci}$$

4.3

4.3 The gamma radiation from 1 mL of a solution containing 370 Bq (0.01 μCi) ^{198}Au and 185 Bq (0.005 μCi) ^{131}I is counted daily over a 16 day period. Assume an equal detection efficiency of the scintillation counter of 10% for all the quantum energies involved. What will be the relative counting rates of the ^{131}I and ^{198}Au at time t = 0, t = 3 days, t=8 days, and t=16 days. Plot the daily total counting rates on semi–log paper, and write the equation of the curve of total count rate vs. time.

^{198}Au emits gammas in 99.5% of the transformations (from ICRP 38) and has a half life of 2.7 days.

$$370\ \text{Bq} \times \frac{1\frac{\text{trans}}{\text{sec}}}{\text{Bq}} \times \frac{99.5}{100} \times \frac{10\ \text{count}}{100\ \text{trans}} = 36.8\ \text{counts per sec at time zero}$$

The ^{131}I decay scheme is on page 83 of "Introduction to Health Physics."

$$185\ \text{Bq} \times \frac{1\frac{\text{trans}}{\text{sec}}}{\text{Bq}} \times \frac{107}{100} \times \frac{10\ \text{count}}{100\ \text{trans}} = 19.8\ \text{counts per sec at time zero}$$

So the total number of counts detected per second at time zero would be:

36.8 + 19.8 = 56.6 counts per sec total

So the ratio of counts for each at time zero is:

$$^{198}\text{Au} = \frac{36.8}{56.5} = 0.65 = 65\%\ \text{of counts were due to}\ ^{198}\text{Au}$$

$$^{131}\text{I} = \frac{19.8}{56.5} = 0.35 = 35\%\ \text{of counts were due to}\ ^{131}\text{I}$$

At t =3 days;

^{198}Au
$T_{1/2} = 2.7$ days

Equation 4.21

$$\lambda = \frac{0.693}{T} = \frac{0.693}{2.7 \text{ days}} = 0.257 \text{ d}^{-1}$$

Equation 4.18:

$t = 3$ days
$\lambda = 0.257$ days^{-1}
$A_0 = 36.8$ cps

$$A = A_0 e^{-\lambda t} = 36.8 \times \text{e}^{-0.257 \times 3} = 17.0 \text{ cps}$$

^{131}I
$T_{1/2} = 8.05$ days

Equation 4.21

$$\lambda = \frac{0.693}{T} = \frac{0.693}{8.05 \text{ days}} = 8.6 \times 10^{-2} \text{ d}^{-1}$$

Replacing the values in equation 4.18:

$t = 3$ days
$\lambda = 8.6 \times 10^{-2}$ d^{-1}
$A_0 = 19.8$ cps

$$A = A_0 e^{-\lambda t} = 19.8 \times \text{e}^{-0.086 \times 3} = 15.3 \text{ cps}$$

Total counts per second on 3rd day:

17.1 cps + 15.3 cps = 32.4 cps

$$^{198}\text{Au} = \frac{17.1}{32.4} = 0.52 = 52\% \text{ of counts were due to } ^{198}\text{Au}$$

$$^{131}\text{I} = \frac{15.2}{32.4} = 0.479 = 48\% \text{ of counts were due to } ^{131}\text{I}$$

At t = 8 days;

^{198}Au

Replacing the values in equation 4.18:

t = 8 days
$\lambda = 0.257\ \text{d}^{-1}$
A_0 = 35.96 cps

$$A = A_0 e^{-\lambda t} = 36.8 \times \text{e}^{-0.257 \times 8} = 4.7 \text{ cps}$$

^{131}I

Equation 4.18:
t = 8 days
$\lambda = 8.6 \times 10^{-2}\ \text{d}^{-1}$
A_0 = 19.8 cps

$$A = A_0 e^{-\lambda t} = 19.8 \times \text{e}^{-0.086 \times 8} = 9.9 \text{ cps}$$

Total counts per second on 8th day: 4.7 cps + 9.9 cps = 14.6 cps

$$^{198}\text{Au} = \frac{4.7}{14.6} = 0.32 = 32\% \text{ of counts were due to } ^{198}\text{Au}$$

$$^{131}\text{I} = \frac{9.9}{14.6} = 0.68 = 68\% \text{ of counts were due to } ^{131}\text{I}$$

At t =16 days;

^{198}Au

^{198}Au

Replacing the values in equation 4.18:

$t = 16$ days
$\lambda = 0.257\ d^{-1}$
$A_0 = 36.8$ cps

$$A = A_0\, e^{-\lambda t} = 36.8 \times e^{-0.257 \times 16} = 0.60 \text{ cps}$$

^{131}I
Equation 4.18:
$t = 16$ days
$\lambda = 8.6 \times 10^{-2}$ days^{-1}
$A_0 = 19.8$ cps

$$A = A_0\, e^{-\lambda t} = 19.8 \times e^{-0.086 \times 16} = 5 \text{ cps}$$

Total counts per second on 16th day: 0.6 cps + 5 cps = 5.6 cps

$$^{198}\text{Au} = \frac{0.6}{5.6} = 0.11 = 11\% \text{ of counts were due to } ^{198}\text{Au}$$

$$^{131}\text{I} = \frac{5}{5.6} = 0.89 = 89\% \text{ of counts were due to } ^{131}\text{I}$$

The decay of the activity of the mixture is given in the table below and plotted graphically:

Day	A(t), cps	% ^{198}Au	%^{131}I
0	56.6	65	35
3	32.4	52	48
8	14.6	32	68
16	5.6	11	89

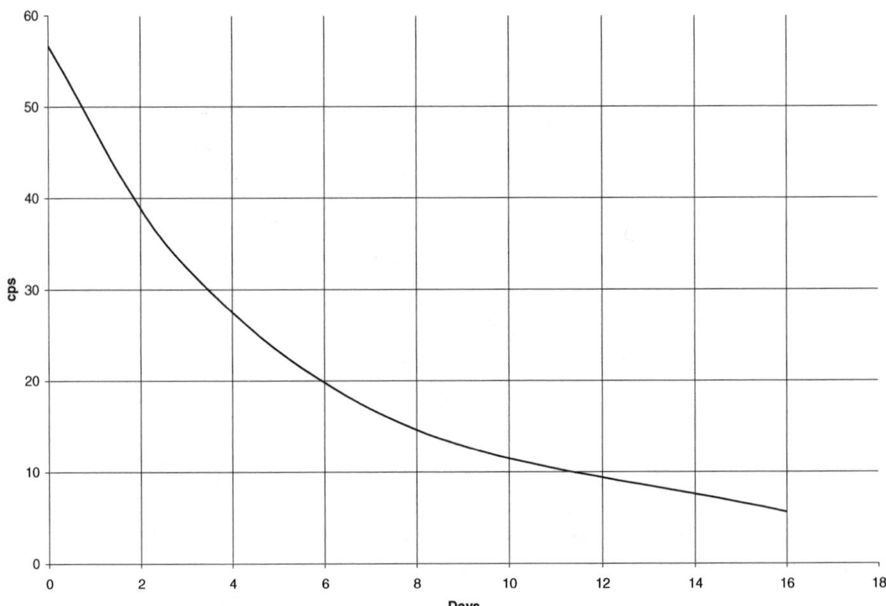

The equation for the curve of the total activity as a function of time is the sum of the activities of each of the two components, ^{198}Au and ^{131}I, The initial count rates, A_0, and the transformation constants for each isotope are:

	^{198}Au	^{131}I
A_0	36.8 cps	19.8 cps
slope, λ	0.257 d^{-1}	0.086 d^{-1}

$$A(t) = A_{01}e^{-\lambda_1 t} + A_{02}e^{-\lambda_2 t}$$
$$A(t) = 36.8e^{-0.257t} + 19.8e^{-0.086t}$$

4.4

4.4 The following counting rates were obtained on a sample that was identified as a pure beta emitter.

Day	0	1	2	3	5	10	20
cpm	5500	5240	5000	4750	4320	3400	2050

(a) Plot the data on semi–log paper.

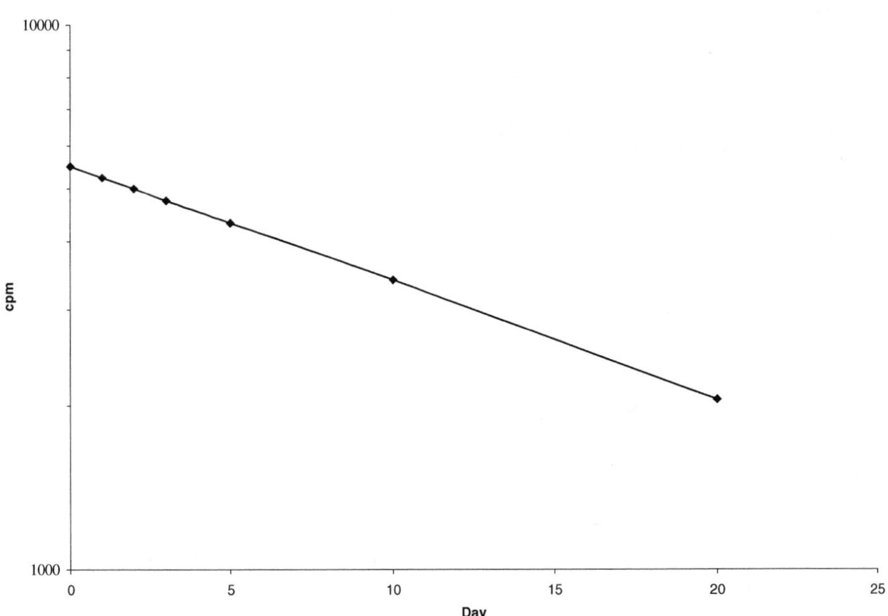

(b) Determine the half life from the graph.

Looking at the graph, it can be seen that the number of counts has decreased by half, to 2750 counts, at approximately 14.3 days.

(c) What is the value of the transformation constant, per day?

Use equation 4.21,

$$\lambda = \frac{0.693}{T} = \frac{0.693}{14.3 \text{ days}} = 4.85 \times 10^{-2} \text{ d}^{-1} \text{ is the transformation constant.}$$

(d) Write the equation for the decay curve.

Equation 4.18 is replaced by the values:

$A_0 = 5500$
$\lambda = 4.85 \times 10^{-2}\ \text{d}^{-1}$

$A = A_0 e^{-\lambda t} = 5500 \times e^{-0.0485 \times t}$

(e) What is the radionuclide?

Looking in the RHH in the table of beta emitters by increasing energy, and for an isotope that emits only a beta, it can be seen that the isotope is ^{32}P.

4.5 **4.5** If we start with 5 mg ^{210}Pb, what would be the activity of this sample 10 years later?

$T_{1/2} = 22$ years

Equation 4.21,

$$\lambda = \frac{0.693}{T} = \frac{0.693}{22\ \text{yr}} = 3.15 \times 10^{-2}\ \text{yr}^{-1}$$ is the transformation constant.

Equation 4.18 is replaced by the values:
$t = 10$ yr
$A_0 = 5$ mg
$\lambda = 3.15 \times 10^{-2}\ \text{yr}^{-1}$

$A = A_0 e^{-\lambda t} = (5\ \text{mg}) \times e^{-0.0315 \times 10} = 3.65$ mg is the amount of ^{210}Pb left after 10 years.

Calculating the specific activity of ^{210}Pb using equation 4.31;
$A_{Ra} = 226$
$T_{Ra} = 1620$ yr
$A_{Pb\text{-}210} = 210$
$T_{Pb\text{-}210} = 22$ yr

$$SA = \frac{A_{Ra} T_{Ra}}{A_{Pb-210} T_{Pb-210}} = \frac{226 \times 1620\ \text{yr}}{210 \times 22\ \text{yr}} = 79.25 \frac{\text{Ci}}{\text{g}}$$ is the specific activity of ^{210}Pb.

Calculating the activity after 10 years:

$$3.65 \text{ mg} \times \frac{\text{g}}{1000 \text{ mg}} \times \frac{79.25 \text{ Ci}}{\text{g}} = 0.2893 \text{ Ci} = 298.3 \text{ mCi}$$

$$0.2893 \text{ Ci} \times \frac{3.7 \times 10^{10} \text{ Bq}}{\text{Ci}} = 1.07 \times 10^{10} \text{ Bq} = 10.7 \text{ GBq}$$

4.6 The decay constant for ^{235}U is 9.72×10^{-10} per year. Compute the number of transformations per second in a 500 mg sample of ^{235}U. **4.6**

$\lambda = 9.72 \times 10^{-10}$ per year

Find the half life with equation 4.21

$$T = \frac{0.693}{\lambda} = \frac{0.693}{9.72 \times 10^{-10} \text{ yr}^{-1}} = 7.13 \times 10^{8} \text{ yr}$$

Using the specific activity equation (4.31):
$A_{Ra} = 226$
$T_{Ra} = 1620$ yrs
$A_{U-235} = 235$
$T_{U-235} = 7.13 \times 10^{8}$ yr

$$SA = \frac{A_{Ra} \times T_{Ra}}{A_i \times T_i} = \frac{226 \times 1620 \text{ yrs}}{235 \times (7.13 \times 10^{8} \text{ yrs})} = 2.19 \times 10^{-6} \text{ Ci/g U–235}$$

Calculate the number of curies present in 500 mg;

$$500 \text{ mg} \times \frac{1 \text{ g}}{1000 \text{ mg}} \times \frac{2.19 \times 10^{-6} \text{ Ci}}{\text{g}} = 1.093 \times 10^{-6} \text{ Ci}$$

Converting curies to transformations per second:

$$1.093 \times 10^{-6} \text{ Ci} \times \frac{3.7 \times 10^{10} \frac{\text{transformations}}{\text{sec}}}{1 \text{ Ci}} = 4 \times 10^{4} \text{ transformations per}$$

second

Alternately;

Activity = λN, where N = number of radioactive atoms.

$$N = \frac{6.02 \times 10^{23}\ \frac{\text{atoms}}{\text{mole}}}{235\ \frac{\text{g}}{\text{mole}}} \times 0.5\ \text{g} = 1.28 \times 10^{21}\ \text{atoms}$$

$$\lambda = \frac{9.72 \times 10^{-10}\ \text{y}^{-1}}{365\ \frac{\text{d}}{\text{y}} \times 8.64 \times 10^{4}\ \frac{\text{s}}{\text{d}}} = 3.082 \times 10^{-17}\ \text{s}^{-1}$$

Activity = 3.08×10^{-17} s^{-1} × 1.28×10^{21} atoms = 4×10^{4} dps

4.7

4.7 Two hundred MBq (5.4 mCi) ^{210}Po are necessary for a certain ionization source. How many grams ^{210}Po does this represent?

$T_{Po\text{–}210}$ = 138 days
$A_{Po\text{–}210}$ =210
A_{Ra} = 226
T_{Ra} = 1620 yrs

Use the specific activity equation (4.31):

$$SA = \frac{A_{Ra} \times T_{Ra}}{A_i \times T_i} = \frac{226 \times 1620\ \text{yrs}}{210 \times 138\ \text{d} \times \frac{1\ \text{yr}}{365\ \text{d}}} = 4.61 \times 10^{3}\ \text{Ci/g Po–210}$$

Converting activity to mCi:

5.4 mCi = 5.4×10^{-3} Ci

Now convert Ci into grams:

$$5.4 \times 10^{-3}\ \text{Ci} \times \frac{1\ \text{g}}{4.61 \times 10^{3}\ \text{Ci}} = 1.17 \times 10^{-6}\ \text{g} = 1.17\ \mu\text{g}$$

4.8 How long would it take for 99.9% of ^{137}Cs to decay, if its half–life is 30 years? 4.8

T = 30 years

Equation 4.21

$$\lambda = \frac{0.693}{T} = \frac{0.693}{30\ \text{yr}} = 0.0231\ \text{yr}^{-1}$$

What fraction is remaining if 99.9% has disappeared?

1.000 – 0.999 = 0.001 is all that would remain.

So that the ratio between what remains and what was started with is:

$$\frac{A}{A_0} = \frac{\text{final}}{\text{initial}} = 0.001$$

Using equation 4.21 and solving for t:

$$\frac{A}{A_0} = e^{-\lambda t} = 0.001$$

$$t = \frac{6.91}{\lambda} = 299\ \text{years}$$

4.9 How long will it take for each of the following radioisotopes to decrease to 0.0001% of its initial activity? 4.9

(a) ^{99}Mo $\quad T_{1/2} = 66$ hr

Equation 4.17 is used to find the number of half lives it takes for any isotope to decay to 0.0001% of its initial value:

n = number of half lives

$$\frac{I}{I_0} = 0.000001 = 10^{-6}$$

$$\frac{I}{I_0} = \frac{1}{2^n}$$

Replacing values

$$10^{-6} = \frac{1}{2^n}$$

$$n = \frac{6}{\log(2)} = 20 \text{ half lives are needed to decrease to 0.0001\% of initial activity.}$$

So for ^{99}Mo: $T_{1/2}$ = 66 hr; 66 hr × 20 = 1320 hr = 55 days

(b) ^{99m}Tc: $T_{1/2}$ = 6 hr; 6 hr × 20 = 120 hr = 5 days

(c) ^{131}I : $T_{1/2}$ = 8 days; 8 days × 20 = 160 days

(d) ^{125}I: $T_{1/2}$ = 60 days; 60 days × 20 = 1200 days

4.10

4.10 For use in carcinogenesis studies, benzo(a)pyrene is tagged with ^{3}H to a specific activity of 4×10^{11} Bq/millimole. If there is only 1 tritium atom on a tagged molecule, what percentage of the benzo(a)pyrene is tagged with ^{3}H?

Remember that tritium is a hydrogen atom with 2 neutrons, and is written ^{3}H. First, find the specific activity of carrier free tritium, using equation 4.31:
A_{Ra} = 226
T_{Ra} = 1620 years
A_{H-3} = 3
T_{H-3} = 12.3 years

$$SA_{H-3} = \frac{A_{Ra}T_{Ra}}{A_H T_H} = \frac{226 \times 1620 \text{ yr}}{3 \times 12.3 \text{ yr}} = 9922 \text{ Ci/g Tritium}$$

$$\frac{9922 \text{ Ci}}{\text{g }^3\text{H}} \times \frac{3 \text{ g}}{\text{mol }^3\text{H}} \times \frac{1 \text{ mol }^3\text{H}}{6.02 \times 10^{23} \text{atoms }^3\text{H}} \times \frac{3.7 \times 10^{10} \text{Bq}}{\text{Ci}}$$

$$= 1.83 \times 10^{-9} \frac{\text{Bq}}{\text{atom }^3\text{H}}$$

Next, calculate the proportion of benzo(a)pyrene molecules tagged:

$$\frac{4\times10^{11}\,\text{Bq}}{\text{mmol Benzo.}}\times\frac{1000\text{ mmol}}{1\text{ mol}}\times\frac{1\text{ mol}}{6.02\times10^{23}\text{ molecules}}$$

$$= 6.64\times10^{-10}\,\frac{\text{Bq}}{\text{Benzo. molecules}}$$

Divide the number of Bq/Benzo atom by Bq/^{3}H atom to find the fraction of benzo(a)pyrene atoms tagged:

$$\frac{\left\{\dfrac{6.64\times10^{-10}\,\text{Bq}}{\text{Benzo. atom}}\right\}}{\left\{\dfrac{1.83\times10^{-9}\,\text{Bq}}{\text{atom }(^{3}\text{H})}\right\}} = 0.363 \text{ is the fraction of benzo(a)pyrene molecules tagged}$$

Thus, 36.3% of the benzo(a)pyrene molecules are tagged with tritium.

4.11 How many alpha particles are emitted per minute by 1 cm^{3} ^{222}Ra at a temperature of 27°C and a pressure of 100,000 Pa? **4.11**

100,000 Pa = 0.987 atmospheres

27 + 273 = 300 K

Assume that the radon is an ideal gas.
Recalling the ideal gas law where $PV=nRT$,
P = pressure in atmospheres
V = Volume in liters
n = number of moles
R= gas constant = 0.082 L·atm/mol·K
T = absolute temperature, kelvin

$$\frac{n}{V}=\frac{P}{RT}=\frac{0.987\text{ atm.}}{0.082\dfrac{\text{L}\cdot\text{atm}}{\text{mole}\cdot\text{K}}\times300\text{ K}}=0.04\frac{\text{moles}}{\text{L}} \text{ of radon gas}$$

Now calculate the specific activity of ^{222}Rn (equation 4.31):

$A_{Ra} = 226$
$T_{Ra} = 1620$ years
$A_{Rn-222} = 222$
$T_{Rn-222} = 3.82$ days $= 0.01$ year

$$SA_{Rn-222} = \frac{A_{Ra}T_{Ra}}{A_{Rn}T_{Rn}} = \frac{226 \times 1620 \text{ yr}}{222 \times 0.01 \text{ yr}} = 1.65 \times 10^5 \text{ Ci/g } ^{222}\text{Ra}$$

Calculate the number of transformations per minute using the specific activity, and the number of moles per liter of ^{222}Rn calculated above. (Note the equation is split into two lines);

$$\frac{1.65 \times 10^5 \text{Ci}}{\text{g } ^{222}\text{Ra}} \times \frac{222 \text{ g } ^{222}\text{Ra}}{\text{mol}} \times \frac{0.04 \text{ mol } ^{222}\text{Ra}}{\text{L } ^{222}\text{Ra}} \times \frac{1 \text{ L}}{1000 \text{ cm}^3} \times$$

$$\times \frac{1 \text{ cm}^3 \ ^{222}\text{Ra}}{\text{sample}} \times \frac{2.22 \times 10^{12} \frac{\text{trans}}{\text{min}}}{1 \text{ Ci}} \times \frac{1\ \alpha}{\text{trans}}$$

$= 3.25 \times 10^{15}$ α per minute emitted from the sample

4.12 **4.12** Calculate the number of beta particles emitted per minute by 1 kg KCl, if ^{40}K emits 1 beta particle per transformation.

Find the specific activity of ^{40}K (equation 4.31):

$A_{Ra} = 226$
$T_{Ra} = 1620$ yr
$A_{K-40} = 40$
$T_{K-40} = 1.29 \times 10^9$ yr

$$SA_{K-40} = \frac{A_{Ra}T_{Ra}}{A_K T_K} = \frac{226 \times 1620 \text{ yr}}{40 \times 1.29 \times 10^9 \text{ yr}} = 7.1 \times 10^{-6} \text{ Ci/g } ^{40}\text{K}$$

Natural abundance of ^{40}K is 0.0117 % of all K.

K = 39.1 grams per mole
Cl = 35.457 grams per mole

$KCl = 39.1 + 35.457 = 74.557$ grams per mole

Solve for the number of curies of ^{40}K per sample, using the specific activity:

$$\frac{1000 \text{ g KCl}}{\text{sample}} \times \frac{1 \text{ mol KCl}}{74.6 \text{ g KCl}} \times \frac{1 \text{ mol K}}{1 \text{ mol KCl}} \times \frac{\left(\frac{0.0117}{100}\right) \text{mol } ^{40}\text{K}}{1 \text{ mol K}} \times \frac{40 \text{ g } ^{40}\text{K}}{1 \text{ mol } ^{40}\text{K}} \times \frac{7.1 \times 10^{-6} \text{ Ci}}{\text{g } ^{40}\text{K}}$$

$= 4.49 \times 10^{-7}$ Ci ^{40}K per sample

Convert to betas per minute:

$$\frac{4.49 \times 10^{-7} \text{ Ci}}{\text{sample}} \times \frac{2.22 \times 10^{12} \frac{\text{trans}}{\text{min}}}{\text{Ci}} \times \frac{1 \, \beta}{\text{trans}} = 9.96 \times 10^{5} \, \frac{\beta}{\text{min}} \text{ in one kg sample}$$

4.13 Iodine 125, a widely used isotope in the practice of nuclear medicine, has a half life of 60 days. **4.13**
(a) How long will it take for 4 MBq (~ 1μCi) to decrease to 0.1% of its initial activity?

$T_{1/2} = 60$ days

Equation 4.21

$$\lambda = \frac{0.693}{T} = \frac{0.693}{60 \text{ d}} = 0.01155 \text{ d}^{-1}$$

Equation 4.21:
$t = 60$ days
$\lambda = 0.01155 \text{ d}^{-1}$

$$\frac{A}{A_0} = 0.001 = e^{-\lambda t}$$

$$t = \frac{\ln \frac{A}{A_0}}{-\lambda} = \frac{\ln 0.001}{-0.01155 \text{ d}^{-1}} = 598 \text{ d}$$

(b) What is the mean life of ^{125}I?

$\lambda = 0.01155\ d^{-1}$ {From part (a)}

Equation 4.24

$$\tau = \frac{1}{\lambda} = \frac{1}{0.01155\ d^{-1}} = 86.6 \text{ days}$$

4.14 **4.14** If uranium ore contains 10% U_3O_8, how many metric tons are necessary to produce 1 g radium if the extraction process is 90% efficient?

First, find the ratio (in grams) of uranium to the radium in the ore using the specific activities of each. Assume that the radium is in secular equilibrium with the uranium, and radium has the specific activity of 1 curie per gram.

Use equation 4.31
$A_{Ra} = 226$
$T_{Ra} = 1620$ years
$A_U = 238$
$T_U = 4.51 \times 10^9$ years

$$SA_{U\text{-}238} = \frac{A_{Ra} T_{Ra}}{A_U T_U} = \frac{226 \times 1620 \text{ yr}}{238 \times 4.51 \times 10^9 \text{ yr}} = 3.4 \times 10^{-7} \text{ Ci/g}$$

Obtain the number of grams of radium per gram of uranium, knowing that in ore, ^{226}Ra is in equilibrium with ^{238}U. Therefore, we have:

3.4×10^{-7} g radium / g uranium

$$\frac{1 \text{ tonne } U_3O_8}{10 \text{ tonnes Ore}} \times \frac{1000 \text{ kg } U_3O_8}{1 \text{ tonne } U_3O_8} \times \frac{1000 \text{ g } U_3O_8}{1 \text{ kg } U_3O_8} \times \frac{1 \text{ mole } U_3O_8}{\{(238 \times 3) + (16 \times 8)\} \text{g } U_3O_8}$$

$= 118.8$ moles U_3O_8/ton

$$\frac{118.8 \text{ mol } U_3O_8}{\text{tonne ore}} \times \frac{3 \text{ mol}^{238}\text{U}}{1 \text{ mol } U_3O_8} \times \frac{238 \text{ g}^{238}\text{U}}{1 \text{ mol}^{238}\text{U}} \times \frac{3.4 \times 10^{-7} \text{ g Ra}}{1 \text{ g }^{238}\text{U}}$$

$= 0.029$ g radium/tonne ore

Inverting this solution to find how many tons ore per one gram:

$$\frac{\text{tonne ore}}{0.029 \text{ g Radium}} = 35 \text{ tonnes per gram of radium}$$

However, the process is only 90% efficient (according to the question), so:

$$\frac{35 \text{ tonns ore}}{1 \text{ g radium}} \times \frac{100}{90} = 39 \text{ tonnes of ore are needed to yield 1 gram of radium.}$$

4.15 How much ^{234}U is there in one ton of the uranium ore containing 10% U_3O_8? **4.15**

The activity of ^{234}U is equal to the activity of ^{238}U since ^{234}U is in secular equilibrium with ^{238}U.

$$SA\left(^{238}U\right) = \frac{1620 \text{ y} \times 226}{4.5 \times 10^9 \text{ y} \times 238} = 3.4 \times 10^{-7} \frac{\text{Ci}}{\text{g}}$$

In one ton (2000 lbs.) uranium ore, we have 200 lbs. U_3O_8, or

$200 \text{ lbs} \times 453.6 \frac{\text{g}}{\text{lb}} = 9.07 \times 10^4 \text{ g } U_3O_8$ and the amount of ^{238}U in this amount of U_3O_8 is

$$0.993 \times 9.07 \times 10^4 \text{ g } U_3O_8 \times \frac{3.4 \times 238}{3.4 \times 238 + 8 \times 16} \frac{\text{g}^{238}\text{U}}{\text{g } U_3O_8} = 7.64 \times 10^4 \text{ g }^{238}\text{U}$$

The activity in this quantity of ^{238}U is

$$7.64 \times 10^4 \text{ g }^{238}\text{U} \times 3.4 \times 10^{-7} \frac{\text{Ci}}{\text{g }^{238}\text{U}} = 2.6 \times 10^{-2} \text{ Ci}$$

The specific activity of ^{234}U is

$$SA\left({}^{234}U\right) = \frac{1620\ y \times 226}{4.58 \times 10^5\ y \times 234} = 6.3 \times 10^{-3}\ \frac{Ci}{g}$$

Since the activities of the two uranium isotopes are equal, the weight of the ^{234}U is

$$w = \frac{2.6 \times 10^{-2}\ Ci}{6.3 \times 10^{-3}\ \frac{Ci}{g}} = 4.1\ g$$

Alternatively;

$^{234}U = 5.5 \times 10^{-5}$ is the fractional abundance of ^{234}U in natural uranium

Calculate the number of grams per mole of U_3O_8:

Uranium
238.0289 × 3 = 714.0867 g/mole

Oxygen
15.9994 × 8 = 127.9952 g/mole

U_3O_8 = 714.0867 g/mole + 127.9952 g/mole = 842.0819 g/mole

Note that the equation is split into two lines below;

$$1\text{ ton ore} \times \frac{10\text{ ton } U_3O_8}{100\text{ tons ore}} \times \frac{2000\text{ lb } U_3O_8}{\text{ton } U_3O_8} \times \frac{0.4536\text{ kg}}{1\text{ lb}} \times \frac{1000\text{ g}}{1\text{ kg}} \times \frac{1\text{ mol } U_3O_8}{842.0819\text{ g } U_3O_8} \times$$

$$\times \frac{3\text{ mol U}}{1\text{ mol } U_3O_8} \times \frac{5.5 \times 10^{-5}\text{ mol}({}^{234}U)}{1\text{ mol U}} = 0.0178\text{ moles } {}^{234}U\text{ per ton ore}$$

$$\frac{0.0178\text{ mol } {}^{234}U}{\text{ton ore}} \times \frac{234\text{ g}\,{}^{234}U}{1\text{ mol}\,{}^{234}U} = 4.18\text{ g } {}^{234}U\text{ per ton of ore}$$

4.16

4.16 Compare the activity of the ^{234}U to that of the ^{235}U and the ^{238}U in the ore of problems 4.14 and 4.15.

The natural abundance of $^{235}U = 0.72\%$, and its half-life = 7.13×10^8 yr. Therefore, in 1 ton (2000 lbs) of 10% U_3O_8 ore, we have

$$\frac{(2000 \times 0.1)\text{lbs } U_3O_8}{\text{ton}} \times 453\frac{\text{g}}{\text{lb}} \times \frac{(3 \times 238)\text{ g U}}{(3 \times 238 + 8 \times 16)\text{ g } U_3O_8} \times 7.2 \times 10^{-3}\,\frac{\text{g } ^{235}U}{\text{g U}} = 554\frac{\text{g } ^{235}U}{\text{ton}}$$

The specific activity of ^{235}U (eq. 4.31) is

$A_{Ra} = 226$
$T_{Ra} = 1620$ yr
$A_{U-235} = 235$
$T_{U-235} = 7.13 \times 10^8$ yr

$$SA = \frac{A_{Ra} \times T_{Ra}}{A_i \times T_i} = \frac{226 \times 1620\text{ yr}}{235 \times (7.13 \times 10^8\text{ yr})} = 2.19 \times 10^{-6}\text{ Ci/g U–235}$$

^{235}U activity in one ton ore is 2.6×10^{-2} Ci/ton (from problem 4.15)
^{234}U activity = ^{238}U activity (secular equilibrium)
Therefore the total activity in 1 ton of this ore is
$1.21 \times 10^{-3} + 2(2.6 \times 10^{-2}) = 5.32 \times 10^{-2}$ Ci/ton

$$^{234}U = \frac{2.6 \times 10^{-2}}{5.32 \times 10^{-2}} \times 100 = 48.87\%$$

$$^{235}U = \frac{1.21 \times 10^{-2}}{5.32 \times 10^{-2}} \times 100 = 2.27\%$$

^{238}U activity = ^{234}U activity = 48.87%
Total activity = 48.87% + 2.27% + 48.87% = 100%

Alternatively,
^{234}U
$A_{Ra} = 226$
$T_{Ra} = 1620$ yrs
$A_{U-234} = 234$
$T_{U-234} = 2.47 \times 10^5$ yr

Equation 4.31:

$$SA = \frac{A_{Ra}T_{Ra}}{A_i T_i} = \frac{226 \times 1620\text{ yr}}{234 \times (2.47 \times 10^5\text{ yr})} = 6.33 \times 10^{-3}\text{ Ci/g U–234}$$

^{235}U

$A_{Ra} = 226$
$T_{Ra} = 1620$ yr
$A_{U-235} = 235$
$T_{U-235} = 7.13 \times 10^8$ yr

Replacing numbers in equation 4.31:

$$SA = \frac{A_{Ra} \times T_{Ra}}{A_i \times T_i} = \frac{226 \times 1620\text{ yr}}{235 \times (7.13 \times 10^8\text{ yr})} = 2.19 \times 10^{-6}\text{ Ci/g U–235}$$

^{238}U

$A_{Ra} = 226$
$T_{Ra} = 1620$ yr
$A_{U-238} = 238$
$T_{U-238} = 4.51 \times 10^9$ yr

Equation 4.31:

$$SA = \frac{A_{Ra} \times T_{Ra}}{A_i \times T_i} = \frac{226 \times 1620\text{ yr}}{238 \times 4.51 \times 10^9\text{ yr}} = 3.41 \times 10^{-7}\text{ Ci/g U–238}$$

Percent abundance

$^{234}U = 0.0055$
$^{235}U = 0.720$
$^{238}U = 99.2745$

From problem 4.14 there are 118.8 moles U_3O_8/ton ore

$$\frac{118.8\text{ mol }U_3O_8}{\text{ton ore}} \times \frac{3\text{ mol U}}{1\text{ mol }U_3O_8} = 356.4\text{ moles Uranium per ton ore.}$$

$$\frac{356.4 \text{ mol U}}{\text{ton ore}} \times \frac{0.0055 \text{ mol}^{234}\text{U}}{100 \text{ mol U}} \times \frac{234 \text{ g}}{1 \text{ mol}^{234}\text{U}} \times \frac{6.33 \times 10^{-3}\text{Ci}}{\text{g}}$$

$= 0.029$ Ci ^{234}U per ton ore

Similarly for U–235

$$\frac{356.4 \text{ mol U}}{\text{ton ore}} \times \frac{0.720 \text{ mol}^{235}\text{U}}{100 \text{ molU}} \times \frac{235 \text{ g}}{1 \text{ mol }^{235}\text{U}} \times \frac{2.19 \times 10^{-6}\text{Ci}}{\text{g}}$$

$= 0.00132$ Ci ^{235}U per ton ore

And U–238

$$\frac{356.4 \text{ mol U}}{\text{ton ore}} \times \frac{99.2745 \text{ mol}^{238}\text{U}}{100 \text{ mol U}} \times \frac{238 \text{ g}}{1 \text{ mol}^{238}\text{U}} \times \frac{3.41 \times 10^{-7}\text{Ci}}{\text{g}}$$

$= 0.0287$ Ci ^{238}U per ton ore

4.17 Calculate the activity in Bq and μCi in each of the uranium isotopes in 1 g of natural U, and then, using these results together with the values for the isotopic abundance's, calculate the activity of 1 g of natural U. **4.17**

^{238}U

The sample activity is equal to the SA times the mass of the sample. The specific activity is (equation 4.31):

$A_{Ra} = 226$

$T_{Ra} = 1620$ yr

$A_{U-238} = 238$

$T_{U-238} = 4.5 \times 10^9$ yr

$$SA = \frac{A_{Ra} T_{Ra}}{A_{U-238} T_{U238}} = \frac{226 \times 1620 \text{ yr}}{238 \times 4.5 \times 10^9 \text{ yr}} = 3.4 \times 10^{-7} \frac{\text{Ci}}{\text{g}}$$

The isotopic abundance of ^{238}U is 99.276% of all uranium, so the activity in one gram of natural uranium due to ^{238}U is:

$$1\text{ g} \times \frac{99.276\text{ g }^{238}\text{U}}{100\text{ g U}} \times \frac{3.4 \times 10^{-7}\text{ Ci}}{\text{g }^{238}\text{U}} \times \frac{10^{6}\ \mu\text{Ci}}{\text{Ci}}$$ = 0.34 μCi (1.26 × 10^4 Bq) in one gram of natural uranium due to ^{238}U.

For ^{235}U we have
$A_{Ra} = 226$
$T_{Ra} = 1620$ yr
$A_{U\text{-}235} = 235$
$T_{U\text{-}235} = 7.13 \times 10^8$ yr

$$SA = \frac{A_{Ra}T_{Ra}}{A_{U-235}T_{U235}} = \frac{226 \times 1620\text{ yr}}{235 \times 7.13 \times 10^{8}\text{ yr}} = 2.19 \times 10^{-6}\ \frac{\text{Ci}}{\text{g}}$$

The isotopic abundance of ^{235}U is 0.7196% of all uranium, so the activity in one gram of natural uranium due to ^{235}U is:

$$1\text{ g} \times \frac{7.2 \times 10^{-3}\text{ g }^{235}\text{U}}{1\text{ g U}} \times \frac{2.19 \times 10^{-6}\text{ Ci}}{\text{g}} \times \frac{10^{6}\ \mu\text{Ci}}{\text{Ci}}$$ = 0.016 μCi (5.9 × 10^2 Bq) in one gram of natural uranium due to ^{235}U.

Since ^{234}U is in secular equilibrium with ^{238}U, the two activities are equal, 0.34 μCi (1.26 × 10^4 Bq)

Adding the activities together, ^{238}U + ^{235}U+^{234}U
0.34 μCi + 0.016 μCi + 0.34 μCi = 0.7 μCi = 2.6 × 10^4 Bq in 1 g natural uranium.

4.18 **4.18** What will be the temperature rise after 24 hours in a well insulated 100 mL aqueous solution containing 1 gram $Na_2{}^{35}SO_4$, if the specific activity of the sulfur is 3.7 × 10^{12} Bq/gram (100 Ci/gram)?

First, find the specific activity of ^{35}S and compare it to the specific activity listed in the problem to find the fraction of sulfur atoms that are ^{35}S;

Equation 4.31

$A_{Ra} = 226$
$T_{Ra} = 1620$ yr
$A_{S-35} = 35$
$T_{S-35} = 87.44$ days $= 0.24$ yr

$$SA = \frac{A_{Ra}T_{Ra}}{A_{S-35}T_{S-35}} = \frac{226 \times 1620 \text{ yr}}{35 \times 0.24 \text{ yr}} = 4.36 \times 10^4 \frac{\text{Ci}}{\text{g}}$$

Now calculate the fraction of the mass of the tagged (*S) sulfur in the compound that is ^{35}S:

$$\frac{100 \frac{\text{Ci}}{\text{g}} \text{ Tagged}^{35}\text{S}}{4.36 \times 10^4 \frac{\text{Ci}}{\text{g}} \text{ S}} = \frac{1 \text{ g}^{35}\text{S}}{439 \text{ g S}}$$

Since only a very small fraction of all the sulfur atoms is tagged as ^{35}S, using 32 grams for the atomic weight of the tagged sulfer is a reasonable assumption.

The atomic weights are as follows:

Na = 23
S = 32
O = 16
$Na_2{}^*SO_4 = (2 \times 23) + 32 + (4 \times 16) = 142$ g/mole

^{35}S activity concentration

$$\frac{1 \text{ g Na}_2{}^*\text{SO}_4}{100 \text{ mL}} \times \frac{32 \text{ g}^*\text{S}}{142 \text{ g Na}_2{}^*\text{SO}_4} \times 100 \frac{\text{Ci}}{\text{g}^*\text{S}} \times \frac{3.7 \times 10^{10} \text{ Bq}}{\text{Ci}} = 8.34 \times 10^9 \frac{\text{Bq}}{\text{mL}}$$

$\overline{E}\,(^{35}\text{S}) = 0.049$ MeV per beta
Specific heat of water = 4.19 J/mL·°C
Temperature rise:

$$\frac{8.34\times10^{9}\ \frac{\text{Bq}}{\text{mL}}\times\frac{1\frac{\beta}{\text{sec}}}{1\text{Bq}}\times\frac{0.049\ \text{MeV}}{\beta}\times\frac{1.6\times10^{-13}\ \text{J}}{1\ \text{MeV}}\times8.64\times10^{4}\ \frac{\text{sec}}{\text{d}}}{4.19\ \frac{\text{J}}{\text{cal}}\times1\ \frac{\text{cal}}{\text{mL}\cdot{}^{\circ}\text{C}}}$$

= 1.3 °C (or K) rise in temp.

4.19 **4.19** The mean concentration of potassium in crustal rocks is 27 g/kg. If ^{40}K constitutes 0.012% of potassium, what is the ^{40}K activity in one metric ton of rock?

Calculate the specific activity of ^{40}K using equation 4.31:

$A_{\text{Ra}} = 226$
$T_{\text{Ra}} = 1620$ yr
$A_{\text{K-40}} = 40$
$T_{\text{K-40}} = 1.3 \times 10^{9}$ yr

$$SA = \frac{A_{Ra}T_{Ra}}{A_{K40}T_{K40}} = \frac{1620\ \text{yr}\times226}{40\times1.3\times10^{9}\ \text{yr}} = 7.04\times10^{-6}\ \text{Ci/g}$$

1 tonne rock

$$\frac{10^{3}\ \text{kg rock}}{\text{tonne rock}}\times\frac{27\ \text{g K}}{1\ \text{kg rock}}\times\frac{0.00012\ \text{g}\ ^{40}\text{K}}{1\ \text{g K}}\times\frac{7.04\times10^{-6}\ \text{Ci}}{\text{g}\ ^{40}\text{K}}\times\frac{1\times10^{6}\ \mu\text{Ci}}{1\ \text{Ci}}$$

= 23 μCi /tonne rock

4.20 **4.20** A solution of ^{203}Hg is received with the following assay: 1MBq/mL on 1 March 1981 at 8:00 am. It is desired to make a solution whose activity will be 0.1 MBq/mL on 1 April 1981. Calculate the dilution factor to give the desired activity. $T_{1/2}$ ^{203}Hg = 46 days.

$\Delta t = 31$ days

Equation 4.21:

$$\lambda = \frac{0.693}{46\ \text{days}} = 0.015\ \text{d}^{-1}$$

Find the activity that would be present on 1 April 1981 using equation 4.18;

$A = A_0\,e^{-\lambda t} = 1$ MBq/ mL $\times\ e^{-0.015\times 31} = 0.628$ MBq/ mL is the activity left in the solution after 31 days.

To find the quantity needed to obtain 0.1 MBq/mL:

$V_1 = 1$ mL
$V_2 = ?$ mL
$C_1 = 0.628$ MBq/mL
$C_2 = 0.1$ MBq/mL

$$C_1V_1 = C_2V_2$$

$$V_2 = \frac{C_1V_1}{C_2} = \frac{0.628\,\frac{\text{MBq}}{\text{mL}} \times 1\text{ mL}}{0.1\,\frac{\text{MBq}}{\text{mL}}} = 6.28\text{ mL}$$

6.28 to 1 is the dilution factor.

4.21 In a mixture of two radioisotopes, 99% of the activity is due to ^{24}Na and 1% is due to ^{32}P. At what subsequent time will the two activities be equal? 4.21

^{24}Na $T_{1/2} = 15$ hours $= 0.625$ days

Using equation 4.21

$$\lambda_{Na} = \frac{0.693}{0.625\text{ d}} = 1.11\text{ d}^{-1}$$

^{32}P $T_{1/2} = 14.3$ days

$$\lambda_P = \frac{0.693}{14.3\text{ d}} = 0.0485\text{ d}^{-1}$$

Use equation 4.18:

$$A = A_0 e^{-\lambda t}$$

Since the activity of the ^{24}Na is 99 times the ^{32}P activity, the two activities will be equal

$$99 \times e^{-1.11 \times t} = 1 \times e^{-0.0485 \times t}$$

$$t = \frac{\ln 99}{1.06} = 4.3 \text{ days} = 104 \text{ hr}$$

4.22

4.22 Low level waste from a biomedical laboratory consists of a mixture of 100 μCi (3.7 MBq) ^{131}I and 10 μCi (0.37 MBq) ^{125}I. Plot the decay curve for the total activity over a period of 365 days and write the equation for the decay curve.

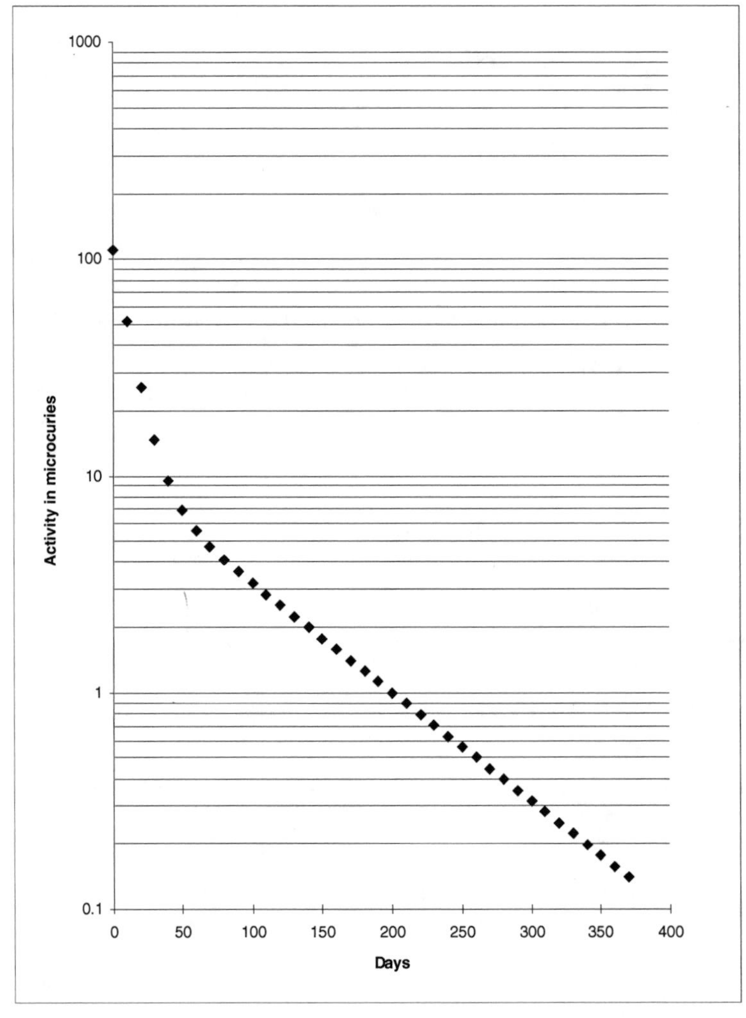

The decay constant for each of the isotopes can be found using equation 4.21:
For ^{131}I,

$T = 8.05$ d

$$\lambda = \frac{0.693}{T} = \frac{0.693}{8.05\ \text{d}} = 0.087\ \text{d}^{-1}$$

For ^{125}I,

$T = 60.14$ days

$$\lambda = \frac{0.693}{T} = \frac{0.693}{60.14\ \text{d}} = 0.0115\ \text{d}^{-1}$$

The total activity is the combination of the decay of the ^{131}I and ^{125}I decay equations using equation 4.18;

$$A = A_0 e^{-\lambda t} = A_{I-131} e^{-\lambda t} + A_{I-125}\, e^{-\lambda t} = 100 \times e^{-0.087 \times t} + 10 \times e^{-0.0115 \times t}$$

4.23 ThB is transformed to ThC at a rate of 6.54% per hour, and ThC is transformed at a rate of 1.15% per min. How long will it take for the two isotopes to reach their equilibrium state? **4.23**

$$\lambda_{ThB} = 0.0654\ \text{hr}^{-1}$$

$$\lambda_{ThC} = 0.0115\ \text{min}^{-1} = \frac{0.0115}{\text{min}} \times \frac{60\ \text{min}}{\text{hr}} = 0.69\ \text{hr}^{-1}$$

Use equation 4.57 to find the time at which the ThC activity reaches its maximum activity:

$$t_m = \frac{\ln\left(\frac{\lambda_{ThC}}{\lambda_{ThB}}\right)}{\lambda_{ThC} - \lambda_{ThB}} = \frac{\ln\left(\frac{0.69}{0.0654}\right)}{0.69 - 0.0654} = 3.78\ \text{hr}$$

So 3.78 hours after the ThB is isolated the activity will be at a maximum, however, looking at the drawing on page 111 of the third edition, it can be seen that they are not in equilibrium until the activity of the ThC moves off of it's "peak", which will occur roughly after 6 to 7 half lives (60.5 min times 7, approximately twice the time it took to reach peak activity), and the two isotopes will then be in "equilibrium".

4.24

4.24 How many grams of ^{90}Y are there when ^{90}Y is equilibrated with 10 mg ^{90}Sr?

^{90}Sr
$T_{1/2} = 28$ yr
Calculate the specific activity of ^{90}Sr using equation 4.31:

$A_{Ra} = 226$
$T_{Ra} = 1620$ yr
$A_{Sr} = 90$
$T_{Sr} = 28$ yr

$$SA = \frac{A_{Ra}T_{Ra}}{A_{Sr}T_{Sr}} = \frac{226 \times 1620 \text{ yr}}{90 \times 28 \text{ yr}} = 145.3 \text{ Ci/g} = 145.3 \text{ mCi/mg}$$

At secular equilibrium, the ^{90}Y activity = ^{90}Sr activity,
10 mg x 145.3 mCi/mg = 1453 mCi = 1.453 Ci

Calculate the specific activity of ^{90}Y using equation 4.31:
$A_{Ra} = 226$
$T_{Ra} = 1620$ yr
$A_Y = 90$

$$SA = \frac{A_{Ra}T_{Ra}}{A_Y T_Y} = \frac{226 \times 1620 \text{ yr}}{90 \times 7.3 \times 10^{-3} \text{ yr}} = 5.57 \times 10^5 \text{ Ci/g}$$

Calculating the ^{90}Y weight after equilibrium:

$$\frac{1.453 \text{ Ci}}{5.57 \times 10^5 \dfrac{\text{Ci}}{\text{g } ^{90}\text{Y}}} = 2.6 \times 10^{-3} \text{ mg} = 2.6 \ \mu\text{g}$$

4.25

4.25 Radiogenic lead constitutes 98.5% of the element as found in lead ore. The isotopic constitution of lead in nature is: ^{204}Pb, 1.5%; ^{206}Pb, 23.6%; ^{207}Pb, 22.6%; ^{208}Pb, 52.3%. How much uranium and thorium decayed completely to produce 985 mg of radiogenic lead?

Assume the total sample had 1000 mg of lead, with only 985 mg radiogenic, so the number of mg of each type of lead would be:

^{206}Pb, 23.6% × 1000 mg = 236 mg

^{207}Pb, 22.6% × 1000 mg = 226 mg

^{208}Pb, 52.3% × 1000 mg = 523 mg

^{206}Pb is the end product of the ^{238}U decay chain,

$$^{238}\text{U: } 236\text{ mg } ^{206}\text{Pb} \times \frac{1\text{ mol}^{206}\text{Pb}}{206\text{ g}} \times \frac{1\text{ mol}^{238}\text{U}}{1\text{ mol}^{206}\text{Pb}} \times \frac{238\text{ g}^{238}\text{U}}{1\text{ mol}^{238}\text{U}} = 272.66\text{ mg}$$

^{207}Pb, 22.6% × 1000 mg = 226 mg

^{207}Pb is the end product of the ^{235}U decay chain,

$$^{235}\text{U: } 226\text{ mg } ^{207}\text{Pb} \times \frac{1\text{ mol}^{207}\text{Pb}}{207\text{ g}} \times \frac{1\text{ mol}^{235}\text{U}}{1\text{ mol}^{207}\text{Pb}} \times \frac{235\text{ g}^{235}\text{U}}{1\text{ mol}^{238}\text{U}} = 256.6\text{ mg}$$

^{208}Pb, 52.3% × 1000 mg = 523 mg

^{208}Pb is the end product of the ^{232}Th decay chain,

$$^{232}\text{Th: } 523\text{ mg } ^{208}\text{Pb} \times \frac{1\text{ mol}^{208}\text{Pb}}{208\text{ g}} \times \frac{1\text{ mol}^{232}\text{Th}}{1\text{ mol}^{208}\text{Pb}} \times \frac{232\text{ g}^{232}\text{Th}}{1\text{ mol}^{232}\text{Th}} = 583\text{ mg}$$

4.26 How long after 1 kg of ^{241}Pu is isolated will the ^{241}Am activity be at its maximum? What will the activity be at that time? **4.26**

^{241}Pu: $T_{1/2} = 13.2$ yr

Using equation 4.21: $\lambda_{Pu} = \frac{0.693}{T} = \frac{0.693}{13.2\text{ yr}} = 0.0525\text{ yr}^{-1}$

^{241}Am: $T_{1/2} = 458$ yr

Using equation 4.21: $\lambda_{Pu} = \frac{0.693}{T} = \frac{0.693}{458\ \text{yr}} = 0.0015\ \text{yr}^{-1}$

The time of maximum activity is found using equation 4.57:

$$t_m = \frac{\ln\left(\frac{\lambda_{Am}}{\lambda_{Pu}}\right)}{\lambda_{Am} - \lambda_{Pu}} = \frac{\ln\left(\frac{0.0015}{0.0525}\right)}{0.0015 - 0.0525} = 70\ \text{yr to max. activity}$$

Calculate the number of atoms of ^{241}Pu in 1 kg:

$$N_{Ao} = 1\ \text{kg Pu} \times \frac{1000\ \text{g}}{1\ \text{kg}} \times \frac{1\ \text{mol}}{241\ \text{g}} \times \frac{6.02 \times 10^{23}\ \text{atoms}}{1\ \text{mol}} = 2.5 \times 10^{24}\ \text{atoms Pu}$$

To find the activity after 70 years, use equation 4.53:

$$\lambda_{Am} N_{Am} = \frac{\lambda_{Am}\lambda_{Pu} N_{Pu(0)}}{\lambda_{Am} - \lambda_{Pu}}\left(e^{-\lambda_{Pu} t} - e^{-\lambda_{Am} t}\right)$$

$$\lambda_{Am} N_{Am} = \frac{0.0015\ \text{yr}^{-1} \times 0.0525\ \text{yr}^{-1} \times 2.5 \times 10^{24}\ \text{atoms}}{0.0015\ \text{yr}^{-1} - 0.0525\ \text{yr}^{-1}}\left(e^{-0.0525 \times 70} - e^{-0.0015 \times 70}\right)$$

$$\lambda_{Am} N_{Am} = 3.37 \times 10^{21}\ \text{transformations/yr}$$

$$\frac{3.37 \times 10^{21}\ \text{transformations}}{\text{yr}} \times \frac{1\ \text{yr}}{365\ \text{d}} \times \frac{1\ \text{d}}{24\ \text{hr}} \times \frac{1\ \text{hr}}{3600\ \text{sec}} \times \frac{1\ \text{Bq}}{\frac{\text{trans}}{\text{sec}}} = 1.1 \times 10^{14}\ \text{Bq}$$

4.27

4.27 How long after 14 minute ^{146}Ce is isolated will the activity of the 24 minute ^{146}Pr daughter be equal to that of the parent?

^{146}Ce: $T_{1/2} = 14$ min

Using equation 4.21: $\lambda_{Ce} = \frac{0.693}{14\ \text{min}} = 0.0495\ \text{min}^{-1}$

^{146}Pr: $T_{1/2} = 24$ min

Using equation 4.21: $\lambda_{\text{Pr}} = \dfrac{0.693}{24\,\text{min}} = 0.0289\ \text{min}^{-1}$

$$A_A(t) = A_0 e^{-\lambda_A t}$$

$$A_0 = \lambda_A N_A$$

The activity of the ^{146}Pr daughter (B), after isolation of its parent is give by equation 4.53

$$A_B(t) = \lambda_B N_B = \frac{\lambda_B \lambda_A N_{A0}}{\lambda_B - \lambda_A}\left(e^{-\lambda_A t} - e^{-\lambda_B t}\right)$$

Since $\lambda_A N_{Ao} = A_{A0}$, the activity of the daughter may be rewritten as

$$A_B(t) = \frac{\lambda_B A_{A0}}{\lambda_B - \lambda_A}\left(e^{-\lambda_A t} - e^{-\lambda_B t}\right)$$

Setting the activity of ^{146}Ce (A) equal to that of ^{146}Pr (B);

$$A_0 e^{-\lambda_A t} = \frac{\lambda_B A_0}{\lambda_B - \lambda_A}\left(e^{-\lambda_A t} - e^{-\lambda_B t}\right)$$

$$e^{-\lambda_A t} = \frac{\lambda_B}{\lambda_B - \lambda_A}\left(e^{-\lambda_A t} - e^{-\lambda_B t}\right)$$

$$e^{-0.0495t} = \frac{0.0289}{0.0289 - 0.0495}\left(e^{-0.0495t} - e^{-0.0289t}\right)$$

$t = 26$ min.

4.28 Thirty seven MBq (1 mCi) ^{99m}Tc are milked from a ^{99}Mo "cow". What will be the activity of the ^{99m}Tc daughter, ^{99}Tc, 1 year after the milking? **4.28**

Since the half-life of ^{99m}Tc is 6 hours (2.16×10^4 seconds), all of it will have decayed to ^{99}Tc atoms one year after milking. The half-life of ^{99}Tc is 2.13×10^5 years (6.72×10^{12} seconds). Since activity is given by

$A = \lambda N$

we can calculate the number of ^{99m}Tc atoms in 37 MBq (37×10^6 disintegrations per second)

$$37 \times 10^{6}\ \text{s}^{-1} = \frac{0.693}{2.16 \times 10^{4}\ \text{s}} \times N$$

$N = 1.16 \times 10^{12}$ atoms ^{99m}Tc

The activity of the ^{99}Tc, therefore is

$$A = \lambda N = \frac{0.693}{6.72 \times 10^{12}\ \text{s}} \times 1.16 \times 10^{12}\ \text{atoms} = 0.12\ \text{s}^{-1} = 0.12\ \text{Bq}$$

4.29

4.29 Calculate the specific activity of ^{85}Kr ($T_{1/2}$ = 10.7 years) in Bq/m^3 and μCi/cm^3 at 25°C and 760 mm Hg.

T= 25°C = 298 K

$$R = 0.082 \frac{\text{L} \cdot \text{atm}}{\text{mole} \cdot \text{K}}$$

P = 760 mm Hg = 1 atm

The ideal gas equation is used to find the number of moles per liter of ^{85}K gas:

$$\frac{n}{V} = \frac{P}{RT} = \frac{1\ \text{atm}}{0.082 \frac{\text{L} \cdot \text{atm}}{\text{mole} \cdot \text{K}} \times 298\ \text{K}} = 4.1 \times 10^{-2}\ \text{moles/L}$$

Calculating the specific activity with equation 4.31:

$A_{Ra} = 226$

$T_{Ra} = 1620$ yr

$A_{Kr} = 85$

$T_{Kr} = 10.7$ yr

$$SA = \frac{A_{Ra} T_{Ra}}{A_{Kr} T_{Kr}} = \frac{226 \times 1620\ \text{yr}}{85 \times 10.6\ \text{yr}} = 406.3\ \text{Ci/g}$$

$$\frac{406.3\ \text{Ci}}{\text{g}} \times \frac{85\ \text{g}}{\text{mol}} \times \frac{4.1 \times 10^{-2}\ \text{mol}}{\text{L}} \times \frac{\text{L}}{1000\ \text{cm}^3} \times \frac{1 \times 10^{6}\ \mu\text{Ci}}{1\ \text{Ci}} = 1.4 \times 10^{6}\ \mu\text{Ci/cm}^3$$

$$\frac{1.4\times10^{6}\ \mu\text{Ci}}{\text{cm}^{3}}\times\frac{3.7\times10^{4}\ \text{Bq}}{1\ \mu\text{Ci}}\times\frac{1\times10^{6}\ \text{cm}^{3}}{\text{m}^{3}}=5.19\times10^{16}\ \text{Bq/m}^{3}$$

4.30 Calculate the specific power of ^{35}S and of ^{14}C in **4.30**
(a) watts per MBq,

The maximum energy of the ^{35}S beta particle is 0.167 MeV, but the average energy of the beta is 0.0488 MeV,
^{35}S= 0.049 MeV/transformation

$$\frac{1\ \text{W}}{1\ \text{J}/\text{sec}}\times\frac{1\frac{\text{trans}}{\text{sec}}}{\text{Bq}}\times\frac{1\times10^{6}\ \text{Bq}}{\text{MBq}}\times\frac{0.0488\ \text{MeV}}{\text{trans}}\times\frac{1.6\times10^{-13}\ \text{J}}{\text{MeV}}=7.8\times10^{-9}\ \frac{\text{W}}{\text{MBq}}$$

The maximum energy of the ^{14}C beta particle is 0.156 MeV, but the average energy of the beta is 0.0494 MeV,
^{14}C= 0.0494 MeV/transformation

$$\frac{1\ \text{W}}{1\ \text{J}/\text{sec}}\times\frac{1\frac{\text{trans}}{\text{sec}}}{\text{Bq}}\times\frac{1\times10^{6}\ \text{Bq}}{\text{MBq}}\times\frac{0.0494\ \text{MeV}}{\text{trans}}\times\frac{1.6\times10^{-13}\ \text{J}}{\text{MeV}}=7.9\times10^{-9}\ \frac{\text{W}}{\text{MBq}}$$

(b) Watts per kg.

The specific activity of ^{35}S is calculated with equation 4.31:
$A_{\text{Ra}} = 226$
$T_{\text{Ra}} = 1620$ yr
$A_{\text{S}} = 35$

$$T_{\text{S}} = 88\ \text{day}\times\frac{1\ \text{yr}}{365\ \text{d}} = 0.24\ \text{yr}$$

$$SA=\frac{A_{Ra}T_{Ra}}{A_{S}T_{S}}=\frac{226\times1620\ \text{yr}}{35\times0.24\ \text{yr}}=4.34\times10^{4}\ \text{Ci/g}=1.61\times10^{9}\ \text{MBq/g}$$

Applying the information from part (a),

$$\frac{7.8\times10^{-9}\,\text{W}}{\text{MBq}}\times\frac{1.61\times10^{9}\,\text{MBq}}{\text{g}}\times\frac{1000\text{ g}}{\text{kg}}=1.3\times10^{4}\ \frac{\text{W}}{\text{kg}}\text{ of }^{35}\text{S}$$

The specific activity of ^{14}C is calculated with equation 4.31:
$A_{Ra} = 226$
$T_{Ra} = 1620$ years
$A_S = 14$
$T_S = 5730$ years

$$\text{SA} = \frac{A_{Ra}T_{Ra}}{A_C T_C} = \frac{226\times1620\text{ yr}}{14\times5730\text{ yr}} = 4.56\text{ Ci/g}$$

$$\frac{4.56\text{ Ci}}{\text{g}}\times\frac{3.7\times10^{10}\,\text{Bq}}{\text{Ci}}\times\frac{1\text{ MBq}}{1\times10^{6}\,\text{Bq}} = 1.69\times10^{5}\text{ MBq/g}$$

Applying the information from part (a),

$$\frac{7.9\times10^{-9}\,\text{W}}{\text{MBq}}\times\frac{1.69\times10^{5}\,\text{MBq}}{\text{g}}\times\frac{1000\text{ g}}{\text{kg}}=1.3\ \frac{\text{W}}{\text{kg}}\text{ of }^{14}\text{C}$$

4.31

4.31 Calculate the specific power of ^{90}Sr in
(a) watts per MBq,

The maximum energy of the ^{90}Sr beta particle is 0.546 MeV, but the average energy of the beta is 0.1958 MeV. However, ^{90}Sr typically is in equilibrium with its short lived (64 hr) daughter, ^{90}Y,which emits a beta whose average energy is 0.9348 MeV
^{90}Y= 0.9348 MeV/transformation

Summing the two average energies gives the average beta energy per ^{90}Sr transformation.

0.1958 + 0.9348 = 1.13 MeV/transformation

$$\frac{1\text{ W}}{1\text{ J/sec}}\times\frac{1\frac{\text{trans}}{\text{sec}}}{\text{Bq}}\times\frac{1\times10^{6}\,\text{Bq}}{\text{MBq}}\times\frac{1.13\text{ MeV}}{\text{trans}}\times\frac{1.6\times10^{-13}\,\text{J}}{\text{MeV}}=1.8\times10^{-7}\ \frac{\text{W}}{\text{MBq}}$$

(b) Watts per kg.

The specific activity of ^{90}Sr is calculated with equation 4.31:
$A_{Ra} = 226$
$T_{Ra} = 1620$ yr
$A_{Sr} = 90$
$T_{Sr} = 28$ yr

$$\text{SA} = \frac{A_{Ra}T_{Ra}}{A_{Sr}T_{Sr}} = \frac{226 \times 1620 \text{ yr}}{90 \times 28 \text{ yr}} = 145.3 \text{ Ci/g}$$

$$\frac{145.3 \text{ Ci}}{\text{g}} \times \frac{3.7 \times 10^{10} \text{ Bq}}{\text{Ci}} \times \frac{1 \text{ MBq}}{1 \times 10^{6} \text{ Bq}} = 5.4 \times 10^{6} \text{ MBq/g}$$

Applying the information from part (a),

$$\frac{1.8 \times 10^{-7} \text{ W}}{\text{MBq}} \times \frac{5.4 \times 10^{6} \text{ MBq}}{\text{g}} \times \frac{1000 \text{ g}}{\text{kg}} = 972 \frac{\text{W}}{\text{kg}} \text{ of } ^{90}\text{Sr}$$

4.32 How many joules of energy are released in 3 hours by an initial volume of 1 liter ^{41}Ar at 0°C and 760 mm Hg? **4.32**

$V = 1$ L
$T = 0°\text{C} = 273$ K

$R = 0.082 \frac{\text{L} \cdot \text{atm}}{\text{mole} \cdot \text{K}}$
$P = 760$ mm Hg $= 1$ atm

The ideal gas equation is used to find the number of moles of gas present:

$$\frac{n}{V} = \frac{P}{RT} = \frac{1 \text{ atm}}{0.082 \frac{\text{L} \cdot \text{atm}}{\text{mole} \cdot \text{K}} \times 273 \text{ K}} = 0.0447 \frac{\text{mol}}{\text{L}}$$

Converting to grams of ^{41}Ar per liter;

$$0.0447\frac{\text{mol}}{\text{L}}\times\frac{41\text{ g}}{1\text{ mol}}=1.8327\frac{\text{g}}{\text{L}}$$

The maximum energy of the ^{41}Ar beta particle is 1.198 MeV, but the average energy of the beta is 0.4593 MeV. Also, ^{41}Ar emits a γ with each transformation, of 1.293 MeV, which contributes to the energy output of ^{41}Ar. Thus, the two energies are summed;

1.293 + 0.4593 = 1.75 MeV/transformation (total)

The specific activity of ^{41}Ar is calculated with equation 4.31:
$A_{\text{Ra}} = 226$
$T_{\text{Ra}} = 1620$ yr
$A_{\text{Ar}} = 41$

$$T_{\text{Ar}} = 1.83\text{ hr}\times\frac{1\text{ d}}{24\text{ hr}}\times\frac{1\text{ yr}}{365\text{ d}}=2.08\times10^{-4}\text{ yr}$$

$$\text{SA} = \frac{A_{Ra}T_{Ra}}{A_{Ar}T_{Ar}} = \frac{226\times1620\text{ yr}}{41\times2.08\times10^{-4}\text{ yr}} = 4.3\times10^{7}\text{ Ci/g}$$

Combining the specific activity with the number of grams per liter of ^{41}Ar;

$$\frac{4.3\times10^{7}\text{ Ci}}{\text{g}}\times\frac{3.7\times10^{10}\ \frac{\text{t}}{\text{s}}}{\text{Ci}}\times\frac{1.7\text{ MeV}}{\text{t}}\times\frac{1.6\times10^{-13}\text{ J}}{\text{MeV}}\times\frac{1.83\text{ g}}{\text{L}}\times\frac{1\text{ W}}{1\frac{\text{J}}{\text{s}}}=7.9\times10^{5}\ \frac{\text{J}/\text{s}}{\text{L}}$$

However, the ^{41}Ar is transformed to stable potassium with a half-life of 110 minutes. The rate of energy emission from the ^{41}Ar will decrease according to the radioactive transformation.
$J = J_0 e^{-\lambda t}$

where λ is the ^{41}Ar transformation constant

$$\lambda = \frac{0.693}{T_{1/2}} = \frac{0.693}{110\text{ min}} = 0.0063\text{ min}^{-1}$$

The total energy release during 3 hours, therefore, is calculated by integrating the energy release rate over 180 minutes (3 hours)

$$J = J_0 \int_0^t e^{-\lambda t} = \frac{J_0}{\lambda}\left(1 - e^{-\lambda t}\right)$$

Substituting the approximate values into this equation yields

$$J = \frac{7.9 \times 10^5 \dfrac{\text{J}}{\text{sec}} \times \dfrac{60 \text{ sec}}{\text{min}}}{0.0063 \text{ min}^{-1}} \times (1 - e^{-0.0063 \times 180}) = 5.1 \times 10^9 \text{ J}$$

4.33 (a) Calculate the specific power, in watts/kg, of ^{41}Ar. 4.33

In problem 4.32, we found that ^{41}Ar emits 1.75 MeV per transformation, and that its specific activity is 4.3 x 10^4 Ci/g. The specific power of ^{41}Ar is calculated with these values:

$$\frac{4.3 \times 10^7 \text{ Ci}}{\text{g}} \times \frac{1000 \text{ g}}{\text{kg}} \times \frac{3.7 \times 10^{10} \dfrac{\text{trans}}{\text{sec}}}{1 \text{ Ci}} \times \frac{1.75 \text{ MeV}}{\text{trans}} \times \frac{1.6 \times 10^{-13} \text{ J}}{\text{MeV}} \times \frac{1 \text{ W}}{1 \dfrac{\text{J}}{\text{sec}}}$$

$= 4.5 \times 10^8$ W/kg

(b) What is the specific power of ^{41}Ar 4 hours after the ^{41}Ar is isolated in a bottle?

The specific power of ^{41}Ar does not change, since specific power is measured on a per kg basis. However, the quantity of ^{41}Ar will decrease to about 22% of its initial value after 4 hours, and the total power output will decrease accordingly.

4.34 What volume of radon 222 (at 0°C and 760 torr) is in equilibrium with 0.1 gram radium 226? 4.34

Since the specific activity of ^{226}Ra is 1 Ci/g, and since the ^{222}Rn is in secular equilibrium with the 0.1 Ci ^{226}Ra, we have 0.1 Ci ^{222}Rn. The specific activity of ^{222}Rn is calculated with equation 4.31:

$A_{Ra} = 226$
$T_{Ra} = 1620$ yr
$A_S = 222$

$$T_S = 3.82 \text{ d} \times \frac{1 \text{ yr}}{365 \text{ d}} = 0.0104 \text{ yr}$$

$$\text{SA} = \frac{A_{Ra}T_{Ra}}{A_{Rn}T_{Rn}} = \frac{226 \times 1620 \text{ yr}}{222 \times 0.0104 \text{ yr}} = 1.58 \times 10^5 \text{ Ci/g}$$

$$0.1 \text{ Ci Rn} \times \frac{1 \text{ g}^{222}\text{Rn}}{1.58 \times 10^5 \text{Ci}} \times \frac{1 \text{ mole}}{222 \text{ g}^{222}\text{Rn}} = 2.8 \times 10^{-9} \text{ mole } ^{222}\text{Rn present in equilib-}$$

rium with ^{226}Ra

According to the ideal gas law, the volume of any gas at 0 °C and 760 mm Hg is 22.4 L (2.24×10^4 mL). The volume of Rn in equilibrium with 0.1 Ci Ra is

Vol (Rn) = 2.8×10^{-9} mole × 2.24×10^4 mL/mole = 6.4×10^{-5} mL

4.35

4.35 One hundred milligrams radium as $RaBr_2$ (specific gravity = 5.79) is in a platinum capsule whose inside dimensions are 2 mm diameter × 4 cm long. What will be the gas pressure, at body temperature, inside the capsule 100 years after manufacture if it originally contained air at atmospheric pressure at room temperature (25°C)?

Careful examination of table 4.3 reveals that when ^{226}Ra decays, its progeny emits alpha particles and since each alpha particle is a helium nucleus, it will eventually capture 2 electrons and form helium gas, which is what will produce the pressure in the capsule.

^{226}Ra emits one alpha ($T_{1/2}$ = 1620 year)
^{222}Rn emits one alpha ($T_{1/2}$ =3.825days)
^{218}Po emits one alpha ($T_{1/2}$ = 3.05 min)
^{214}Po emits one alpha ($T_{1/2} = 1.64 \times 10^{-4}$ sec)
^{210}Po emits one alpha ($T_{1/2}$ = 138.4 days)

Pure radium when isolated does not quickly attain transient equilibrium with all of its progeny. The half life of ^{210}Pb (19.4 years) limits the rate that determines the establishment of equilibrium between radium and all its progeny. The first four alpha emitters in the chain of radium progeny attain secular equilibrium within a very short period of time relative to the 100 years required for ^{210}Pb to attain (for practical purposes) equilibrium. Thus, assume that ^{226}Ra emits 4 alpha particles per decay (since in secular equilibrium almost immediately), and there is a buildup with a fifth alpha particle (from ^{210}Po) which is also emitted.

The fraction of alphas from ^{210}Po can be determined by comparing the area under the "built up"curve to the total area of the dashed rectangle.

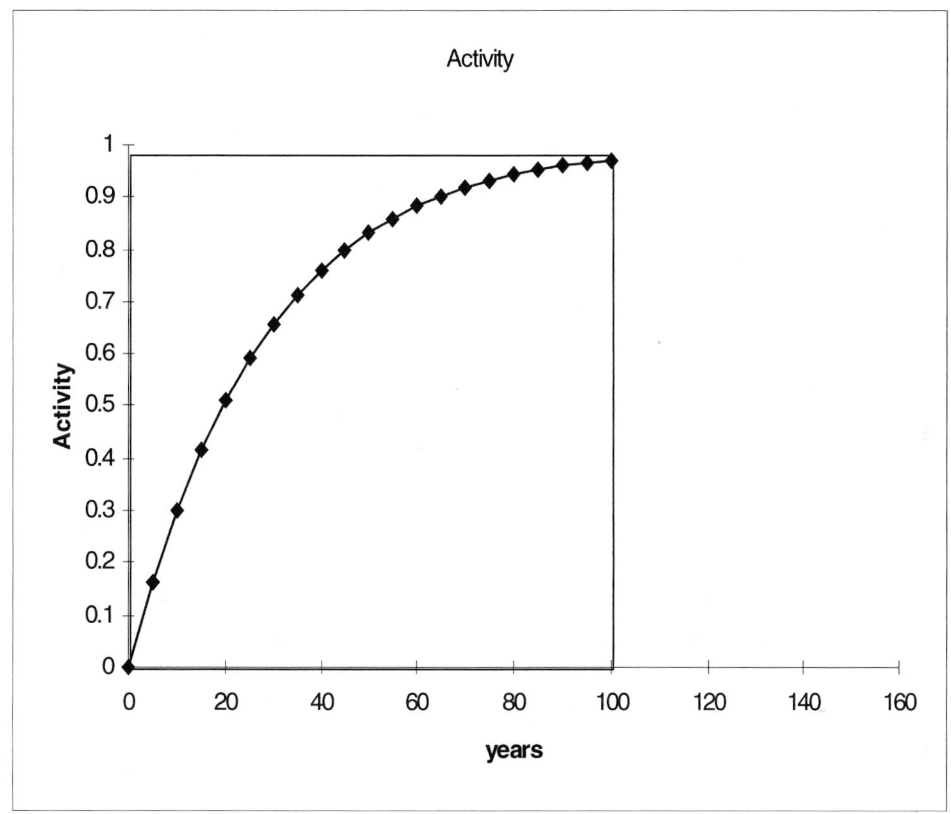

Fraction of α from ^{210}Po contributing to the helium over 100 years:

If A_E = equilibrium activity, then

$$\text{fraction} = \frac{\text{area}_{\text{undercurve}}}{\text{area}_{\text{rectangle}}} = \frac{\int_0^{100} A_E\left(1-e^{-\lambda t}\right)dt}{A_E \times T} = \frac{A_E\left[\int_0^T dt - \int_0^T e^{-\lambda T}dt\right]}{A_E \times T}$$

Integrating from $T = 0$ to $T = 100$:

$$\text{fraction} = \frac{T - \left[\frac{1}{\lambda}\left(1-e^{-\lambda T}\right)\right]}{T} = \frac{100 - \left[\frac{1}{0.0359}\left(1-e^{-0.0359(100)}\right)\right]}{100} = 0.73$$

Thus the effective number of α particles emitted over 100 years is 4 + 0.73 = 4.73 α particles per decay of ^{226}Ra.

Now calculate the amount of ^{226}Ra transformed during the 100 year period. Since equation 4.18 gives the amount left:

$$A = A_0\, e^{-\lambda t}$$

To find the fraction that decays, modify equation 4.18;

$$A_{decayed} = A_0\,(1 - e^{-\lambda t})$$

Rearrange this equation;

$$\frac{A_{decayed}}{A_0} = (1 - e^{-\lambda t})$$

Put in the values:

$$\lambda = \frac{0.693}{1620\ \text{yr}} = 0.000428\ \text{yr}^{-1}\ \text{(equation 4.21)}$$

$T = 100$ years

$$\frac{A_{decayed}}{A_0} = (1 - e^{-\lambda t}) = (1 - e^{-0.000428 \times 100}) = 0.042$$

0.042 is the fraction of the ^{226}Ra activity which decays over 100 years. So the quantity of radium decaying over 100 years is:

$0.042 \times 100 \text{ mg} = 4.2 \text{ mg}$

Converting this to decays, and knowing that there are 4.73 α particles emitted per decay (from above) on average, over 100 years;

$$4.2 \text{ mg} \times \frac{1 \text{ g}}{1000 \text{ mg}} \times \frac{1 \text{ mol}\,^{226}\text{Ra}}{226 \text{ g}} \times \frac{6.02 \times 10^{23} \text{ atoms decayed}}{1 \text{ mol}\,^{226}\text{Ra}} \times \frac{4.73\alpha}{\text{atom decay}}$$

$= 5.3 \times 10^{19}$ atoms of helium formed over 100 years.

Converting into moles:

$$5.3 \times 10^{19} \text{ atoms He} \times \frac{1 \text{ mol}}{6.02 \times 10^{23} \text{ atoms}} = 8.8 \times 10^{-5} \text{ moles He formed}$$

Volume of the capsule is:
$L = 4$ cm
$r = 1$ mm $= 0.1$ cm

$$V = L\pi r^2 = 4 \times \pi \times 0.1^2 = 0.126 \text{ cm}^3 \times \frac{1 \text{ L}}{1000 \text{ cm}^3} = 1.26 \times 10^{-4} \text{ L}$$

The volume that the $RaBr_2$ occupies is now calculated to determine what volume the gas may occupy;
Molecular Weight of $RaBr_2 = 226 + 2 \times 79.916 = 385.832$ grams per mole

$\rho_{RaBr_2} = 5.79$ (given in problem)

$$\frac{\frac{385.832 \text{ g RaBr}_2}{226 \text{ g Ra}} \times 0.1 \text{ g}\,^{226}\text{Ra}}{5.79 \frac{\text{g RaBr}_2}{\text{cm}^3} \times 1000 \frac{\text{cm}^3}{\text{L}}} = 2.95 \times 10^{-5} \text{ L is the RaBr}_2 \text{ volume}$$

Thus the volume available for the gas is:
$1.26 \times 10^{-4} \text{ L} - 2.95 \times 10^{-5} \text{ L} = 9.65 \times 10^{-5} \text{ L}$

The ideal gas equation is used to find the pressure of the helium gas formed at room temperature in the needle;

$T = 298$ K
$V = 9.65 \times 10^{-5}$ L
$n = 8.8 \times 10^{-5}$ moles He

$$R = 0.082 \frac{\text{L} \cdot \text{atm}}{\text{mole} \cdot \text{K}}$$

$$P = \frac{nRT}{V} = \frac{8.8 \times 10^{-5} \text{ mol} \times 0.082 \frac{\text{L} \cdot \text{atm}}{\text{mole} \cdot \text{K}} \times 298 \text{ K}}{9.65 \times 10^{-5} \text{ L}} = 22.3 \text{ atm}$$

Thus 22.3 atmospheres is the pressure due to the helium gas formed by the decay of the radium alone. The initial gas pressure when the needle was manufactured must also be considered.

22.3 + 1 = 23.3 atm.

4.36

4.36 A volume of 10 cm^3 tritium gas $^3H_2$ at NTP dissipates 3.11 joules per hour. (a) What is the mean activity of the tritium?
$V = 10$ cm^3 = 0.01 L
$T = 0°C = 273$ K

$$R = 0.082 \frac{\text{L} \cdot \text{atm}}{\text{mole} \cdot \text{K}}$$

$P = 760$ torr = 1 atm
The ideal gas equation is used to find the number of moles of gas present:

$$n = \frac{PV}{RT} = \frac{1 \text{ atm} \times 0.01 \text{ L}}{0.082 \frac{\text{L} \cdot \text{atm}}{\text{mole} \cdot \text{K}} \times 273 \text{ K}} = 4.47 \times 10^{-4} \text{ moles tritium gas present}$$

$$4.47 \times 10^{-4} \text{ mol} \times \frac{6.02 \times 10^{23} \text{ molecules}}{1 \text{ mol}} \times \frac{2 \text{ atoms}}{1 \text{ molecule}} = 5.38 \times 10^{20} \text{ atoms tritium}$$

The decay constant for tritium is found using equation 4.21:
$T_{1/2} = 12.3$ years

$$\lambda_H = \frac{0.693}{12.3 \text{ yr}} = 0.0563 \text{ yr}^{-1} = \frac{0.0563}{\text{yr}} \times \frac{1 \text{ yr}}{3.2 \times 10^7 \text{ sec}} = 1.76 \times 10^{-9} \text{ sec}^{-1}$$

Activity $= \lambda N = 1.76 \times 10^{-9} \text{ sec}^{-1} \times 5.38 \times 10^{20}$ atoms tritium $= 9.47 \times 10^{11}$ Bq

(b) What is the mean beta ray energy, if one beta particle is emitted per transition?

$$\frac{3.11 \text{ J}}{\text{hr}} \times \frac{1 \text{ hr}}{3600 \text{ sec}} \times \frac{1 \text{ MeV}}{1.6 \times 10^{-13} \text{ J}} \times \frac{1 \text{ sec}}{9.47 \times 10^{11} \text{ trans}} = 5.7 \times 10^{-3} \frac{\text{MeV}}{\text{trans}}$$

4.37 Barium 140 decays to ^{140}La with a half–life of 12.8 days, and the ^{140}La decays to stable ^{140}Ce with a half–life of 40.5 hours. A radiochemist, after precipitating ^{140}Ba, wishes to wait until he has a maximum amount of ^{140}La before separating the ^{140}La from the ^{140}Ba. (a) How long must he wait? **4.37**

$$^{140}\text{Ba} \xrightarrow[\text{A}]{12.8 \text{ d}} {}^{140}\text{La} \xrightarrow[\text{B}]{40.5 \text{ hr}} {}^{140}\text{Ce}$$

Using equation 4.21:

$$\lambda_{Ba} = \frac{0.693}{12.8 \text{ d}} = 0.054 \text{ d}^{-1} \qquad \lambda_{La} = \frac{0.693}{1.69 \text{ d}} = 0.41 \text{ d}^{-1}$$

Equation 4.57:

$$t_m = \frac{\ln\left(\frac{\lambda_{La}}{\lambda_{Ba}}\right)}{\lambda_{La} - \lambda_{Ba}} = \frac{\ln\left(\frac{0.41}{0.054}\right)}{0.41 - 0.054} = 5.69 \text{ d} = 136.5 \text{ hr}$$

(b) If he started with 1000 MBq (27mCi) before separating the ^{140}La from the ^{140}Ba, how many micrograms ^{140}La will he collect?

Equation 4.53 relates the activity of the daughter (A_{La}) to the initial activity of the parent (A_{Ba})at time t after isolation of the parent.

$$A_{La} = A_{Ba}\frac{\lambda_{La}}{\lambda_{La} - \lambda_{Ba}}\left(e^{-\lambda_{Ba}t} - e^{-\lambda_{La}t}\right)$$

$$A_{La} = 27\ \text{mCi}\frac{0.41\ \text{d}^{-1}}{0.41\ \text{d}^{-1} - 0.054\ \text{d}^{-1}}\left(e^{-0.054\times 5.69} - e^{-0.41\times 5.6}\right) = 19.9\ \text{mCi}$$

The specific activity of ^{140}La ($T_{1/2} = 1.69$ d) is

$$SA = \frac{1620\ \text{y}\times 365\frac{\text{d}}{\text{y}}\times 226}{1.69\ \text{d}\times 140} = 5.65\times 10^{5}\ \frac{\text{Ci}}{\text{g}}$$

Therefore the weight of ^{140}La is

$$\frac{19.9\times 10^{-3}\ \text{Ci}}{5.65\times 10^{5}\ \frac{\text{Ci}}{\text{g}}} = 3.5\times 10^{-8}\ \text{g}$$

Alternatively:
From part (a)

$$\lambda_{Ba} = 0.054\ \text{d}^{-1} = \frac{0.054}{\text{d}}\times\frac{1\ \text{d}}{24\ \text{hr}}\times\frac{1\ \text{hr}}{3600\ \text{sec}} = 6.25\times 10^{-7}\ \text{sec}^{-1}$$

$$\lambda_{Ba}N_{BaO} = 10^{9}\ \text{Bq}$$

$$t_m = 136.6\ \text{hr} = 4.92\times 10^{5}\ \text{sec}$$

Placing the terms in equation 4.53:

$$\lambda N_{La} = \frac{\lambda_{Ba}N_{Ba0}\lambda_{La}}{\lambda_{La} - \lambda_{Ba}}\left(e^{-\lambda_{Ba}t} - e^{-\lambda_{La}t}\right)$$

$$\lambda N_{La} = \frac{4.75\times 10^{6}\ \text{sec}^{-1}\times 10^{9}\ \text{sec}^{-1}}{(4.75\times 10^{-6}\ \text{sec}^{-1}) - (6.25\times 10^{-7}\ \text{sec}^{-1})}$$

$$\times\left(e^{-6.25\times 10^{-7}\ \text{sec}^{-1}\times 4.92\times 10^{5}\ \text{sec}} - e^{-4.75\times 10^{-6}\ \text{sec}^{-1}\times 4.92\times 10^{5}\ \text{sec}}\right)$$

$$\lambda N_{La} = 7.36\times 10^{8}\ \text{Bq}$$

$$7.18\times10^{8}\,\text{Bq}\times\frac{1\ \text{Ci}}{3.7\times10^{10}\,\text{Bq}}=2.0\times10^{-2}\ \text{Ci}$$ is the maximum activity of the ^{140}La.

Next, convert to grams:
From above,
$\lambda_{La}=4.75\times10^{-6}\ \text{sec}^{-1}$
$(\lambda N)_{La}=7.36\times10^{8}\ \text{Bq}$

Solve for N_{La}

$$N_{La}=\frac{7.36\times10^{8}\,\text{Bq}}{\lambda_{La}}=\frac{7.36\times10^{8}\,\frac{\text{atoms}}{\text{sec}}}{4.75\times10^{-6}\,\text{sec}}=1.5\times10^{14}\ \text{atoms}\ ^{140}\text{La}$$

$$1.5\times10^{14}\ \text{atoms}\ ^{140}\text{La}\times\frac{1\ \text{mol}\ ^{140}\text{La}}{6.02\times10^{23}\,\text{atoms}\ ^{140}\text{La}}\times\frac{140\ \text{g}\ ^{140}\text{La}}{1\ \text{mol}\ ^{140}\text{La}}=3.5\times10^{-8}\ \text{g}\ ^{140}\text{La}$$

4.38 Strontium 90 is to be used as a heat source for generating electrical energy in a satellite, (a) How much ^{90}Sr activity is required to generate 50 watts of electrical power, if the conversion efficiency from heat to electricity is to 30%? **4.38**

Since the process of energy conversion is only 30% efficient, the required power (gross) needed is:

$$50\ \text{W}\times\frac{100}{30}=166.67\ \text{W}$$ are actually needed.

The maximum energy of the ^{90}Sr beta particle is 0.546 MeV, so the average energy of the beta would be roughly 1/3 of 0.546 MeV, as described in chapter 4,

$$\overline{E}_{\beta}(^{90}\text{Sr})=0.546\ \text{MeV}\left(\frac{1}{3}\right)=0.182\ \text{MeV/transformation}$$

However, since ^{90}Sr typically is in equilibrium with its short lived (64 hr) daughter, ^{90}Y, it's beta is also taken into account, as it is has 2.27 MeV and contributes significantly to the power,

$$\overline{E}_{\beta}(^{90}\text{Y})\ 2.27\ \text{MeV}\left(\frac{1}{3}\right)=0.76\ \text{MeV/transformation}$$

Summing the two energies,

0.182 + 0.76 = 0.94 MeV/transformation

$$\frac{1\ \text{W}}{1\ \text{J}/\text{sec}} \times \frac{1\frac{\text{trans}}{\text{sec}}}{\text{Bq}} \times \frac{0.94\ \text{MeV}}{\text{trans}} \times \frac{1.6\times10^{-13}\ \text{J}}{\text{MeV}} = 1.5\times10^{-13}\ \frac{\text{W}}{\text{Bq}}$$

$$166.67\ \text{W} \times \frac{1\ \text{Bq}}{1.5\times10^{-13}\ \text{W}} \times \frac{1\ \text{Ci}}{3.7\times10^{10}\ \text{Bq}} = 3.0\times10^{4}\ \text{Ci}\ ^{90}\text{Sr}$$

(b) Weight of the isotopic heat source is an important factor in the design of the power source. If weight is to be kept to a minimum, and if the source is to generate 50 watts after 1 year of operation, would there be an advantage to using ^{210}Po?

The energy of the ^{210}Po alpha particle is 5.3 MeV, but as noted on p.77 of the text, including the recoil energy yields 5.4 MeV/transformation; the ^{210}Po half-life is 138 days.

$$\frac{1\ \text{W}}{1\ \text{J}/\text{sec}} \times \frac{1\frac{\text{trans}}{\text{sec}}}{\text{Bq}} \times \frac{5.4\ \text{MeV}}{\text{trans}} \times \frac{1.6\times10^{-13}\ \text{J}}{\text{MeV}} = 8.64\times10^{-13}\ \frac{\text{W}}{\text{Bq}}$$

$$166.67\ \text{W} \times \frac{1\ \text{Bq}}{8.64\times10^{-13}\ \text{W}} \times \frac{1\ \text{Ci}}{3.7\times10^{10}\ \text{Bq}} = 5.2\times10^{3}\ \text{Ci}$$ is needed at the end of the year to allow for decay. At the beginning of the year the required ^{210}Po activity according to equation 4.18 is

$$A_0 = \frac{A}{e^{-\lambda t}} = \frac{5.2\times10^{3}\ \text{Ci}}{e^{-\frac{0.693}{138\ \text{d}}\times 365\ \text{d}}} = 3.3\times10^{4}\ \text{Ci}$$ needed at the start of the year, so that at the end of the year, there is enough activity present to provide the 166.67 (gross) watts of power to the unit.

Calculate the number of grams of ^{210}Po to which this quantity corresponds:

$T_{\text{Po-210}}$ = 138 days

$A_{\text{Po-210}}$ =210

A_{Ra} = 226

T_{Ra} = 1620 yrs

Substituting these values into the equation for specific activity equation (4.31), we have:

$$SA = \frac{A_{Ra}T_{Ra}}{A_iT_i} = \frac{226 \times 1620 \text{ yr}}{210 \times (138 \text{ d} \times \frac{1 \text{ yr}}{365 \text{ d}})} = 4.61 \times 10^3 \text{ Ci/g Po–210}$$

$3.3 \times 10^4 \text{ Ci} \times \frac{1 \text{ g}}{4.61 \times 10^3 \text{ Ci}} = 7.2 \text{ g}$ ^{210}Po needed at the start of the year.

Now calculate how many grams of ^{90}Sr would be needed, based on the 3.0×10^4 Ci ^{90}Sr calculated in part (a), and assuming that the decay would be negligible over a one year period, since ^{90}Sr has a 28 year half life:

The specific activity of ^{90}Sr is calculated with equation 4.31:
$A_{Ra} = 226$
$T_{Ra} = 1620$ yr
$A_S = 90$
$T_S = 28$ yr

$$SA = \frac{A_{Ra}T_{Ra}}{A_{Sr}T_{Sr}} = \frac{226 \times 1620 \text{ yr}}{90 \times 28 \text{ yr}} = 145.3 \text{ Ci/gram}$$

$3.0 \times 10^4 \text{ Ci } ^{90}\text{Sr} \times \frac{1 \text{ g}}{145.3 \text{ Ci}} = 206.5 \text{ g}$ ^{90}Sr required.

Compare the 7.2 g ^{210}Po with 206.5 g ^{90}Sr required, and there is an advantage to using ^{210}Po.

4.39 Carbon 14 is produced naturally by the ^{14}N(n,p)^{14}C interaction of cosmic radiation with the nitrogen in the atmosphere at a rate of about 1.4×10^{14} Bq/year. If the half life of ^{14}C is 5700 years, what is the steady state global inventory of ^{14}C? **4.39**

Q = global inventory
rate of formation of ^{14}C = 1.4×10^{15} Bq/yr
rate of decay of ^{14}C = λQBq/yr

Equation 4.21

$$\lambda = \frac{0.693}{T} = \frac{0.693}{5700\text{ yr}} = 1.2 \times 10^{-4}\text{ yr}^{-1}\ {}^{14}\text{C}$$

Under steady state conditions

Rate of formation = Rate of decay

1.4×10^{15} Bq/yr = λ yr^{-1} × Q Bq

$$Q = \frac{1.4 \times 10^{15}\ \frac{\text{Bq}}{\text{yr}}}{1.2 \times 10^{-4}\text{ yr}} = 1.15 \times 10^{19}\text{ Bq}$$

4.40

4.40 The global steady state inventory of naturally produced tritium from the interaction of cosmic rays with the atmosphere is estimated by the United Nations Scientific Committee on the Effects of Atomic Radiation to be 1.26×10^{18} Bq (34×10^{6} Ci). If the half life of tritium if 12.3 years, what is the annual production of natural tritium?

Q = global inventory of ^{3}H = 1.26×10^{18} Bq/yr
λ = rate constant of ^{3}H
$T_{1/2}$ = 12.3 yr

Equation 4.21

$$\lambda_B = \frac{0.693}{T} = \frac{0.693}{12.3\text{ yr}} = 5.6 \times 10^{-2}\text{ yr}^{-1}\ {}^{3}\text{H}$$

Under steady state conditions,

Production per year = decay per year

Production per year = $\lambda Q = \frac{5.6 \times 10^{-2}}{\text{yr}} \times 1.26 \times 10^{18}\text{ Bq} = 7.1 \times 10^{16}\ \frac{\text{Bq}}{\text{yr}}$ is the rate of production of ^{3}H in the atmosphere.

Solutions for Chapter 5

INTERACTION OF RADIATION WITH MATTER

5.1 The density of Hg is 13.6 grams/cm^3 and its atomic weight is 200.6. Calculate the number of Hg atoms/cm^3. **5.1**

$$\frac{13.6\text{ g}}{\text{cm}^3} \times \frac{\text{mol}}{200.6\text{ g}} \times \frac{6.02 \times 10^{23}\text{ atoms}}{1\text{ mol}} = 4.08 \times 10^{22}\text{ atoms/cm}^3$$

5.2 The density of quartz (SiO_2) crystals is 2.65 gm/cm^3. What is the atomic density (atoms/cm^3) of silicon and oxygen in quartz? **5.2**

Atomic Weights: Si = 28.09, O = 16

28.09 + (2 × 16) = 60.09 g/mol SiO_2

First, Silicon:

$$\frac{2.65\text{ g}}{\text{cm}^3} \times \frac{1\text{ mol SiO}_2}{60.09\text{ g}} \times \frac{1\text{ mol Si}}{1\text{ mol SiO}_2} \times \frac{6.02 \times 10^{23}\text{ atoms}}{\text{mol}} = 2.65 \times 10^{22}\text{ atoms/cm}^3$$

Oxygen:

$$\frac{2.65\text{ g}}{\text{cm}^3} \times \frac{1\text{ mol SiO}_2}{60.09\text{ g}} \times \frac{2\text{ mol O}}{1\text{ mol SiO}_2} \times \frac{6.02 \times 10^{23}\text{ atoms}}{\text{mol}} = 5.3 \times 10^{22}\text{ atoms/cm}^3$$

5.3 Compare the electronic densities of a piece of aluminum 5 mm thick and a piece of iron of the same density thickness. **5.3**

t = 5 mm = 0.5 cm

$\rho_{Al} = 2.7\ g/cm^3$

Density thickness of 0.5 cm thick Al:

$$0.5\ cm \times \frac{2.7\ g}{cm^3} = 1.35\ g/cm^2$$

Computing the electronic density (knowing that z = 13 and molecular weight = 27):

$$\frac{1.35\ g}{cm^2} \times \frac{1\ mol}{27\ g} \times \frac{6.02 \times 10^{23}\ atoms}{1\ mol} \times \frac{13\ electrons}{1\ atom\ Al} = 3.913 \times 10^{23}\ electrons/cm^2$$

The density thickness of 5 mm of aluminum was computed above as 1.35 g/cm^2. Computing the electron density of a piece of iron with the same density thickness, 1.35 g/cm^2 (the iron would, of course, not be as thick).

Fe = 55.85 g/mole

Fe = 26 electrons per atom

Fe electronic density:

$$\frac{1.35\ g}{cm^2} \times \frac{1\ mol}{55.85\ g} \times \frac{6.02 \times 10^{23}\ atoms}{1\ mol} \times \frac{26\ electrons}{1\ atom\ Fe} = 3.78 \times 10^{23}\ electrons/cm^2$$

5.4 **5.4** In surveying a laboratory, a health physicist wipes a contaminated surface, and runs an absorption curve using a thin end window counter and aluminum absorbers. The range of the beta rays (no gamma rays were found) was found to be 800 mg/cm^2 aluminum. What could the contaminant be?

Compute the energy using equation 5.3, where R is in units of mg/cm^2

$R = 800\ mg/cm^2$

$\ln E = 6.63 - 3.2376\,(10.2146 - \ln R)^{1/2}$

$\ln E = 6.63 - 3.2376\,(10.2146 - \ln (800))^{1/2}$

$E = 1.73$ MeV

The Radiological Health Handbook (1970) has a table of energies of beta emitters arranged by energy on page 91 which can be used to determine the isotope from the beta energy. A maximum of 1.73 MeV beta particle corresponds to P–32.

5.5 A health physicist finds an unknown contaminant that proves to be a pure beta emitter. To help identify the contaminant, he runs an absorption curve to determine the maximum energy of the beta rays. He uses an end window G.M. counter whose mica window (density = 2.7 gm/cm^2) is 0.1 mm thick, and he finds that 1.74 mm Al stops all the beta particles. The distance between the sample and the G.M. counter was 2 cm. What was the energy of the beta particle? What is the contaminant? **5.5**

Calculate the density of each of the components in the beta particle's path: the air, aluminum, and the mica window:

Air
thickness of air = 2 cm
$\rho_{air} = 1.293 \times 10^{-3}$ g/cm^3

$$\frac{1.293 \times 10^{-3}\,\text{g}}{\text{cm}^3} \times 2\text{ cm} = 0.002586\text{ g/cm}^2$$

Aluminum
thickness of aluminum = 1.74 mm
$\rho_{Al} = 2.7$ g/cm^3

$$1.74\text{ mm} \times 2.7\frac{\text{g}}{\text{cm}^3} \times \frac{1\text{ cm}}{10\text{ mm}} = 0.4698\text{ g/cm}^2$$

Mica
thickness of mica = 0.1 mm
$\rho_{mica} = 2.7$ g/cm^3

$$0.1 \text{ mm} \times \frac{1 \text{ cm}}{10 \text{ mm}} \times 2.7 \frac{\text{g}}{\text{cm}^3} = 0.027 \text{ g/cm}^2$$

The density thicknesses are now added together to find the total amount of material that stops the beta:

$$R = 0.002586 \text{ g/cm}^2 + 0.4698 \text{ g/cm}^2 + 0.027 \text{ g/cm}^2 = 0.4994 \text{ g/cm}^2$$

Convert this to mg/cm^2

$$R = \frac{0.4994 \text{ g}}{1 \text{ cm}^2} \times \frac{1000 \text{ mg}}{1 \text{ g}} = 499.4 \text{ mg/cm}^2$$

Putting $R = 499.4 \text{ mg/cm}^2$ into the range to energy equation (5.3) to find the energy:

$$\ln E = 6.63 - 3.2376 \, (10.2146 - \ln (R))^{1/2}$$

$$\ln E = 6.63 - 3.2376 \, (10.2146 - \ln (499.4))^{1/2}$$

$$E = 1.17 \text{ MeV}$$

The table for ascending beta emitters in the RHH shows that Bi–210 emits a 1.17 MeV beta with no gamma

5.6 **5.6** A 5 MeV photon produces a positron electron pair in a Pb shield. If both particles are of equal energy, how far will they travel in the shield?

From the text in Chapter 5, it can be seen that the mass energy equivalence of a positron is 0.511 MeV and 0.511 MeV for the electron. Subtracting the energy of formation from the initial photon energy:

5 MeV – (2) 0.511 = 3.98 MeV is the energy left to contribute to the kinetic energy of the positron and electron. If each particle has equal energy, the remaining energy is divided between the two particles:

$\frac{3.98 \text{ MeV}}{2}$ = 1.99 MeV is the kinetic energy associated with each particle.

The range of an electron can be found using equation 5.2, since an electron with kinetic energy is indistinguishable from a beta;

$$R = 412E^{\,1.265 - 0.0954(\ln E)}$$

$$R = 412\,(1.99)^{\,1.265 - 0.0954(\ln(1.99))} = 940\frac{\text{mg}}{\text{cm}^2}$$

The density of lead is 11.35 g/cm^3

$$\frac{940\text{ mg}}{\text{cm}^2} \times \frac{1\text{ g}}{1000\text{ mg}} \times \frac{1\text{ cm}^3}{11.35\text{ g}} = 0.083\text{ cm is the range in lead of the electrons.}$$

Note that the annihilation radiation from the positron is not addressed in this problem.

5.7 A Compton electron that was scattered straight forward ($\phi = 0°$) was completely stopped by an aluminum absorber 460 mg/cm^2 thick. **5.7**
a) What was the kinetic energy of the Compton electron?

Using the range energy equation (5.3), where $R = 460$ mg/cm^2

$$\ln E = 6.63 - 3.2376\,(10.2146 - \ln R)^{1/2}$$

$$E = \ln^{-1}\{6.63 - 3.2376\,(10.2146 - \ln(460))^{1/2}\} = 1.09\text{ MeV}$$

b. What was the energy of the incident photon?

Since the Compton electron is scattered directly forward ($\phi = 0°$), the photon had to be scattered directly backward, $\theta = 180°$ (since this reaction can be thought of as a classical physics collision problem), so that momentum is conserved. Also, conservation of energy applies in this reaction, so that the energy of the Compton electron (1.09 MeV from part a) , and the energy of the scattered photon E', added together must equal the energy of the incident photon (E):

$$E = 1.09 + E'$$

Using this information, as well as equation 5.31A,

$$E' = \frac{E}{1 + (E / m_0c^2)(1 - \cos\theta)}$$

Solve for E' in the equation $E = 1.09 + E'$

$E' = E - 1.09$

Now substitute in for E'

$$E - 1.09 = \frac{E}{1 + (E / m_0c^2)(1 - \cos\theta)}$$

Since it is an electron which is scattered, the mass energy equivalence of an electron (0.51 MeV)can be used in the equation, and $\theta = 180°$. Substituting values:

$$E - 1.09 = \frac{E}{1 + (E / 0.51 \text{ MeV}) \times (1 - \cos\ 180)}$$

Solving for E, we get the quadratic equation

$(3.6 \times E^2) - (3.92 \times E) - 1 = 0$

This is of the form $ax^2 + bx + c$, where

$a = 3.6$
$b = -3.92$
$c = -1$

Solve for E

$$E = \frac{-b \pm \sqrt{b^2 - 4ac}}{2a} = \frac{3.9 \pm \sqrt{-3.9^2 - 4 \times (3.6) \times (-1)}}{2 \times (3.6)} = 0.542 \pm 0.76$$

$E = 1.30$ MeV is the solution which satisfies this equation.

5.8

5.8 Monochromatic 0.1MeV gamma rays are scattered through an angle of 120° by a carbon block.

(a) What is the energy of the scattered photon?

$E = 0.1$ MeV
$m_0c^2 = 0.511$ MeV
$\theta = 120°$

Equation 5.31A:

$$E' = \frac{E}{1+(E/m_0c^2)(1-\cos\theta)} = \frac{0.1}{1+(0.1/0.511)\times(1-\cos(120))} = 0.077 \text{ MeV}$$

(b) What is the kinetic energy of the Compton electron?

$E - E' = E_{e-}$

0.1 MeV – 0.077 MeV = 0.023 MeV

5.9 A 1.46 MeV gamma from naturally occurring ^{40}K is scattered two times: first through an angle of 30° and then through an angle of 150°. **5.9**
(a) What is the energy of the photon after the second scattering?

Calculating the energy of the first scattered photon:
$E = 1.46$ MeV
$\theta = 30°$
$m_0c^2 = 0.51$ MeV (the rest mass energy of an electron)

Using this information, 5.31A,

$$E' = \frac{E}{1+(E/m_0c^2)(1-\cos\theta)} = \frac{1.46}{1+(1.46/0.511)\times(1-\cos(30))} = 1.056 \text{ MeV}$$

This is the energy of the first scattered photon. Now it is scattered again:

Substitute in the variables for the second scatter (Equation 5.31A),

$$E'' = \frac{1.056}{1+(1.056/0.511)\times(1-\cos(150))} = 0.22 \text{ MeV}$$

(b) What is the energy of the photon if the angular sequence is reversed?

Using the same formulas, only reversing that the order the angles are input:

$$E' = \frac{1.46}{1 + (1.46/0.511) \times (1 - \cos(150))} = 0.23 \text{ MeV}$$

This is the energy of the first scattered photon. Now it is scattered again:

$$E'' = \frac{0.23}{1 + (0.23/0.511) \times (1 - \cos(30))}$$ = 0.22 MeV is the energy of the second scattered photon.

5.10

5.10 What is the energy of the Compton edge for the 0.661MeV gamma from Cs–137?

$E = 0.661$ MeV
$\theta = 180°$ for maximum energy Compton electron (definition of Compton edge)
$m_0c^2 = 0.51$ MeV (the rest mass energy of an electron)

Using this information, (Equation 5.31A)

$$E' = \frac{E}{1 + (E/m_0c^2)(1 - \cos\theta)} = \frac{0.661}{1 + (0.661/0.511) \times (1 - \cos(180))} = 0.184 \text{ MeV}$$ is the energy of the scattered photon.

Using the relationship that

$E_{e-} = E - E' = 0.661 - 0.184 = 0.48$ MeV for the Compton edge.

5.11

5.11 The energy of a scattered photon is 0.2 MeV after it was scattered through an angle of 135°. What was the photon's energy before the scattering collision?

$E' = 0.2$ MeV
$m_0c^2 = 0.51$ MeV
$\theta = 135°$

Equation 5.31A:

$$E' = \frac{E}{1 + (E / m_0 c^2)(1 - \cos\theta)}$$

$$0.2 = \frac{E}{1 + (E / 0.511) \times (1 - \cos(135))}$$

$E = 0.61$ MeV

5.12 What is the energy of the Compton edge for the following gammas? **5.12**
(a) 0.136 MeV from ^{57}Co,

The Compton edge occurs when the maximum amount of energy is transferred from the incoming photon to the scattered electron. The scattered photon is scattered at an angle of 180° to the scattered electron. There are many ways to solve for the energy of the Compton edge electron; for this solution one technique will be used, and answer (b) will be solved using another technique.

$\theta = 180°$

Use equation 5.30:

$\Delta\lambda = 0.0242\ (1 - \cos\theta)$ Å $= 0.0242\ (1 - \cos(180)) = 4.8 \times 10^{-2}$ Å is the change in wavelength of the incident photon compared to the scattered photon.

Calculating the initial wavelength of the incident photon:

$$\lambda = \frac{12400}{E_{eV}} = \frac{12400}{0.136\ \text{MeV} \times \dfrac{1 \times 10^6\ \text{eV}}{\text{MeV}}} = 9.12 \times 10^{-2}\ \text{Å}$$

Adding the change to the initial wavelength:

4.84×10^{-2} Å $+ 9.12 \times 10^{-2}$ Å $= 0.1396$ Å

Converting the scattered photon wavelength back to MeV:

$E' = \frac{12400}{\lambda} = \frac{12400}{0.1396} = 88840$ eV = 0.089 MeV is the energy of the scattered photon. Now subtract it from the initial energy of the photon (incident photon):

$E_{\text{compton electron}} = E(\gamma) - E'(\gamma) = 0.136\ \text{MeV} - 0.089\ \text{MeV} = 0.047$ MeV is the energy of the most energetic (Compton edge) electron.

(b) 0.811 MeV from ^{58}Co,

Using equation 5.31A to find the energy of the scattered photon (E'):
m_0c^2 = rest mass energy equivalence of electron = 0.51 MeV
$\theta = 180°$
$E = 0.811$ MeV

$E' = \frac{E}{1+\left(\frac{E}{m_0c^2}\right)(1-\cos\theta)} = \frac{0.811}{1+\left(\frac{0.811}{0.51}\right)\times(1-\cos(180))} = 0.194$ MeV is the energy of the scattered photon.

Subtract it from the initial energy of the photon (incident photon):

$E(\gamma) - E'(\gamma) = E_{\text{compton electron}}$

$0.811 - 0.194 = 0.617$ MeV is the energy of the most energetic (Compton edge) electron.

(c) 1.33 MeV from ^{60}Co.

Using equation 5.31A to find the energy of the scattered photon (E'):
m_0c^2 = rest mass energy equivalence of electron = 0.51 MeV
$\theta = 180°$
$E = 1.33$ MeV

$$E' = \frac{E}{1+\left(\frac{E}{m_0c^2}\right)(1-\cos\theta)} = \frac{1.33}{1+\left(\frac{1.33}{0.51}\right)\times(1-\cos(180))} = 0.214 \text{ MeV is the}$$

energy of the scattered photon.

Subtract it from the initial energy of the photon (incident photon):

$E_{\text{compton electron}} = E(\gamma) - E'(\gamma) = 1.33 - 0.214 = 1.12$ MeV is the energy of the most energetic (Compton edge) electron.

5.13 The following gamma–ray absorption data were taken with lead absorbers: **5.13**

Absorber thickness, mm	0	2	4	6	8	10	15	20	25
Counts per minute	1000	880	770	680	600	530	390	285	210

(a) Determine the linear, mass, and atomic attenuation coefficients.

The attenuation coefficient may be determined graphically. Plot the data on semi-log paper, with the count rate on the logarithmic scale. If the data fall on a single straight line, as in this case, then the attenuation coefficient is the slope of the line. The absorber half thickness (HVL) is determined from the curve and the slope is calculated. From the absorption curve, we find the half thickness to be 11 mm (1.1 cm).

$$\mu_\ell = \frac{0.693}{\text{HVL}} = \frac{0.693}{1.1 \text{ cm}} = 0.63 \text{ cm}^{-1}$$

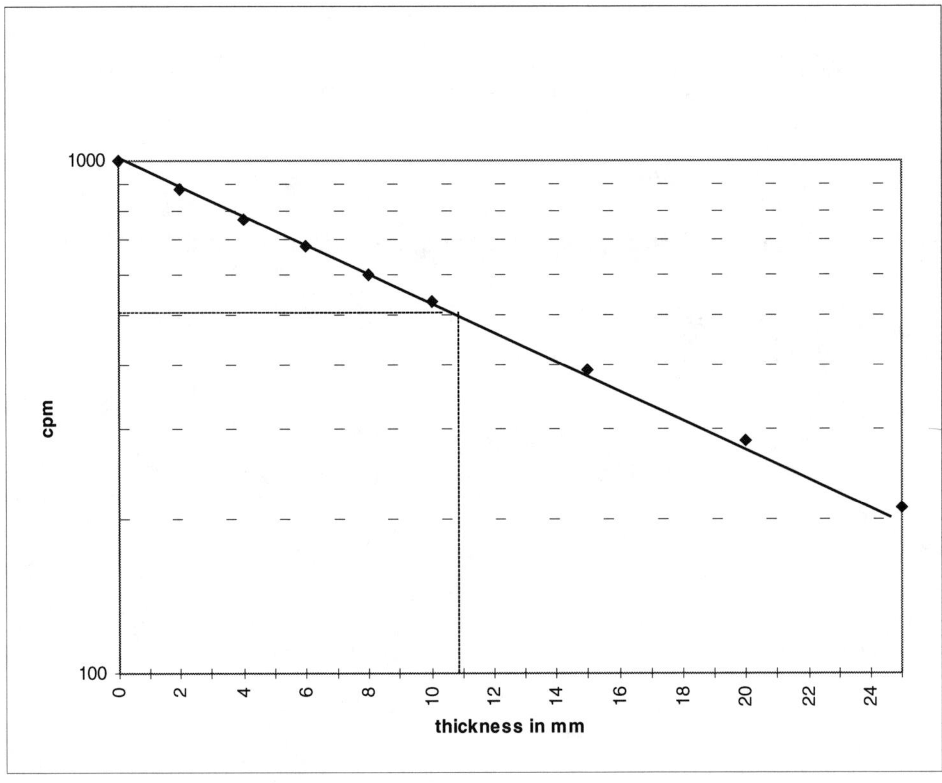

Calculating the mass attenuation coefficient:

$\rho_{Pb} = 11.35$ g/cm^3

$$\mu_m = \frac{\mu_{linear}}{\rho} = \frac{0.63}{\text{cm}} \times \frac{\text{cm}^3}{11.3 \text{ g}} = 0.056 \text{ cm}^2/\text{g}$$

Calculating the atomic attenuation coefficient:

Since the atomic weight of Pb is 207.21, there are 207.21 g Pb per mole.

$$\mu_a = \frac{\mu_l}{N \dfrac{\text{atoms}}{\text{cm}^2}} = \frac{0.63 \, \text{cm}^{-1}}{\dfrac{6.02 \times 10^{23} \dfrac{\text{atoms}}{\text{mole}}}{207.21 \dfrac{\text{g}}{\text{mole}} \times \dfrac{\text{cm}^3}{11.3 \, \text{g}}}} = 19.2 \times 10^{-24} \text{ cm}^2/\text{atom}$$

(b) What was the energy of the gamma ray?

Check in Appendix E, under lead attenuation, to determine the energy. From part (a), the mass attenuation coefficient is 0.055 cm²/g. Looking carefully in Appendix E, a value of 0.0569 cm²/g is close to the value calculated in part (a), and this corresponds to a value of 1.25 MeV. So the gamma ray energy is approximately 1.25 MeV.

5.14 The following absorption data were taken with aluminum absorbers: 5.14

Absorber Thickness, cm	0	0.02	0.04	0.06	0.08	0.1	0.12	0.14	0.16	0.2	0.4	0.8	1.5	2	2.8
Counts per minute	1000	576	348	230	168	134	120	107	96	95	90	82	68	60	50

(a) Plot the data. What types of radiations do the curve suggest?

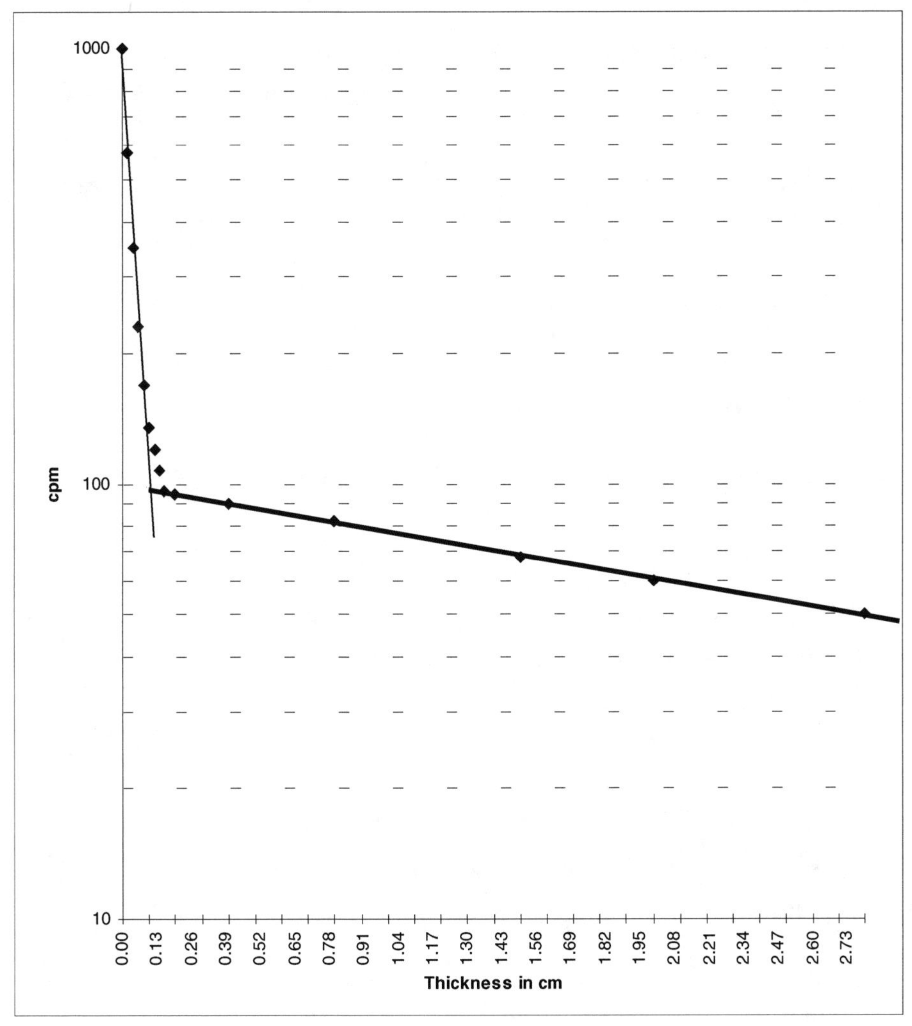

Because the curve falls rapidly for the first 0.08 cm, it appears that there is a β emitter present. Since counts above background are still detected after all the betas have been stopped, a γ must also be emitted.

The data points, after the betas have been stopped, fall on a straight line on semi–log paper; these points probably represent a gamma ray.
The line intersects the y axis at 100 cpm, the gamma count rate from the sample due to the gamma emitter is 100 cpm.

(b) If a beta particle is present, what is its energy?

A line representing the beta portion of the absorption curve intersects the gamma portion at 0.16 cm. This thickness represents the range, in aluminum, of the beta radiation.

Expressing the 0.16 cm range in aluminum in units of density thickness:
Density of aluminum, $\rho = 2.7\ \text{g/cm}^3$

$$0.16\ \text{cm} \times \frac{2.7\ \text{g}}{\text{cm}^3} \times \frac{1000\ \text{mg}}{1\ \text{g}} = 432\ \text{mg/cm}^2$$

and using the range equation (5.3) to find the energy of the β:
$\ln E = 6.63 - 3.2376 \times (10.2146 - \ln R)^{1/2}$

$\ln E = 6.63 - 3.2376 \times (10.2146 - \ln (432))^{1/2}$

$E = 1\text{MeV}$ is the approximate energy of the β

(c) If a gamma ray is present, what is its energy?

The slope of the “hard” straight line component of the absorption curve, which represents the gamma component, is

$$\mu = \frac{0.693}{\text{HVL}} = \frac{0.693}{2.8\ \text{cm} \times 2.7 \dfrac{\text{g}}{\text{cm}^3}} = 0.92 \frac{\text{cm}^2}{\text{g}}$$

From Appendix E, we find the gamma energy to be 0.4 MeV for a mass attenuation coefficient of 0.0922 cm^2/g

(d) Looking up the 0.6 MeV β in a table of energy vs. isotope (in the Radiological Health Handbook, 1970), Au-198 is found to be the most likely isotope because it emits a 0.41 MeV gamma and a 1.37 MeV beta. Computer programs also exist which can be used to determine the isotope based solely on energies.

(e) Write the equation that fits the absorption data.

The absorption curve can be resolved into 2 components. First, the "hard" portion, which is a straight line representing gamma radiation, is extrapolated to the y axis. Then, the various y values of the extrapolated straight line are subtracted from the total absorption curve, to give the y values for the "soft" component, which represents possible beta radiation. In this manner, the intercept of the gamma component is 100 cpm and its slope is 0.25 cm^{-1}. The intercept of the beta component is 1000 – 100, or 900 cpm, and its slope is 24 cm^{-1}. The equation of the absorption curve, therefore is

$$A = 900e^{-24t} + 100e^{-0.25t}$$

The frequency of betas and gammas from ^{198}Au is about equal. The higher beta count rate is due to the higher counter efficiency for betas than for gammas.

5.15 A collimated gamma ray beam consists of equal numbers of 0.1 MeV and 1.0 MeV photons. If the beam enters a 15 cm thick concrete shield, what is the relative portion of 1 MeV photons to 0.1 MeV photons in the emergent beam? **5.15**

$\mu_{0.1\text{ MeV}} = 0.169\ cm^2/g$ (Appendix E)
$\mu_{1.0\text{ MeV}} = 0.0635\ cm^2/g$ (Appendix E)
$\rho_{concrete} = 2.35\ g/cm^3$ (Table 5.2)

Convert the thickness to density thickness:

$$t = 15\ cm \times \frac{2.35\ g}{cm^3} = 35.25\ g/cm^2$$

Use equation 5.19:

$$I/I_0 = e^{-\mu t}$$

$$I_0 = \frac{I_{0.1\text{ MeV}}}{e^{-\mu_{0.1\text{ MeV}}t}} = \frac{I_{1\text{ MeV}}}{e^{-\mu_{1\text{ MeV}}t}}$$

$$\frac{I_{1\text{ MeV}}}{I_{0.1\text{MeV}}} = \left(\frac{e^{-\mu_{1\text{ MeV}}t}}{e^{-\mu_{0.1\text{ MeV}}t}}\right) = \left(\frac{e^{-0.0635\cdot35.25}}{e^{-0.169\cdot35.25}}\right) = 41.3$$

5.16

5.16 Three collimated gamma–ray beams of equal flux, whose quantum energies are 2, 5, and 10 MeV, respectively, pass through a 5 cm thickness of lead. What is the ratio of the emergent fluxes?

$\mu_{2\text{MeV}} = 0.0455\text{ cm}^2/\text{g}$
$\mu_{5\text{MeV}} = 0.0424\text{ cm}^2/\text{g}$
$\mu_{10\text{MeV}} = 0.0484\text{ cm}^2/\text{g}$
$\rho_{\text{Pb}} = 11.35\text{ g/cm}^3$

Use equation 5.24A:

For 2 MeV photons

$$e^{-\mu t} = e^{-0.0455\text{ cm2/g} \times 5\text{ cm} \times 11.35\text{ g/cm3}} = e^{-2.58} = 0.0756$$

For 5 MeV photons:

$$e^{-\mu t} = e^{-0.0424\text{ cm2/g} \times 5\text{ cm} \times 11.35\text{ g/cm3}} = e^{-2.41} = 0.09$$

For 10 MeV photons:

$$e^{-\mu t} = e^{-0.0484\text{ cm2/g} \times 5\text{ cm} \times 11.35\text{ g/cm3}} = e^{-2.75} = 0.064$$

Calculating the ratios:

$$\frac{0.0756}{0.0756}:\frac{0.0756}{0.09}:\frac{0.0756}{0.0641} = 1 : 0.8 : 1.2$$

5.17

5.17 A collimated beam of 0.2 MeV gamma radiation delivers an incident energy flux of 2 J/m^2/sec to a Pb shield 1 g/cm^2 thick.
(a) What is the incident photon flux, photons/cm^2/sec?

$$\frac{1 \text{ photon}}{0.2 \text{ MeV}} \times \frac{\text{MeV}}{1.6 \times 10^{-13} \text{J}} \times \frac{2 \text{ J}}{\text{m}^2 \cdot \text{s}} \times \frac{1 \text{ m}^2}{10^4 \text{ cm}^2} = 6.25 \times 10^9 \frac{\text{photons}}{\text{cm}^2 \cdot \text{s}}$$

(b) What is the rate of energy absorption in the shield, ergs/g/sec and J/kg/sec?

$\mu_{en} = 0.821 \frac{\text{cm}^2}{\text{g}}$ is the energy absorption coefficient for Pb for 0.2 MeV gamma (Appendix F)

$$I_0 = 2 \frac{\text{J}}{\text{m}^2 \cdot \text{s}} = 2 \times 10^{-4} \frac{\text{J}}{\text{cm}^2 \cdot \text{s}}$$

$$I = I_0 \, \text{e}^{-\mu t}$$

Incident energy absorbed $= I_0 - I = I_0 - I_0 \, \text{e}^{-\mu t} = I_0 (1 - \text{e}^{-\mu t})$

$$\Delta I = 2 \times 10^{-4} \frac{\text{J}}{\text{cm}^2 \cdot \text{s}} \left(1 - e^{-0.821 \frac{\text{cm}^2}{\text{g}} \times 1 \frac{\text{g}}{\text{cm}^2}} \right)$$

$$\Delta I = 1.12 \times 10^{-4} \frac{\text{J}}{\text{g} \cdot \text{s}} = 0.112 \frac{\text{J}}{\text{kg} \cdot \text{s}}$$

$$1.12 \times 10^{-1} \frac{\text{J}}{\text{kg} \cdot \text{s}} \times \frac{1 \times 10^7 \text{erg}}{\text{J}} = 1.12 \times 10^3 \frac{\text{ergs}}{\text{g} \cdot \text{s}}$$

5.18 Calculate the thickness of Al and Cu required to attenuate narrow, collimated, monochromatic beams of 0.1 MeV and 0.8 MeV gamma rays to **5.18**

(a) one half the incident intensity (HVL),

(b) one–tenth the incident intensity (TVL). Express your answer in cm and grams/cm^2.

(c) What is the relationship between a half–value layer and a tenth–value layer?

Gamma ray attenuation is given by equation 5.19

$$I = I_0 \, \text{e}^{-\mu t}$$

The linear attenuation coefficients, μ_l cm^{-1}, as listed in Table 5.2, and the mass attenuation coefficients, μ_m cm^2/g, as listed in Appendix E are:

	μ_l cm^{-1}		μ_m cm^2/g	
	0.1 MeV	0.8 MeV	0.1 MeV	0.8 MeV
Al	0.435	0.185	0.161	0.068
Cu	3.8	0.58	0.427	0.065

By definition, a half value layer, HVL, is that absorber thickness that transmits one half the incident radiation, and a tenth value layer, TVL, transmits one tenth the incident radiation.

HVL: $\frac{I}{I_0} = \frac{1}{2} e^{-\mu t}$ TVL: $\frac{I}{I_0} = \frac{1}{10} e^{-\mu t}$

$$t(\text{HVL}) = \frac{\ln\left(\frac{1}{2}\right)}{-\mu} \qquad t(\text{TVL}) = \frac{\ln\left(\frac{1}{10}\right)}{-\mu}$$

$$\text{HVL} = \frac{0.693}{\mu} \qquad \text{TVL} = \frac{2.3}{\mu}$$

$$\frac{\text{TVL}}{\text{HVL}} = \frac{2.3/\mu}{.693/\mu}$$

Therefore, TVL = 3.3 HVL

If we substitute the appropriate values for the attenuation coefficients into the equations above, we have for 0.1 MeV, the linear (HVL_l) and the mass (HVL_m) half value layers and tenth value layers, in Al:

$$\text{HVL}_\ell = \frac{0.693}{0.435\ \text{cm}^{-1}} = 1.59\ \text{cm} \qquad \text{HVL}_m = \frac{0.693}{0.161\ \frac{\text{cm}^2}{\text{g}}} = 4.3\frac{\text{g}}{\text{cm}^2}$$

The TVL = 3.3 HVL
Therefore,
$\text{TVL}_l = 3.3 \times 1.59\ \text{cm} = 5.25\ \text{cm}$ $\text{TVL}_m = 3.3 \times 4.3\ \text{g/cm}^2 = 14.2\ \text{g/cm}^2$

Other HVL's and TVL's are calculated in a similar manner, and the results are tabulated below:

HVL	0.1 MeV		0.8 MeV	
	Linear, cm	Mass, cm²/g	Linear, cm	Mass, cm²/g
Al	1.59	4.3	3.75	10.2
Cu	0.18	1.62	1.12	10.7

TVL	0.1 MeV		0.8 MeV	
	Linear, cm	Mass, cm²/g	Linear, cm	Mass, cm²/g
Al	5.25	14.2	12.4	33.7
Cu	0.59	5.35	3.7	35.3

5.19 The mass attenuation coefficient for muscle for 1 MeV γ radiation is 0.070 cm^2/g. What is the mean free path of a 1 MeV photon in muscle? **5.19**

The mean free path is simply the reciprocal of the attenuation coefficient.

$$\mu_m = 0.070\frac{\text{cm}^2}{\text{g}}$$

$$\rho_m = 1\frac{\text{g}}{\text{cm}^3}$$

$$\text{MFP} = \frac{1}{\mu} = \frac{1}{0.07\frac{\text{cm}^2}{\text{g}} \times 1\frac{\text{g}}{\text{cm}^3}} = 14.29 \text{ cm}$$

5.20 A laminated shield consists of two layers each of alternating thickness of aluminum and lead, each layer having a density thickness of 1.35 g/cm^2. The shield is irradiated with a narrow collimated beam of 0.2 MeV photons. **5.20**
(a) What is the overall thickness of the laminated shield in cm?

The shield consists of 1 sheet Al, a sheet of Pb, a sheet of Al, and a sheet of Pb. This makes a total of 2 layers of each type of material in the shield. Since there are two layers of each material, multiply each density thickness by two;

$1.35\ \text{g/cm}^2 \times 2 = 2.7\ \text{g/cm}^2$ is the total density thickness contributed by each material layer.

Using the density of each material, the thickness of each layer of material can be determined:

Aluminum has a density of $2.7\ \text{g/cm}^3$

$$\frac{2.7\frac{\text{g}}{\text{cm}^2}}{2.7\frac{\text{g}}{\text{cm}^3}} = 1\ \text{cm}$$ is the thickness of the aluminum in the shield.

Lead has a density of $11.3\ \text{g/cm}^3$

$$\frac{2.7\frac{\text{g}}{\text{cm}^2}}{11.3\frac{\text{g}}{\text{cm}^3}} = 0.24\ \text{cm}$$ is the thickness of the lead in the shield.

Adding together the two layers:

$1 + 0.24 = 1.24$ cm thick is the total thickness

(b) Calculate the shield attenuation factor when the (1) aluminum layer is first, (2) lead layer is first.

From table 5.2:
$\mu_{Al} = 0.324\ \text{cm}^{-1}$
$\mu_{Pb} = 10.15\ \text{cm}^{-1}$

From part (a), the thicknesses are:
$t_{Al} = 1$ cm Al
$t_{Pb} = 0.24$ cm Pb

Combining this into equation 5.19;

$$I/I_0 = e^{-\mu t} = e^{-\{(1 \times 0.324) + (0.24 \times 10.15)\}} = 0.063$$

Putting the lead or aluminum first does not make a difference in the result.

5.21 Calculate the probability that a 2 MeV photon in a narrow collimated beam will be removed from the beam by each of the following shields, **5.21**
(a) Lead, 1 cm thick

$$\frac{I}{I_0} = \text{Probability of transmission}$$

$$1 - \frac{I}{I_0} = 1 - e^{-\mu t} = \text{Probability of removal}$$

$t = 1$ cm

$\mu_{Pb} = 0.516 \text{ cm}^{-1}$ (table 5.2)

$$\frac{I}{I_0} = 1 - e^{-\mu t} = 1 - e^{-0.516 \times 1} = 0.403$$

(b) Iron, 1 cm thick

$t = 1$ cm

$\mu_{Fe} = 0.335 \text{ cm}^{-1}$ (table 5.2)

$$\frac{I}{I_0} = 1 - e^{-\mu t} = 1 - e^{-0.535 \times 1} = 0.285$$

(c) Lead, 1 g/cm² thick

ρ_{Pb}=11.35 g/cm³

$$t = \frac{1 \text{ g}}{\text{cm}^2} \times \frac{\text{cm}^3}{11.35 \text{ g}} = 8.8 \times 10^{-2} \text{cm}$$

$\mu_{Pb} = 0.516 \text{ cm}^{-1}$ (table 5.2)

$$\frac{I}{I_0} = 1 - e^{-\mu t} = 1 - e^{-0.516 \times 0.088} = 0.044$$

(d) Iron, 1 g/cm² thick

ρ_{Fe}=7.86 g/cm³

$$t = \frac{1\text{ g}}{\text{cm}^2} \times \frac{\text{cm}^3}{7.86\text{ g}} = 0.127\text{ cm}$$

$$\mu_{Pb} = 0.335\text{ cm}^{-1}\ \text{(table 5.2)}$$

$$\frac{I}{I_0} = 1 - e^{-\mu t} = 1 - e^{-0.535 \times 0.127} = 0.0416$$

5.22

5.22 Calculate the neutron threshold energy for the reaction $^{11}C(n,\gamma)\ ^{12}C$, if the prompt capture gamma ray is 21.5 MeV.

$$^{11}C + {}^{1}n + E_n \rightarrow {}^{12}C + \gamma$$

Calculating the mass lost by the neutron absorption (From CRC), and adding the energy equivalent of the prompt gamma ray to the ^{12}C;

^{11}C = 11.01143 amu
^{1}n = 1.008665 amu
^{12}C = 12.00000 amu

931 MeV = 1 amu

$$\gamma = 21.5\text{ MeV} \times \frac{\text{amu}}{931\text{ MeV}} = 2.309435 \times 10^{-2}\text{ amu}$$

$$12.00000\text{ amu} + 1.008665\text{ amu} + E_n = 11.01143\text{ amu} + 2.309345 \times 10^{-2}\text{ amu}$$

$$E_n = 2.998 \times 10^{-3}\text{ amu}$$

$$\frac{931\text{ MeV}}{\text{amu}} \times 2.998 \times 10^{-3}\text{ amu} = 2.8\text{ MeV}$$

5.23

5.23 X–rays are generated as bremsstrahlung by causing high–speed electrons to be stopped by a high atomic numbered target. If the electrons are accelerated by a constant high voltage of 250 kV, and if the electron beam current is 10 mA, calculate the X–ray energy flux at a distance of 1 m from the tungsten target. Neglect absorption by the glass tube, and assume that the bremsstrahlung are emitted isotropically.

For mono–energetic electrons, equation 5.11b applies to determine the fraction of energy in the electron beam which is converted into bremsstrahlung:

E = 250 keV = 0.25 MeV, the kinetic energy of the electron hitting the target
Z = 74 (the atomic number for Tungsten)

$f = 1 \times 10^{-3}\, Z E = 1 \times 10^{-3} \times 74 \times 0.25 = 0.0185$ is the fraction of the electron's energy converted to photons.

Calculating the energy input:
P = power in watts
I = current in amps = 10 mA = 10×10^{-3} A
E = Voltage = 250 kV = 250×10^{3} V

$P = I E = 10 \times 10^{-3}\ \text{A} \times (250 \times 10^{3}\ \text{V}) = 2500\ \text{W}$
Therefore, the rate at which the energy is converted to bremsstrahlung is:
2500 W × 0.0185 = 46.25 W is the rate energy is converted to bremsstrahlung.
Since the bremsstrahlung is spread over the surface of a sphere whose radius is 100 cm:

$$\text{X–ray energy flux} = \frac{46.25\ \text{W} \times 10^{3}\ \dfrac{\text{mW}}{\text{W}}}{4 \times \pi \times (100\ \text{cm})^{2}} = 0.37\ \text{mW/cm}^{2}$$

5.24 If the most energetic photon results from the instantaneous stopping of an electron in a single collision, what voltage must be applied across an X-ray tube in order to generate X-rays whose shortest wavelength approaches 0.124 angstroms? **5.24**

λ = 0.124 angstroms = 0.124×10^{-8} cm
$h = 6.63 \times 10^{-27}$ erg/sec
$c = 3 \times 10^{10}$ cm/sec

Equation 2.76;

$$E = \frac{hc}{\lambda} = \frac{6.63 \times 10^{-27}\ \text{erg} \cdot \text{sec} \times 3 \times 10^{10}\ \dfrac{\text{cm}}{\text{sec}} \times 6.25 \times 10^{5}\ \dfrac{\text{MeV}}{\text{erg}}}{0.124 \times 10^{-8}\ \text{cm} \times 1.6 \times 10^{-12}\ \dfrac{\text{erg}}{\text{eV}}} = 0.1\ \text{MeV}$$

Since 1 eV is the energy gained by an electron accelerated by a potential of 1 volt, a potential of 100,000 V the required wavelength.

5.25

5.25 A beta particle whose kinetic energy is 0.159 MeV passes through a 4 mg/cm^2 window into a helium–filled Geiger tube. How many ion pairs will the beta particle produce inside the tube?

First, determine the range of the β (0.159 MeV) using equation 5.2;

$R = 412\, E^{\,1.265 - 0.0954 \ln E} = 412 \times (0.159)^{1.265 - 0.0954 \times \ln(0.159)} = 29.145$ mg/cm^2 is the range of the electron.

Since the thin window partly attenuates the β, subtract the thin window density (4 mg/cm^2) thickness from the total range:

29.145 mg/cm^2 – 4 mg/cm^2 = 25.145 mg/cm^2

Now find the fraction of energy left in the beta after going through the window;

$$\frac{25.145 \dfrac{\text{mg}}{\text{cm}^2}}{29.145 \dfrac{\text{mg}}{\text{cm}^2}} = 0.863$$

Multiplying by the initial energy:

0.863 × (0.159MeV) = 0.137 MeV is the energy left after going through the window.

From table 5.1, ^{4}He consumes 41.5 eV per ion pair:

$$0.137 \text{ MeV} \times \frac{1 \times 10^6 \text{eV}}{1 \text{ MeV}} \times \frac{\text{ion pair He}}{41.5 \text{ eV}} = 3305 \text{ ion pairs}$$

5.26

5.26 If the neutron emission rate from ^{252}Cf is 2.31 × 10^6 neutrons per second per μg, and the transformation rate constant for alpha emission is 0.25 per year, what is the neutron emission rate per MBq and per μCi?

$\lambda = 0.25 \text{ yr}^{-1}$

$$T_{Cf} = \frac{0.693}{0.25} = 2.772 \text{ yr}$$

Calculate the specific activity of ^{252}Cf, use equation 4.31 in order to determine the number of μCi in 1 μg :

$A_{Ra} = 226$
$T_{Ra} = 1620$ yr
$A_{Cf} = 252$
$T_{Cf} = 2.772$ yr

$$SA = \frac{A_{Ra}T_{Ra}}{A_{Cf}T_{Cf}} = \frac{226 \times 1620 \text{ yr}}{252 \times 2.772 \text{ yr}} = 524.12 \text{ Ci/g} = 524 \ \mu\text{Ci}/\mu\text{g}$$

To find the neutron emission rate per μCi:

$$\frac{2.31 \times 10^6 \frac{\text{neutron}}{\text{sec}}}{\mu\text{g}} \times \frac{1 \ \mu\text{g}}{524 \ \mu\text{Ci}} = 4.4 \times 10^3 \frac{\text{n}}{\text{sec}/\mu\text{Ci}}$$

$$\frac{4.4 \times 10^3 \frac{\text{neutrons}}{\text{sec}}}{\mu\text{Ci}} \times \frac{27 \mu\text{Ci}}{\text{MBq}} = 1.2 \times 10^5 \frac{\text{n}}{\text{sec}/\text{MBq}}$$

5.27 Calculate the speed of a "slow" neutron whose kinetic energy is 0.1 eV. To what temperature does this energy correspond? **5.27**

Substituting neutrons kinetic energy and mass (Appendix A) into the equation for kinetic energy (equation 2.3).

$$\text{Kinetic Energy} = \frac{1}{2}mv^2$$

$$0.1 \text{ eV} \times 1.6 \times 10^{-19} \frac{\text{J}}{\text{eV}} = \frac{1}{2} \times 1.675 \times 10^{-27} v^2$$

$v = 4.4 \times 10^3$ m/s $= 4.4 \times 10^5$ cm/s

Alternatively, knowing that the velocity of a 0.025 eV neutron = 2200 m/s (p.152), and that

$$\frac{E_1}{E_2} = \frac{v_1^2}{v_2^2}$$

Calculating the velocity with equation 5.42:
$E_1 = 0.025$ eV
$E_2 = 0.1$ eV
$v_1^2 = (2200 \text{ m/s})^2 = 4.84 \times 10^6 \text{ m}^2/\text{s}^2$

$$v_2 = \sqrt{\frac{E_2 v_1^2}{E_1}} = \sqrt{\frac{0.1 \times (4.84 \times 10^6)}{0.025}} = 4.4 \times 10^3 \text{ m/s} = 4.4 \times 10^5 \text{ cm/s}$$

Use Equation 5.42

$E = kT$

$k = 8.625 \times 10^{-5} \dfrac{\text{eV}}{\text{K}}$ (p. 152)

$E = 0.1$ eV

$$T = \frac{E}{k} = \frac{0.1 \text{ eV}}{8.6 \times 10^{-5} \dfrac{\text{eV}}{\text{K}}} = 1159 \text{ K} = 886 \text{ °C}$$

5.28 **5.28** When ^{9}Be is irradiated with deuterons, neutrons are produced according to the reaction $^{9}_{4}\text{Be (d,n)}\ ^{10}_{5}\text{B}$. The cross section for this reaction for 15 MeV deuterons is 0.12 barns. What is the neutron flux at a distance of 25 cm from a 1 g beryllium target that is irradiated with 100 μA beam of deuterons, 1.13 cm diameter, assuming an isotropic distribution of neutrons?

Find the number of Be atoms available to react with:

$$N = 1 \text{ g Be} \times \frac{1 \text{ mol}}{9 \text{ g Be}} \times \frac{6.02 \times 10^{23} \text{ atoms Be}}{1 \text{ mol}} = 6.69 \times 10^{22} \text{ atoms } ^{9}\text{Be in the target}$$

Next, determine the number of deuterons available to react with the target:

$$\frac{100 \ \mu\text{A} \times 10^6 \dfrac{\mu\text{A}}{1 \text{ A}} \times 1 \dfrac{\text{C}}{\text{sec}}}{1.6 \times 10^{-19} \text{ C}/\text{deuteron}} = 6.25 \times 10^{14} \text{ deut/sec}$$

Since the area of the deuteron beam is

$$A = \frac{\pi}{4}d^2 = \frac{\pi}{4}(1.13\text{ cm})^2 = 1\text{ cm}^2$$

The deuteron flux at the target is 6.25×10^{14} deut/sec/cm^2

Use equation 5.59, and ignore the decay portion (^{10}B is stable) to find the rate of production of the neutrons:

Reactions per second = $N\phi\sigma$ = neutrons produced per second
$N = 6.69 \times 10^{22}$ atoms ^{9}Be in the target
$\sigma = 0.12$ b
$\phi = 6.25 \times 10^{14}$ deut/sec/cm^2

$$6.69 \times 10^{22}\text{ atoms} \times 6.25 \times 10^{14}\,\frac{\text{deut}}{\text{cm}^2\text{ sec}} \times 0.12\text{ b} \times \frac{1 \times 10^{-24}\,\frac{\text{cm}^2}{\text{atom}}}{1\text{ b}}$$

$= 5.0175 \times 10^{12}$ neutrons/sec

Since the neutrons are isotropically distributed, the neutron flux at a distance of 25 cm will be distributed over a surface area of

$S = 4\pi r^2 = 4 \times \pi \times 25^2 = 7854$ cm^2 and the neutron flux is

$$\frac{5.0175 \times 10^{12}\,\frac{\text{neutrons}}{\text{sec}}}{7854\text{ cm}^2} = 6.4 \times 10^8\text{ neutrons/cm}^2\text{ per sec}$$

5.29 What is the thickness of Cd that will absorb 50% of an incident beam of thermal neutrons? The capture cross section for the element Cd is 2550 barns for thermal neutrons; the specific gravity of Cd is 8.65 and its atomic weight is 112.4. **5.29**

$\sigma = 2550\text{ b} = 2550 \times 10^{-24}\text{ cm}^2$

$$N = \frac{8.65\text{ g}}{\text{cm}^3} \times \frac{1\text{ mol}}{112.4\text{ g}} \times \frac{6.02 \times 10^{23}\text{ atoms}}{1\text{ mol}} = 4.63 \times 10^{22}\text{ atoms Cd}$$

Use equation 5.43;

$$I/I_0 = e^{-\sigma N t}$$

$I/I_0 = 0.5 = e^{-2550 \times 10^{-24}\, cm^2 \times 4.63 \times 10^{22}\, atoms\, Cd \times t}$

$t = 0.0059$ cm thick

5.30

5.30 A small ^{124}Sb gamma ray source, whose activity is 3.7×10^{10} Bq (1 Ci), is completely surrounded by a 25 g sphere of beryllium. Calculate the number of neutrons per second from the ^{9}Be (γ, n) ^{8}Be reaction if the cross section is 1 millibarn, and if the diameter of the spherical cavity enclosing the gamma ray source is 1 cm. The density of Be = 1.8 g/cm^3.

The neutron production rate, R, is
$R = N\phi\sigma$,

Where
N = number of target atoms
ϕ = photon flux
σ = reaction cross section

However, since the gamma source is inside the Be sphere, the gamma flux will continuously decrease as the gammas penetrate into the sphere (Neglecting the very small fraction of the photons that react with a Be nucleus, since σ = 1 mb). We must therefore calculate the neutron production rate, dr, in each successive volume dV (= $4\pi r^2 dr$), and integrate these rates over the thickness of the Be sphere. The neutron production rate dR in an infinitesimal volume dV, is given by

$$dR = dN \text{ atoms} \times \phi \frac{\text{photons}}{\text{cm}^2 \cdot s} \times \sigma \frac{\text{cm}^2}{\text{atom}}$$

$$dN = \frac{6.02 \times 10^{23} \text{ atoms Be}}{9 \text{ g Be}} \times 1.8 \frac{\text{g}}{\text{cm}^3} \times dV \text{ cm}^3$$

$dN = 1.2 \times 10^{23}$ atoms ^{9}Be $\times$ ($4 \times \pi \times r^2$) dr

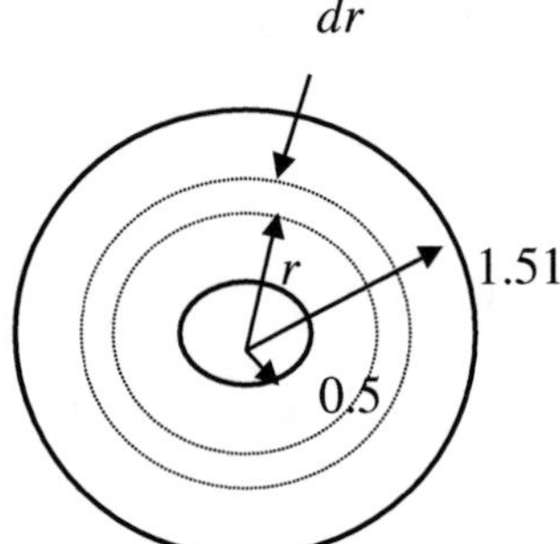

The sphere's outer radius is:

$$\frac{4}{3}\pi\left(r^3 - 0.5^3\right)\text{cm}^3 \times 1.8 \frac{\text{g}}{\text{cm}^3} = 25 \text{ g}$$

$r = 1.51$ cm

$$\phi = \frac{S\ \text{photons/s}}{4\pi r^2}$$

S = gamma ray source activity, photons per second

$$dR = 1.2\times10^{23}\ \frac{\text{atoms}}{\text{cm}^3}\times\left(4\pi r^2 dr\right)\text{cm}^3\times\frac{S\ \text{photons/s}}{4\pi r^2\text{cm}^2}\times\sigma\frac{\text{cm}^2}{\text{atom}}$$

Since the threshold for the (γ, n) reaction is 1.67 MeV, only photons whose energy is equal to or greater than 1.67 MeV can initiate the reaction. Examination of the ^{124}Sb decay scheme (ICRP 38) shows that only 57% of the photons have energies greater than or equal to 1.67 MeV. The effective transformation rate in the 1 Ci ^{124}Sb source is

$$0.57\times3.7\times10^{10}\ \frac{\text{photons}}{\text{s}\cdot\text{Ci}}\times1\ \text{Ci} = 2.11\times10^{10}\ \frac{\text{photons}}{\text{s}}$$

The total neutron production rate is

$$R = \int_{0.5}^{1.51}\left(1.2\times10^{23}\ \frac{\text{atoms}}{\text{cm}^3}\times2.11\times10^{10}\ \frac{\text{photons}}{\text{s}}\times1\times10^{-27}\ \frac{\text{cm}^2}{\text{atom}}\right)dr$$

$$R = 2.53\times10^{6}\int_{0.5}^{1.51}dr = 2.6\times10^{6}\ \frac{\text{neutrons}}{\text{s}}$$

5.31 Cadmium is used as a thermal neutron shield in an average flux of 10^{12} neutrons per cm^2/sec. How long will it take to use up 10% of the ^{113}Cd atoms at 20°C? **5.31**

$$\frac{\text{reactions}}{\text{sec}} = \phi\frac{\text{neutrons}}{\text{cm}^2\cdot\text{sec}}\times\sigma\frac{\text{cm}^2}{\text{target atom}}\times N\ \text{target atoms}$$

$$\frac{dN}{dt} = -\phi\sigma n$$

$$dN = -(\phi\sigma n)dt$$

Integrating between the original and final numbers of ^{113}Cd atoms.

$$N_0 = N e^{-\phi\sigma t}$$

$\phi = 10^{12}$ neutrons/cm^2/sec
$\sigma = 20600$ b $= 2.1 \times 10^{-20}$ cm^2

Equation 5.57

$N/N_0 = 0.9$

$N = N_0 e^{-\phi\sigma t}$

$N/N_0 = e^{-\phi\sigma t}$

$0.9 = e^{-10E12 \times (2.1E-20) \times t}$

$t = 5.02 \times 10^6$ sec

$$5.02 \times 10^6 \text{ sec} \times \frac{\text{hr}}{3600 \text{ sec}} \times \frac{\text{d}}{24 \text{ hr}} = 58.1 \text{ days}$$

5.32

5.32 The cross section for the $^{32}S(n, p)\,^{32}P$ reaction is 300 millibarns for neutrons greater than 2.5 MeV. How many microcuries of ^{32}P activity can we expect if 100 mg of ^{32}S is irradiated in a fast flux of 10^2 neutron/cm^2 sec for 1 week?

$$\sigma = 300 \text{ mb} \times \frac{1 \text{ b}}{1 \times 10^3 \text{ mb}} \times \frac{1 \times 10^{-24} \frac{\text{cm}^2}{\text{atom}}}{1 \text{ b}} = 3 \times 10^{-25} \frac{\text{cm}^2}{\text{atom}}$$

$$n = 100 \text{ mg} \times \frac{1 \text{ g}}{10^3 \text{ mg}} \times \frac{1 \text{ mol}}{32 \text{ g}} \times \frac{6.02 \times 10^{23} \text{ atoms}}{1 \text{ mol}} = 1.88 \times 10^{21} \text{ atoms } ^{32}\text{S}$$

$\phi = 10^2$ neutrons/cm^2 sec

^{32}P half life is 14.3 days:

$$\lambda = \frac{0.693}{14.3} = 0.0485 \text{ d}^{-1}$$

$t = 7$ days

Using equation 5.59:

$$\lambda N = \phi\sigma n(1 - e^{-\lambda t})$$

$$\lambda N = \frac{10^2 \text{ neutrons}}{\text{cm}^2 \cdot \text{sec}} \times \frac{3 \times 10^{-25} \text{cm}^2}{\text{atom}} \times 1.88 \times 10^{21} \text{ atoms} \times (1 - e^{-0.0485 \times 7})$$

$$\lambda N = 0.016 \text{ d/sec} = 0.016 \frac{\text{d}}{\text{sec}} \times \frac{1 \mu\text{Ci}}{3.7 \times 10^4 \text{ d/sec}} = 4.4 \times 10^{-7} \mu\text{Ci}$$

5.33 If the absorption coefficient of the high energy component of cosmic radiation is 2.5×10^{-3} per meter water, calculate the reduction in intensity of these cosmic rays at the bottom of the ocean, at the depth of 10,000 m. **5.33**

Equation 5.19
$\mu = 2.5 \times 10^{-3}\ \text{m}^{-1}$ (given)
t = 10,000 m

$$I/I_0 = e^{-\mu t} = e^{-(2.5E-3) \times (10{,}000)} = 1.39 \times 10^{-11}$$

5.34 If deuterium is irradiated with 2.62 MeV gamma rays from ^{208}Tl(ThC″), the nucleus disintegrates into its component parts of 1 proton and 1 neutron. If the neutron and proton each has 0.225 MeV of kinetic energy, and if the proton has a mass of 1.007593 atomic mass units, calculate the mass of the neutron. **5.34**

First, write the reaction:

$$2.62 \text{ MeV} + {}^2_1\text{H} \rightarrow {}^1_1\text{p} + {}^1_0\text{n} + 2 \times 0.225 \text{ MeV}$$

Based on Appendix A, there are 931 MeV per amu

$$\left(\frac{2.62 \text{ MeV}}{931 \text{ MeV}/1 \text{ amu}}\right) + 2.013928 \text{ amu} = 1.007593 + {}^1_0\text{n} + 2\left(\frac{0.225 \text{ MeV}}{931 \text{ MeV}/1 \text{ amu}}\right)$$

$${}^1_0\text{n} = 1.0089 \text{ amu}$$

5.35 A beam of fast neutrons includes two energy groups. One group, of 1 MeV neutrons, includes 99% of the total neutron flux. The remaining 1% of the neutrons have an energy of 10 MeV. **5.35**

The removal cross sections are in barns as follows:

	1 MeV	10 MeV
H	4.2b	0.95b
O	8b	1.5b
Pb	5.5b	5.1b

(a) What will be the relative proportions of the two groups after passing through 25 cm of water?

In this problem we wish to find the shielding effectiveness (I/I_0) of Pb and H_2O.

Calculate the number of atoms per cm^3 for hydrogen:

Water has a density of 1 g/cm^3, and the molar density of water is 18 g/mole.

$$N_H = \frac{1\text{ g H}_2\text{O}}{\text{cm}^3} \times \frac{1\text{ mol H}_2\text{O}}{18\text{ g H}_2\text{O}} \times \frac{2\text{ mol H}}{1\text{ mol H}_2\text{O}} \times \frac{6.02 \times 10^{23}\text{ atoms H}}{\text{mol H}}$$

$N_H = 6.69 \times 10^{22}$ atoms H / cm^3

A similar calculation is done for oxygen:

$$N_O = \frac{1\text{ g H}_2\text{O}}{\text{cm}^3} \times \frac{1\text{ mol H}_2\text{O}}{18\text{ g H}_2\text{O}} \times \frac{1\text{ mol O}}{1\text{ mol H}_2\text{O}} \times \frac{6.02 \times 10^{23}\text{ atoms O}}{\text{mol O}}$$

$N_H = 3.34 \times 10^{22}$ atoms O / cm^3

Information given in the problem:

$\sigma_{\text{H, 1 MeV}} = 4.2\text{ b} = 4.2 \times 10^{-24}\text{ cm}^2$
$\sigma_{\text{H, 10 MeV}} = 0.95\text{ b} = 0.95 \times 10^{-24}\text{ cm}^2$
$\sigma_{\text{O, 1 MeV}} = 8\text{ b} = 8 \times 10^{-24}\text{ cm}^2$
$\sigma_{\text{O, 10 MeV}} = 1.5\text{ b} = 1.5 \times 10^{-24}\text{ cm}^2$

$t = 25$ cm

Equation 5.43 can now be solved for 1.0 and also 10 MeV neutrons to obtain the attenuation factor.

$$\frac{I}{I_0} = e^{-\sigma N t}$$

Substituting in values:

Solve for the exponent first:

1 MeV neutrons

$$\sigma Nt_{H} = 4.2 \times 10^{-24}\ \text{cm}^2 \times 6.69 \times 10^{22}\ \frac{\text{atoms H}}{\text{cm}^3} \times 25\ \text{cm} = 7.0245$$

$$\sigma Nt_{O} = 8 \times 10^{-24}\ \text{cm}^2 \times 3.34 \times 10^{22}\ \frac{\text{atoms H}}{\text{cm}^3} \times 25\ \text{cm} = 6.68$$

$$\sigma Nt_{H} + \sigma Nt_{O} = 7.0245 + 6.68 = 13.7045$$

Replacing the exponent in the equation:

$$\frac{I}{I_0} = e^{-\sigma Nt} = \text{e}^{-13.7045} = 1.12 \times 10^{-6} \text{ for 1 MeV neutrons}$$

Performing a similar calculation for 10 MeV neutrons:

$$\sigma Nt_{H} = 0.95 \times 10^{-24}\ \text{cm}^2 \times 6.69 \times 10^{22}\ \frac{\text{atoms H}}{\text{cm}^3} \times 25\ \text{cm} = 1.59$$

$$\sigma Nt_{O} = 1.5 \times 10^{-24}\ \text{cm}^2 \times 3.34 \times 10^{22}\ \frac{\text{atoms H}}{\text{cm}^3} \times 25\ \text{cm} = 1.25$$

$$\sigma Nt_{H} + \sigma Nt_{O} = 1.59 + 1.25 = 2.84$$

Replacing the exponent in the equation:

$$\frac{I}{I_0} = e^{-\sigma Nt} = \text{e}^{-\sigma Nt} = \text{e}^{-2.84} = 5.8 \times 10^{-2} \text{ for 10 MeV neutrons}$$

Multiply each by its attenuation factor and initial abundance:
1.12×10^{-6} for 1 MeV neutrons $\times\ 0.99 = 1.11 \times 10^{-6}$
5.8×10^{-2} for 10 MeV neutrons $\times\ 0.01 = 5.8 \times 10^{-4}$
The proportion of the 1 MeV to 10 MeV neutrons in the emergent beam is

$$\frac{1.11 \times 10^{-6}}{5.8 \times 10^{-4}} = 0.0019 : 1 \text{ is the ratio.}$$

5.35(b) What would be the relative proportion of the two groups after passing through a slab of lead of the same density thickness?
Find the density thickness of 25 cm of water:

$\frac{1\text{ g}}{\text{cm}^3} \times 25\text{ cm} = 25\text{ g/cm}^2$ is the density thickness of the water shield.

Now calculate the linear thickness of a 25 g/cm^2 lead shield using equation 5.1.

$$t = \frac{\text{density thickness}}{\text{density}} = \frac{25\ \text{g/cm}^2}{11.3\ \text{g/cm}^3} = 2.21\text{ cm}$$

$$N = \frac{11.3\text{ g}}{\text{cm}^3} \times \frac{1\text{ mol Pb}}{207.21\text{ g}} \times \frac{6.02 \times 10^{23}\text{ atoms Pb}}{1\text{ mol Pb}} = 3.28 \times 10^{22}\text{ atoms/cm}^3\text{ Pb}$$

The attenuation factor is given by equation 5.43:

$$\frac{I}{I_0} = e^{-\sigma Nt}$$

Using the given removal cross sections for Pb for 1 and 10 MeV neutrons, we find the value for the exponent to be:

$$N\sigma\, t\,(1\text{ MeV}) = \frac{3.2 \times 10^{22}\text{ atoms}}{\text{cm}^3} \times 5.5\text{ b} \times \frac{1 \times 10^{-24}\text{ cm}^2}{\text{b}} \times 2.21\text{ cm} = 0.4$$

$$N\sigma\, t\,(10\text{ MeV}) = \frac{3.28 \times 10^{22}\text{ atoms}}{\text{cm}^3} \times 5.1\text{ b} \times \frac{1 \times 10^{-24}\text{ cm}^2}{\text{b}} \times 2.21\text{ cm} = 0.37$$

The Pb attenuation factors, therefore are:

$$\frac{I}{I_0}(1\text{ MeV}) = e^{-\sigma Nt} = e^{-0.4} = 0.67$$

$$\frac{I}{I_0}(10\text{ MeV}) = e^{-\sigma Nt} = e^{-0.37} = 0.69$$

Now multiply by the proportion given in the problem:

1 MeV $\quad 0.67 \times 0.99 = 0.6633$
10 MeV $\quad 0.69 \times 0.01 = 0.0069$
Dividing the two values to obtain the ratio: 0.6633/0.0069 = 96:1

5.36 Boral is an aluminum boron carbide alloy used as a shield against thermal neutrons. If the boron content is 35% by weight, and if the density of boral is 2.7 g/cm^3, calculate the half–thickness of boral for thermal neutrons at room temperature. The capture cross sections are; boron = 755 barns, aluminum = 230 millibarns, carbon = 3.2 millibarns. **5.36**

The ASME Boiler and Pressure Vessel Code, Section II, Materials, gives the carbon content of boral as 2%, and an aluminum content of 63%.

Use equation 5.43:

$$\frac{I}{I_0} = e^{-\sigma Nt}$$

The half value layer means that the intensity would be reduced by one half, so that the ratio of $\frac{I}{I_0} = 0.5$, giving the formula:

$$0.5 = e^{-\sigma Nt}$$

Solve for t;

$$t = \frac{0.693}{\sigma N}$$

σ is given in the question, so find the number of atoms for each component of boral, and then solve for the thickness in the above equation:

$$N_B = \frac{2.7\text{ g}}{\text{cm}^3} \times \frac{1\text{ mol B}}{10.82\text{ g}} \times \frac{6.02 \times 10^{23}\text{ atoms B}}{1\text{ mol B}} \times 0.35 = 5.26 \times 10^{22}\ \frac{\text{atoms B}}{\text{cm}^3}$$

$$N_{Al} = \frac{2.7\text{ g}}{\text{cm}^3} \times \frac{1\text{mol Al}}{26.98\text{ g}} \times \frac{6.02 \times 10^{23}\text{ atoms Al}}{1\text{ mol Al}} \times 0.63 = 3.8 \times 10^{22}\ \frac{\text{atoms Al}}{\text{cm}^3}$$

$$N_C = \frac{2.7\text{ g}}{\text{cm}^3} \times \frac{1\text{ mol Al}}{12.011\text{ g}} \times \frac{6.02 \times 10^{23}\text{ atoms Al}}{1\text{ mol Al}} \times 0.02 = 2.7 \times 10^{21}\ \frac{\text{atoms C}}{\text{cm}^3}$$

Now calculate σN, the macroscopic cross section, Σ, for each material:

$$\sigma N_B = \frac{5.26 \times 10^{22}\text{ atoms B}}{\text{cm}^3} \times \frac{755\text{ b}}{\text{atom B}} \times \frac{1 \times 10^{-24}\text{ cm}^2}{\text{b}} = 39.7\text{ cm}^{-1}$$

$$\sigma N_{Al} = \frac{3.8 \times 10^{22}\text{ atoms Al}}{\text{cm}^3} \times \frac{230\text{ mb}}{\text{atom B}} \times \frac{1 \times 10^{-24}\text{ cm}^2}{1000\text{ mb}} = 0.0087\text{ cm}^{-1}$$

$$\sigma N_C = \frac{2.7\times10^{21}\text{ atoms Al}}{\text{cm}^3}\times\frac{3.2\text{ mb}}{\text{atom B}}\times\frac{1\times10^{-24}\text{ cm}^2}{1000\text{ mb}} = 8.64\times10^{-6}\text{ cm}^{-1}$$

Adding together the contributions:

$$\Sigma = \sigma N = 39.7\text{ cm}^{-1}$$

$$t_{1/2} = \frac{0.693}{\sigma N} = \frac{0.693}{39.7\text{ cm}^{-1}} = 0.0175\text{ cm}$$

Examination of the cross sections and abundance of each of the elements in boral shows that Al and C contribute very little to the total attenuation, and could have been ignored. The complete calculations are included here for reference.

5.37

5.37 The scattering cross sections for N and O for thermal neutrons are 10 and 4.2 barns, respectively. (a) Calculate the macroscopic cross section for air at STP. Air consists of 79 volume percent nitrogen and 21 volume percent oxygen.

$$\sigma_N = 10\text{ b}\times\frac{1\times10^{-24}\,\frac{\text{cm}^2}{\text{atom}}}{1\text{ b}} = 10\times10^{-24}\,\frac{\text{cm}^2}{\text{atom N}}$$

$$N_N = 1.293\times10^{-3}\,\frac{\text{g}}{\text{cm}^3}\times0.79\,\frac{\text{N}_2}{\text{air}}\times\frac{2\text{ atoms}}{\text{molecule}}\times\frac{6.02\times10^{23}\text{ molecules}}{\text{mol}}\times\frac{1\text{ mol}}{28\text{ g}} =$$

$$N_N = 4.39\times10^{19}\,\frac{\text{atoms}}{\text{cm}^3}$$

$$\sigma_O = 4.2\text{ b}\times\frac{1\times10^{-24}\,\frac{\text{cm}^2}{\text{atom}}}{1\text{ b}} = 4.2\times10^{-24}\,\frac{\text{cm}^2}{\text{atom O}}$$

$$N_O = 1.293\times10^{-3}\,\frac{\text{g}}{\text{cm}^3}\times0.21\,\frac{\text{O}_2}{\text{air}}\times\frac{2\text{ atoms}}{\text{molecule}}\times\frac{6.02\times10^{23}\text{ molecules}}{\text{mol}}\times\frac{1\text{ mol}}{32\text{ g}}$$

$$N_O = 1.02\times10^{19}\,\frac{\text{atoms}}{\text{cm}^3}$$

From example 5.11:

$$\Sigma_{air} = \Sigma\,(\sigma_N N_N + \sigma_O N_O)$$

$\Sigma_{air}=$

$$1\times10^{-23}\frac{\text{cm}^2}{\text{atom N}}\times 4.39\times10^{19}\frac{\text{atoms}}{\text{cm}^3}+4.2\times10^{-24}\frac{\text{cm}^2}{\text{atom O}}\times1.02\times10^{19}\frac{\text{atoms}}{\text{cm}^3}$$

$\Sigma_{air} = 4.82 \times 10^{-4}\ \text{cm}^{-1}$

b) What is the scattering mean free path of thermal neutrons in air?

$$\text{MFP} = \frac{1}{\Sigma} = \frac{1}{4.82\times10^{-4}\,\text{cm}^{-1}} = 2075 \text{ cm} = 21 \text{ meters}$$

5.38 How many scattering collisions in graphite are required to reduce the energy of 2.5 MeV neutrons to **5.38**
(a) 0.1% of the initial energy?

If the mean logarithmic energy decrement is ζ per collision (equation 5.46), the number of collisions required to reduce a neutron from an initial energy E_i to a final energy E_f is

$$n = \frac{\ln E_i - \ln E_f}{\zeta} = \frac{1}{\varsigma}\ln\frac{E_i}{E_f}$$

and the mean logarithmic energy decrement is given by equation 5.47

$$\zeta = 1 + \frac{\alpha\ln(\alpha)}{1-\alpha}$$

$\alpha = \left[(M - m)/(M + m)\right]^2$
$E_i = 2.5$ MeV
$E_f = 0.001 \times 2.5 \text{ MeV} = 0.0025$ MeV
M (Carbon) = 12 amu
m (neutron) = 1.008665 amu

Using equation 5.47 information and information in the text following equation 5.47, solving for α:

$$\alpha = \left(\frac{M-m}{M+m}\right)^2 = \left(\frac{12-1.008665}{12+1.008665}\right)^2 = 0.714$$

$$\zeta = 1 + \frac{\alpha\ln(\alpha)}{1-\alpha} = 1 + \frac{(0.714)\times\ln(0.714)}{1-0.714} = 0.158$$

With these values we find the logarithmic energy decrement, ζ, to be 0.158 and the number of collisions to be:

$$n = \frac{1}{\varsigma}\ln\frac{E_i}{E_f} = \frac{1}{0.158}\times\ln\frac{2.5\ \text{MeV}}{0.0025\ \text{MeV}} = 44\ \text{collisions}$$

(b) 0.25 eV?
0.025 eV = 0.025 × 10^{-6} MeV

$$n = \frac{1}{\varsigma}\ln\frac{E_i}{E_f} = \frac{1}{0.158}\times\ln\frac{2.5\ \text{MeV}}{0.025\times10^{-6}\ \text{MeV}} = 117\ \text{collisions}$$

5.39

5.39 A cobalt foil , 1 cm diameter x 0.1 mm thick, is irradiated in a mean thermal flux of 1 × 10^{11} neutrons/cm^2 per second for a period of 7 days. If the activation cross section is 36 barns, and if the density of cobalt is 8.9 grams/cm^3, what is the activity, in Bq and in microcuries, at the end of the irradiation period? Note that natural cobalt is 100% ^{59}Co.

$V = h\pi r^2 = 0.01\ \text{cm} \times \pi \times (0.5\ \text{cm})^2 = 7.854 \times 10^{-3}\ \text{cm}^3$

$$n = \frac{8.9\ \text{grams}}{\text{cm}^3}\times 7.9\times10^{-3}\,\text{cm}^3\times\frac{1\ \text{mole}\ ^{59}\text{Co}}{59\ \text{g}}\times\frac{6.02\times10^{23}\,\text{atoms}}{\text{mole}}$$

$n = 7.17 \times 10^{20}$ atoms
$\phi = 1 \times 10^{11}$ neutrons/cm^{2}sec
$\sigma = 36$ b $= 36 \times 10^{-24}$ cm^2/atom

$$\lambda = \frac{0.693}{5.27\ \text{yr}} = 0.1315\ \text{yr}^{-1}$$

$$t = 7\ \text{d}\times\frac{1\ \text{yr}}{365\ \text{d}} = 0.0192\ \text{yr}$$

Substituting these values into the neutron activation equation 5.59:

$$\lambda N = \phi\sigma n(1-e^{-\lambda t})$$

$$\lambda N = \frac{1\times10^{11}\text{neutrons}}{\text{cm}^2\text{sec}}\times\frac{36\times10^{-24}\,\text{cm}^2}{\text{atom}}\times 7.17\times10^{20}\ \text{atoms}\times(1-e^{-0.1315\times0.0192})$$

$\lambda N = 6.5 \times 10^6$ trans/sec $= 6.5 \times 10^6$ Bq $= 6.5$ MBq

$$6.5 \times 10^6 \text{ Bq} \times \frac{\text{Ci}}{3.7 \times 10^{10} \text{ Bq}} \times \frac{1 \times 10^6 \mu\text{Ci}}{1 \text{ Ci}} = 175 \ \mu\text{Ci}$$

5.40 Type 304 stainless steel consists of 71 weight percent Fe, 19% Cr, and 10% Ni. The isotopic abundance, percentage, and the respective 2200 m/s capture cross sections (barns) are given below: **5.40**

Fe	Fe	Fe	Cr	Cr	Cr	Ni	Ni	Ni
A	Abund	σ_c	A	Abund	σ_c	A	Abund	σ_c
54	5.84	2.9	50	4.31	17	58	67.76	4.4
56	91.68	2.7	52	83.76	0.8	60	26.16	2.6
57	2.17	2.5	53	9.55	18	61	1.25	2
58	0.31	1.1	54	0.38	0.38	62	3.66	15
						64	1.16	1.5

a) Calculate the macroscopic capture cross section.

To calculate the macroscopic cross section, the macroscopic cross section is calculated for each element, and then each macroscopic cross section for each element is then multiplied by the abundance of each element (see example 5.11).

$$\Sigma = \rho \times \frac{1 \text{ mole}}{\text{gram atomic wt}} \times \sigma \times (\text{percent abundance of element})$$

$$\Sigma = \frac{\text{g}}{\text{cm}^3} \times \frac{6.02 \times 10^{23} \text{atoms}}{\text{g}/\text{mol}} \times \text{b} \times \frac{1 \times 10^{-24} \text{ cm}^2/\text{atom}}{\text{b}} \times \text{fractional abundance}$$

Multiply column 2 by (1/column 3) by column 4 by column 5 by Avogadro's number to obtain column 6.

Column 1	Column 2	Column 3	Column 4	Column 5	Column 6	Column 7
	Density SS ρ, g/cm³	A g/mole	Abund	Cap. Cross σ, barns	Macro (ea)	
Fe	7.8196	54	0.0584	2.9	0.014764	
Fe	7.8196	56	0.9168	2.7	0.20808	
Fe	7.8196	57	0.0217	2.5	0.00448	
Fe	7.8196	58	0.0031	1.1	0.000277	
				sum	0.227601	sum × 0.71
					Fe total	0.161597
Cr	7.8196	50	0.0431	17	0.068982	
Cr	7.8196	52	0.8376	0.8	0.06066	
Cr	7.8196	53	0.0955	18	0.15268	
Cr	7.8196	54	0.0238	0.38	0.000788	
				sum	0.283111	sum × 0.19
					Cr total	0.053791
Ni	7.8196	58	0.6776	4.4	0.24198	
Ni	7.8196	60	0.2616	2.6	0.053363	
Ni	7.8196	61	0.0125	2	0.001929	
Ni	7.8196	62	0.0366	15	0.041683	
Ni	7.8196	64	0.0116	1.5	0.00128	
				sum	0.340235	sum × 0.1
					Ni total	0.034024
					Sum Total	0.249411

Yielding a macroscopic cross section of 0.249 cm^{-1}

(b) If a 1 cm diameter collimated beam of 2200 m/s neutrons is incident on a 2 mm thick sheet of type 304 stainless steel, how many neutrons per sec will be captured if the flux is 5×10^{11} n/cm^2 per second?

$I_0 = 5 \times 10^{11}$ n/cm^2 sec
$t = 0.2$ cm
$\Sigma = 0.249$ cm^{-1}

$$\frac{\text{Reactions}}{\text{s}} = \phi\sigma n$$

Find the amount of flux that is transmitted first, using equation 5.43:

$$I = I_0 e^{-\sigma N t}$$

Remembering that $\Sigma = N\sigma$ (from example 5.11)

$$I/I_0 = e^{-\Sigma t} = 5 \times 10^{11}\ \mathrm{e}^{-0.249 \times (0.2)} = 0.95$$

$1 - 0.95 = 0.05$ are captured.

1 cm diameter beam = 0.7854 cm^2 area, so;

$$0.05 \times 5 \times 10^{11} \frac{n}{cm^2 \cdot sec} \times 0.7854\ cm^2 = 1.96 \times 10^{10} \frac{n}{sec} \text{ captured}$$

5.41 A 1 M solution of boric acid, H_3BO_3, is irradiated for 7 days in a thermal flux 10^{11} n/cm²/sec at a temperature of 40°C. What is the concentration of Li, moles/liter, after the irradiation? **5.41**

$$\sigma_{B-10} = 4010\ b = \frac{4010\ b}{atom\ ^{10}B} \times \frac{1 \times 10^{-24}\ cm^2}{b} = 4010 \times 10^{-24} \frac{cm^2}{atom} \text{ is the cross section}$$

at 293K

Calculate the cross section at 40°C using a modification of equation 5.53, because ϕ is assumed to be a Maxwellian distribution, and not a monoenergetic beam of neutrons. The average cross section is given below:

T_0 = 293 K (Chapter 5, reference temperature for thermal neutrons)

T = 273 + 40 = 313 K

$$\sigma = \frac{\sigma_0}{1.128}\sqrt{\frac{T_0}{T}} = \frac{4010 \times 10^{-24}\ cm^2}{1.128} \times \sqrt{\frac{293\ K}{313\ K}} = 3.44 \times 10^{-21} \frac{cm^2}{atom}$$

Only 19.6% of all the boron atoms are ^{10}B, and the other boron atoms cross sections for absorption are not significant. Calculating the number of ^{10}B atoms in the solution:

$$n = \frac{1\ mol\ H_3BO_3}{L} \times \frac{6.02 \times 10^{23}\ molecules\ B}{1\ mol\ H_3BO_3} \times \frac{19.6\ atoms\ ^{10}B}{100\ atoms\ B}$$

$$n = 1.18 \times 10^{23} \frac{atoms\ ^{10}B}{L}$$

Each ^1n reaction with boron results in the production of one lithium atom:

$${}^{10}_{5}B + {}^{1}_{0}n \rightarrow {}^{7}_{3}Li + {}^{4}_{2}He$$

Equation 5.58 can be modified so that the rate of production can be represented. Since Li does not decay, it reduces from

$$\frac{\text{number reactions}}{\text{time}} = \phi\sigma n$$

$$\sigma = 3.44 \times 10^{-21}\,\frac{\text{cm}^2}{\text{atom}}$$

$$n = 1.18 \times 10^{23}\,\frac{\text{atoms}\,^{10}\text{B}}{\text{L}}$$

$$\phi = 1 \times 10^{11}\,\frac{\text{n}}{\text{cm}^2 \cdot \text{sec}}$$

$$t = 7\text{ d} = 7\text{ d} \times \frac{24\text{ hrs}}{1\text{ d}} \times \frac{3600\text{ sec}}{1\text{ hr}} = 6.05 \times 10^5\text{ sec}$$

$$\text{number reactions} = \phi\sigma n(\text{time}) = \text{number of Li atoms}$$

$$1 \times 10^{11}\,\frac{\text{n}}{\text{cm}^2 \cdot \text{sec}} \times 3.44 \times 10^{-21}\,\frac{\text{cm}^2}{\text{atom}} \times 1.18 \times 10^{23}\,\frac{\text{atoms}\,^{10}\text{B}}{\text{L}} \times 6.05 \times 10^5\text{ sec} =$$

$$\text{number of Li atoms} = 2.46 \times 10^{19}\,\frac{\text{atoms Li}}{\text{L}}$$

$\dfrac{2.46 \times 10^{19}\text{ atoms Li}}{\text{L}} \times \dfrac{\text{mol}}{6.02 \times 10^{23}\text{ atoms}} = 4.1 \times 10^{-5}\,\dfrac{\text{mol Li}}{\text{L}}$ is the final concentration.

Solutions for Chapter 6

RADIATION DOSIMETRY

6.1 A 50 μC/kg (~200mR) pocket dosimeter with air equivalent wall has a sensitive volume whose dimensions are 0.5 in. diameter and 2.5 in. long; the volume is filled with air at atmospheric pressure. The capacitance of the dosimeter is 10 pFd. If 200 V are required to charge the chamber, what is the voltage across the chamber when it reads 50 μC/kg (~200 mR)? **6.1**

$$\frac{\Delta Q}{m} = 50 \frac{\mu\text{C}}{\text{kg}}$$

Calculate the volume of the chamber first:
2.54 cm = 1 in.
$L = 2.5 \text{ in} = 6.35 \text{ cm}$

$$r = \frac{0.5 \text{ in}}{2} \times 2.54 \frac{\text{cm}}{\text{in}} = 0.635 \text{ cm}$$

$v = \pi r^2 L = \pi \times 0.635^2 \times 6.35 = 8.04 \text{ cm}^3$
The density of standard air is:
$\rho_{air} = 1.293 \times 10^{-3} \text{ g/cm}^3 = 1.29 \times 10^{-6} \text{ kg/cm}^3$ (Table 5.2)

Therefore, the amount of charge produced in the chamber, ΔQ, is :

$$\Delta Q = \frac{50 \ \mu\text{C}}{\text{kg}_{\text{air}}} \times \frac{1 \times 10^{-6} \text{C}}{1 \ \mu\text{C}} \times \frac{1.293 \times 10^{-6} \text{kg}_{\text{air}}}{1 \text{ cm}^3_{\text{air}}} \times \frac{8.04 \text{ cm}^3_{\text{air}}}{\text{chamber}} = 5.2 \times 10^{-10} \text{ C}$$

C = Capacitance = 10 pF = 10×10^{-12} F

The initial voltage = $V_i = 200$ V

Putting values into equation 6.8;

$$\Delta Q = C \times \Delta V = C \times (V_i - V_f) = 10 \times 10^{-12}\,\text{F} \times (200\ \text{V} - V_f) = 5.2 \times 10^{-10}\ \text{C}$$

$$(200\ \text{V} - V_f) = \frac{5.2 \times 10^{-10}\ \text{C}}{10 \times 10^{-12}\ \text{F}}$$

$V_f = 148$ V

6.2 **6.2** An air ionization chamber whose volume is 1 liter is used as an environmental monitor at a temperature of 27°C and a pressure of 700 torr. What is the exposure rate, in μC/kg per hour and in mR/hr if the saturation current is 10^{-13} amperes?

T = 27°C + 273°C = 300 K
Current = 1×10^{-13} A = 1×10^{-13} C/sec
Volume = 1 liter

Convert to C/kg. This is simply charge per unit mass, so divide the charge produced in the air by the mass of the air. Since the air is given as a volume, it is converted into mass, using the density of air, and multiplying by the appropriate correction factors to account for the different pressure and temperature:

Density of standard air: 1.293×10^{-6} kg/cm^3 (Table 6.2)

Calculating the mass of air in 1 liter first, in kg:

$$1\ \text{L} \times \frac{1000\ \text{cm}^3}{1\ \text{L}} \times \frac{1.293 \times 10^{-6}\,\text{kg}}{\text{cm}^3} = 1.293 \times 10^{-3}\ \text{kg air in 1 liter volume}$$

Convert to the new temperature and pressure:

$$1.293 \times 10^{-3}\ \text{kg} \times \frac{273\ \text{K}}{300\ \text{K}} \times \frac{700\ \text{torr}}{760\ \text{torr}} = 1.1 \times 10^{-3}\ \text{kg at the new temp. and press.}$$

Now divide the charge, in coulombs, by the mass of air in which the charge was produced:

$$\frac{1 \times 10^{-13}\,\frac{\text{C}}{\text{sec}}}{1.1 \times 10^{-3}\,\text{kg}_{\text{air}}} \times \frac{3600\ \text{sec}}{\text{hr}} = 0.33 \times 10^{-6}\ \text{C/kg per hr} = 0.33\ \mu\text{C/kg per hr}$$

$$0.33 \times 10^{-6} \frac{\text{C}}{\text{kg}} \times \frac{1000 \text{ mR}}{2.58 \times 10^{-4} \text{C/kg}} = 1.3 \text{ mR/hr}$$

6.3 A beam of 1 MeV gamma rays and another of 0.1 MeV gamma rays each produce the same ionization density in air. What is the ratio of 1 : 0.1 MeV photon flux? **6.3**

Equal ionization density implies equal energy absorption per cc of air.

$$\text{Energy absorbed per cm}^3 = \phi \frac{\text{photons}}{\text{cm}^2 \cdot \text{sec}} \times E \frac{\text{MeV}}{\text{photon}} \times \mu_a \text{cm}^{-1}$$

where μ_a = energy absorption coefficient

$$\phi_{0.1} \frac{\text{photons}}{\text{cm}^2\text{sec}} \times 0.1 \frac{\text{MeV}}{\text{photon}} \times \mu_{0.1}\text{cm}^{-1} = \phi_1 \frac{\text{photons}}{\text{cm}^2\text{sec}} \times 1.0 \frac{\text{MeV}}{\text{photon}} \times \mu_{1.0}\text{cm}^{-1}$$

From Appendix F;
$\mu_{0.1} = 0.0233 \text{ cm}^{-1}$
$\mu_{1.0} = 0.0280 \text{ cm}^{-1}$

Performing algebra:

$$\frac{\phi_1 \dfrac{\text{photons}}{\text{cm}^2\text{sec}}}{\phi_{0.1} \dfrac{\text{photons}}{\text{cm}^2\text{sec}}} = \frac{0.1 \dfrac{\text{MeV}}{\text{photon}} \times \mu_{0.1}\text{cm}^{-1}}{1.0 \dfrac{\text{MeV}}{\text{photon}} \times \mu_{1.0}\text{ cm}^{-1}} = \frac{0.1 \dfrac{\text{MeV}}{\text{photon}} \times 0.0233 \text{ cm}^{-1}}{1.0 \dfrac{\text{MeV}}{\text{photon}} \times 0.0280 \text{ cm}^{-1}} = 0.083$$

6.4 Assuming a specific heat of the body of 1 calorie/g, calculate the temperature rise due to a total body dose of 5 Gy. **6.4**

$$5 \text{ Gy} \times 1 \frac{\text{J/kg}}{\text{Gy}} \times \frac{1 \text{ kg}}{1000 \text{ g}} \times \frac{1 \text{ calorie}}{4.186 \text{ J}} \times \frac{1^0\text{C}}{\dfrac{\text{calorie}}{\text{gram}}} = 1.19 \times 10^{-3} \text{ °C}$$

6.5

6.5 Compute the exposure rate, in mGy/hr at a distance of 50 cm from a small vial containing 10 mL of an aqueous solution of
(a) 2 GBq (54.1 mCi) ^{51}Cr,

From basic principles, equation 6.15 gives the exposure rate

$$\dot{X} = \frac{f\,\frac{\text{phot}}{\text{t}} \times E\,\frac{\text{MeV}}{\text{phot}} \times 1.6\times10^{-13}\,\frac{\text{J}}{\text{MeV}} \times A\,\frac{\text{tps}}{\text{MBq}} \times 3600\,\frac{\text{s}}{\text{h}} \times \mu_a\ \text{m}^{-1}}{4\times\pi\times d^2\,\text{m}^2 \times \rho\,\frac{\text{kg}}{\text{m}^3} \times 1\,\frac{\text{J/kg}}{\text{Gy}}}$$

f = 0.09 phot/t
E = 0.323 MeV/phot
$A = 2 \times 10^9$ Bq $= 2 \times 10^9$ tps = 2000 MBq
d = 0.5 m
$\rho = 1.293$ kg/m^3

$$\mu_a = 0.0288\,\frac{\text{cm}^2}{\text{g}} \times 1.293\times10^{-3}\,\frac{\text{g}}{\text{cm}^3} \times 100\,\frac{\text{cm}}{\text{m}} = 3.7 \times 10^{-3}\ \text{m}^{-1}\ \text{(Appendix F)}$$

$$\dot{X} = \frac{\frac{0.09\ \text{phot}}{\text{t}} \times \frac{0.323\ \text{MeV}}{\text{phot}} \times 1.6\times10^{-13}\,\frac{\text{J}}{\text{MeV}} \times 2\times10^9\,\frac{\text{t}}{\text{s}} \times 3600\,\frac{\text{s}}{\text{hr}} \times 3.7\times10^{-3}\,\text{m}^{-1}}{4\times\pi\times(0.5\ \text{m})^2 \times 1.293\,\frac{\text{kg}}{\text{m}^3} \times 1\,\frac{\text{J/kg}}{\text{Gy}}}$$

$\dot{X} = 3 \times 10^{-5}$ Gy/hr = 0.03 mGy/hr

Alternatively, the exposure rate can be calculated with the specific gamma ray emission constant, Table 6.3, which gives the exposure rate at 1 meter from a unit quantity of activity. The exposure rate from any quantity of activity at any distance is then calculated from

$$\dot{X} = \frac{\frac{\text{C/kg}\cdot\text{m}^2}{\text{MBq}\cdot\text{hr}} \times A\ \text{MBq}}{(d,\ \text{m})^2}$$

For ^{51}Cr, $\Gamma = 1.11\times10^{-10}\,\frac{\text{C/kg}\cdot\text{m}^2}{\text{MBq}\cdot\text{hr}}$

$$\dot{X}\left({}^{51}\text{Cr}\right) = \frac{1.11\times10^{-10}\,\dfrac{\text{C}/\text{kg}\cdot\text{m}^2}{\text{MBq}\cdot\text{hr}}\times 2\times10^{3}\ \text{MBq}}{(0.5\ \text{m})^2} = 8.88\times10^{-7}\,\frac{\text{C}/\text{kg}}{\text{hr}}$$

To convert to mGy/hr

$$\dot{X}\left({}^{51}\text{Cr}\right) = 8.88\times10^{-7}\,\frac{\text{C}/\text{kg}}{\text{hr}}\times 34\,\frac{\text{Gy}}{\text{C}/\text{kg}}\times 10^{3}\,\frac{\text{mGy}}{\text{Gy}} = 0.03\,\frac{\text{mGy}}{\text{hr}}$$

(b) 2 GBq (54.1 mCi) ^{24}Na, based on the transformation schemes shown below:

For ^{24}Na, $\Gamma = 12.8\times10^{-9}\,\dfrac{\text{C}/\text{kg}\cdot\text{m}^2}{\text{MBq}\cdot\text{hr}}$

$$\dot{X}\left({}^{24}\text{Na}\right) = \frac{12.8\times10^{-9}\,\dfrac{\text{C}/\text{kg}\cdot\text{m}^2}{\text{MBq}\cdot\text{hr}}\times 2\times10^{3}\ \text{MBq}}{(0.5\ \text{m})^2}\times 34\,\frac{\text{Gy}}{\text{C}/\text{kg}}\times 10^{3}\,\frac{\text{mGy}}{\text{Gy}} = 3.5\,\frac{\text{mGy}}{\text{hr}}$$

Alternatively, the exposure rate may also be calculated from basic principles,

$$\dot{X} = \frac{\sum f_i E_i \mu_i \times 1.6\times10^{-13}\,\dfrac{\text{J}}{\text{MeV}}\times A\ \text{GBq}\times 10^{9}\,\dfrac{\text{tps}}{\text{GBq}}\times 3600\,\dfrac{\text{s}}{\text{h}}}{4\pi d^2\ \text{m}^2\times 1\,\dfrac{\text{J}/\text{kg}}{\text{Gy}}}$$

f_1 = 100% = 1
f_2 = 100% = 1
E_1 = 2.75 MeV/phot
E_2 = 1.37 MeV/phot
$A = 2\times10^{9}$ Bq $= 2\times10^{9}$ tps = 2000 MBq
d = 0.5 m
ρ = 1.293 kg/m^3

$$\mu_{a1} = 0.0212 \frac{\text{cm}^2}{\text{g}} \times 10^{33} \frac{\text{g}}{\text{kg}} \times 1 \frac{\text{m}^2}{10^4\,\text{cm}^2} = 2.12 \times 10^{-3}\ \text{m}^2/\text{kg}$$

$$\mu_{a2} = 0.027 \frac{\text{cm}^2}{\text{g}} \times 10^{33} \frac{\text{g}}{\text{kg}} \times 1 \frac{\text{m}^2}{10^4\,\text{cm}^2} = 2.7 \times 10^{-3}\ \text{m}^2/\text{kg}$$

$$\sum f_i E_i \mu_{ai} = 1 \frac{\gamma}{\text{t}} \times 2.75 \frac{\text{MeV}}{\gamma} \times 0.00212 \frac{\text{m}^2}{\text{kg}} + 1 \frac{\gamma}{\text{t}} \times 1.37 \frac{\text{MeV}}{\gamma} \times 0.0027 \frac{\text{m}^2}{\text{kg}}$$

$$\sum f_i E_i \mu_{ai} = 9.53 \times 10^{-3} \frac{\text{MeV} \cdot \text{m}^2}{\text{t}}$$

$$\dot{X} = \frac{9.53 \times 10^{-3} \frac{\text{MeV} \cdot \text{m}^2}{\text{t}} \times 1.6 \times 10^{-13} \frac{\text{J}}{\text{MeV}} \times 2\ \text{GBq} \times 10^9 \frac{\text{tps}}{\text{GBq}} \times 3600 \frac{\text{s}}{\text{hr}}}{4 \times \pi \times (0.5\ \text{m})^2 \times 1 \frac{\text{J}/\text{kg}}{\text{Gy}}}$$

$$\dot{X} = 3.5 \times 10^{-3}\ \text{Gy/hr} = 3.5\ \text{mGy/hr}$$

6.6

6.6 What is the dose rate to the flesh during exposure to 25.4 μC/hr (100mR/hr) of 0.5 MeV gamma radiation?

Exposure in C/kg is a measure of dose to air. Tissue absorbs more energy, by a factor of $\mu_{energy}(\text{tissue}) / \mu_{energy}(\text{air})$, than does air from the same exposure. The tissue dose rate is calculated by converting the exposure to air dose, and then multiplying the air dose by the tissue factor (μ for 0.5 MeV from Table 5.3).

$$\dot{D} = 25.4 \frac{\mu\text{C}/\text{kg}}{\text{hr}} \times 34 \frac{\mu\text{Gy}}{\mu\text{C}/\text{kg}} \times \frac{0.0327\ \text{cm}^2/\text{g}}{0.0297\ \text{cm}^2/\text{g}} \times \frac{1\ \text{mGy}}{1000\ \mu\text{Gy}}$$

$$\dot{D} = 0.95\ \text{mGy/hr}$$

6.7 A collimated beam of 0.3 MeV gamma radiation, whose energy flux is 5 J/m²/s, is shielded by 2 cm Pb. **6.7**
(a) What is the incident particle flux, photons/cm²/sec?

$$\frac{\text{photon}}{0.3\text{ MeV}} \times \frac{\text{MeV}}{1.6\times10^{-13}\text{J}} \times \frac{5\text{ J}}{\text{m}^2\cdot\text{sec}} \times \frac{1\text{ m}^2}{1\times10^4\text{cm}^2} = 1.04\times10^{10}\frac{\text{photons}}{\text{cm}^2\cdot\text{sec}}$$

(b) What is the exposure rate in mR/hr and C/kg/hr, in the incident and emergent beams?
Equation 6.9 is used to find the incident exposure rate:

$E = 0.3$ MeV
$\phi = 1.04 \times 10^{10}$ photons/cm²/sec
$\mu_a = 0.0288$ cm²/g (Table 5.3 for absorption)

$$\dot{X} = \frac{\phi\frac{\text{photons}}{\text{cm}^2\cdot\text{sec}} E\frac{\text{MeV}}{\text{photon}} 1.6\times10^{-13}\frac{\text{J}}{\text{MeV}} \mu_a \frac{\text{cm}^2}{\text{g}}}{34\frac{\text{J}/\text{kg}}{\text{C}/\text{kg}}}$$

$$\dot{X} = \frac{1.04\times10^{10}\frac{\text{photons}}{\text{cm}^2\cdot\text{sec}}\times0.3\frac{\text{MeV}}{\text{photon}}\times1.6\times10^{-13}\frac{\text{J}}{\text{MeV}}\times0.0288\frac{\text{cm}^2}{\text{g}}\times\frac{1000\text{ g}}{\text{kg}}}{34\frac{\text{J}/\text{kg}}{\text{C}/\text{kg}}}$$

$$\dot{X} = 4.23\times10^{-4}\frac{\text{C}/\text{kg}}{\text{sec}} = 4.23\times10^{-4}\frac{\text{C}/\text{kg}}{\text{sec}}\times\frac{3600\text{ sec}}{\text{hr}} = 1.52\frac{\text{C}/\text{kg}}{\text{hr}}$$ is the incident exposure rate.

Converting to R/hr with equation 6.7;

$$1.52\frac{\text{C}/\text{kg}}{\text{hr}}\times\frac{3881\text{ R}}{1\text{C}/\text{kg}}\times\frac{1000\text{ mR}}{1\text{ R}} = 5.91\times10^6\frac{\text{mR}}{\text{hr}}$$ is the incident exposure rate

To find the emergent beam exposure rates, use equation 5.19;
$t = 2$ cm
$\mu = 4.02$ cm^{-1} (table 5.2 for attenuation)

$$\frac{I}{I_0} = e^{-\mu t} = e^{-4.02\ \text{cm}^{-1} \times 2\ \text{cm}} = 3.22 \times 10^{-4}$$ is the reduction in intensity.

So the emergent exposure rates will be:

$$1.52 \frac{\text{C}/\text{kg}}{\text{hr}} \times 3.22 \times 10^{-4} = 4.9 \times 10^{-4} \frac{\text{C}/\text{kg}}{\text{hr}}$$

$$5.91 \times 10^{6} \frac{\text{mR}}{\text{hr}} \times 3.22 \times 10^{-4} = 1.9 \times 10^{3} \frac{\text{mR}}{\text{hr}}$$

(c) What is the tissue dose rate, mGy/hr, in the incident and emergent beams?

To convert to tissue dose rates, use equation 6.11, incident dose first;

$$\mu_m/\rho_m = 0.0317 \text{ (Table 5.3)}$$

$$\mu_a/\rho_a = 0.0288 \text{ (Table 5.3)}$$

$$\dot{D} = 34 \frac{\mu_m/\rho_m}{\mu_a/\rho_a} \dot{X} = 34 \frac{\text{Gy}}{\text{C}/\text{kg}} \times \frac{0.0317\ \text{cm}^2/\text{g}}{0.0288\ \text{cm}^2/\text{g}} \times 1.52 \frac{\text{C}/\text{kg}}{\text{hr}} = 57 \frac{\text{Gy}}{\text{hr}}$$

$$\dot{D} = 57 \frac{\text{Gy}}{\text{hr}} \times \frac{1000\ \text{mGy}}{1\ \text{Gy}} = 5.7 \times 10^{4} \frac{\text{mGy}}{\text{hr}}$$ is the incident beam exposure rate.

Calculating the emergent beam exposure rate with equation 6.11:

$$\dot{D} = 34 \times \frac{0.0317}{0.0288} \times 4.9 \times 10^{-4} \frac{\text{C}/\text{kg}}{\text{hr}} \times \frac{1000\ \text{mGy}}{1\ \text{Gy}} = 18 \frac{\text{mGy}}{\text{hr}}$$

6.8 The exposure rate in a beam of 100 keV gamma rays is 25.8 μC/kg (100 mR) per hour. What is 6.8
(a) photon flux, photons/cm²/sec?

Equation 6.9 can be used to solve for the photon flux. However, the linear absorption coefficient μ_a, which is divided by the air density, ρ_a in equation 6.9, is the mass absorption coefficient for air. Equation 6.9 may therefore be rewritten as

$$\dot{X}\,\frac{\mathrm{C/kg}}{\mathrm{hr}} = \frac{\phi\,\dfrac{\text{photons}}{\mathrm{cm^2\cdot sec}}\times 3600\,\dfrac{\mathrm{s}}{\mathrm{hr}}\times E\,\dfrac{\mathrm{MeV}}{\mathrm{phot}}\times 1.6\times 10^{-13}\,\dfrac{\mathrm{J}}{\mathrm{MeV}}\times \mu_a\,\dfrac{\mathrm{cm^2}}{\mathrm{g}}\times 1000\,\dfrac{\mathrm{g}}{\mathrm{kg}}}{34\,\dfrac{\mathrm{J/kg}}{\mathrm{C/kg}}}$$

Table 5.3 lists the mass energy absorption as μ (air, 0.1 MeV) = 0.0231 cm²/g. Substituting this, the photon energy, and the exposure rate into the equation yields

$$25.8\times 10^{-6}\,\frac{\mathrm{C/kg}}{\mathrm{hr}} = \frac{\phi\,\dfrac{\text{phot}}{\mathrm{cm^2\cdot sec}}\times 3600\,\dfrac{\mathrm{s}}{\mathrm{hr}}\times 0.1\,\dfrac{\mathrm{MeV}}{\mathrm{phot}}\times 1.6\times 10^{-13}\,\dfrac{\mathrm{J}}{\mathrm{MeV}}\times 0.231\,\dfrac{\mathrm{cm^2}}{\mathrm{g}}\times 1000\,\dfrac{\mathrm{g}}{\mathrm{kg}}}{34\,\dfrac{\mathrm{J/kg}}{\mathrm{C/kg}}}$$

$$\phi = 6.6\times 10^{5}\,\frac{\text{photons}}{\mathrm{cm^2\cdot sec}}$$

(b) Power density, W/m² and mW/cm²?

$$6.6\times 10^{5}\,\frac{\text{photons}}{\mathrm{cm^2\cdot sec}}\times\frac{0.1\ \mathrm{MeV}}{\text{photon}}\times\frac{1.6\times 10^{-13}\,\mathrm{J}}{\mathrm{MeV}}\times\frac{1\ \mathrm{W}}{1\,\mathrm{J/sec}}\times\frac{1\times 10^{4}\,\mathrm{cm^2}}{\mathrm{m^2}} = 1.06\times 10^{-4}\,\frac{\mathrm{W}}{\mathrm{m^2}}$$

$$1.06 \times 10^{-4}\ \frac{\text{W}}{\text{m}^2} \times \frac{1\ \text{m}^2}{1 \times 10^4\ \text{cm}^2} \times \frac{1000\ \text{mW}}{\text{W}} = 1.06 \times 10^{-5}\ \frac{\text{mW}}{\text{m}^2}$$

6.9

6.9 In an experiment, a 250 g rat is injected with 10 μCi ^{203}Hg in the form of $Hg(NO_3)_2$. The rat was counted daily in a total body counter, and the following equation was fitted to the whole body counting data

$$Y = 0.55e^{-0.345t} + 0.45e^{-0.0346t},$$

where Y is the fraction of the injected dose retained t days after injection. If the long lived component of the curve represents clearance from the kidneys, while the short lived component represents clearance from the rest of the body, calculate the radiation absorbed dose to the whole body and the kidneys. Assume each kidney weighs 0.7 g, and that the Hg is uniformly distributed in the kidneys and in the body. Base the calculation on the transformation scheme given in Fig. 6.13.

Dose to the body from distributed ^{203}Hg:
The dose to the body includes two components: The dose due to the ^{203}Hg in the body, and the dose to the body from the ^{203}Hg concentrated in the kidneys.

First find the dose rate for Body ← Body. The decay scheme and the Input Data in Fig. 6.13 show that in ^{203}Hg, a 0.213 MeV beta and a 0.279 MeV gamma are emitted from the nucleus in each transformation. The Output Data show that only 81.7% of the 0.279 MeV gammas are seen; The other 18.3% are internally converted. Thus, in addition to the betas, whose mean energy is 0.058 MeV, we also have 3 groups of monoenergetic conversion electrons. We also have characteristic x-rays from the internal conversion electrons. Energy is absorbed from each of these radiations. In the case of the betas, conversion electrons, and the very low energy (average = 0.011 MeV) of the characteristic L X-rays, it is assumed that all the energy is absorbed, i.e. the absorbed fraction $\phi = 1$. Assuming that the 250 g rat can be approximated by a thick ellipsoid, interpolation and extrapolation of the data in Table 6.5 to 0.25 kg shows that only about 9% of the gamma and characteristic x-ray energy is absorbed. The energy of each of these radiations, their frequency, and the absorbed fraction are listed in the table below. The amount of energy absorbed from each of these radiaitons is the product of these 3, and the amount of energy absorbed per ^{203}Hg transformation is the sum of the individual contributions.

Radiation	MeV ×	f ×	ϕ	Absorbed Energy
β	0.058	1.00	1	0.05800
γ	0.2791	0.817	0.09	0.02052
Conv. e^- K	0.1936	0.132	1	0.02556
Conv. e^- L	0.2648	0.039	1	0.01033
Conv. e^-M	0.2761	0.0117	1	0.00323
X-rays, K_α	0.0722	0.0984	0.09	0.00064
X-rays, K_β	0.0833	0.0286	0.09	0.00021
X-rays, L	0.0112	0.0533	1	0.00060
			Total	0.12 MeV/t

The given retention equation shows that 0.55 of the activity is deposited in the body, and that it is cleared from the body at a rate of 0.345 per day. The activity initially deposited in the body is:

$q_{body} = 0.55 \times 10\ \mu\text{Ci} = 5.5\ \mu\text{Ci} = 2.035 \times 10^5\ \text{Bq}$

The dose rate due to this activity is calculated with equation 6.76.

$$\dot{D}_{Body\leftarrow Body} = \frac{q\ \text{Bq} \times 1\frac{\text{tps}}{\text{Bq}} \times E_e\frac{\text{MeV}}{\text{t}} \times 1.6 \times 10^{-13}\frac{\text{J}}{\text{MeV}} \times 8.64 \times 10^4\frac{\text{s}}{\text{day}}}{m\ \text{kg} \times \frac{1\ \text{J}}{\text{kg}}\Big/\text{Gy}}$$

$$\dot{D}_{Body\leftarrow Body} = \frac{2.035 \times 10^5\ \text{Bq} \times 1\frac{\text{tps}}{\text{Bq}} \times 0.12\frac{\text{MeV}}{\text{t}} \times 1.6 \times 10^{-13}\frac{\text{J}}{\text{MeV}} \times 8.64 \times 10^4\frac{\text{s}}{\text{day}}}{0.25\ \text{kg} \times \frac{1\ \text{J}}{\text{kg}}\Big/\text{Gy}}$$

$\dot{D}_{Body\leftarrow Body} = 1.35 \times 10^{-3}$ Gy/day is the initial dose rate to the body from ^{203}Hg in the body.

^{203}Hg:

$\lambda_E = 0.345\ \text{d}^{-1}$ is the effective clearance rate for the body (as given)

$$D_{Body \leftarrow Body} = \frac{D_0}{\lambda_E} = \frac{1.35 \times 10^{-3}\ \frac{\text{Gy}}{\text{day}}}{0.345 \frac{1}{\text{day}}} = 3.91 \times 10^{-3}\ \text{Gy} = 0.391\ \text{rad}$$

Now find the ^{203}Hg dose rate from Body←Kidneys. Consider only the γ and K x-rays (since no betas or L X-rays are considered to escape).

To estimate the dose to the rat's body from the ^{203}Hg in the kidneys, let us approximate the rat as a 250 g sphere whose density is 1 g/cm^3, and therefore has a radius of 3.9 cm. Furthermore, let us assume the activity in the kidneys to be a "point" source in the center of the "sphere." We will consider only the gamma and K x-rays, since the betas and the L X-rays will be absorbed within the kidneys. Under these assumed conditions, the fraction of the emitted energy, ϕ, that is absprbed from the source is given by

$$\phi = \frac{\text{Absorbed Energy}}{\text{Emitted Energy}} = 1 - e^{-\mu r}$$

Where μ is the energy absorption coefficient (Table 5.3). For the 0.279 MeV gammas

$$\phi(0.279\ \text{MeV}) = 1 - e^{-0.0312 \frac{\text{cm}^2}{\text{g}} \times 3.9 \frac{\text{g}}{\text{cm}^2}} = 0.12$$

The initial dose rate to the body due to the 0.279 MeV gamma from the kidneys is (Equation 6.76). (Note: The given retention equation shows that 0.45 of the activity is deposited in the kidneys.)

$$\dot{D}(\gamma)_{Body \leftarrow kidney} = \frac{q\ \text{Bq} \times 1 \frac{\text{tps}}{\text{Bq}} \times E_e \frac{\text{MeV}}{\text{t}} \times 1.6 \times 10^{-13} \frac{\text{J}}{\text{MeV}} \times 8.64 \times 10^4 \frac{\text{s}}{\text{day}}}{m\ \text{kg} \times 1 \frac{\text{J}}{\text{kg}} \Big/ \text{Gy}}$$

$\dot{D}(\gamma)_{Body\leftarrow kidney} =$

$$\frac{0.45\times 3.7\times 10^{5}\ \text{Bq}\times 1\frac{\text{tps}}{\text{Bq}}\times 0.817\frac{\gamma}{\text{t}}\times 0.279\frac{\text{MeV}}{\gamma}\times 0.12\times 1.6\times 10^{-13}\frac{\text{J}}{\text{MeV}}\times 86400\frac{\text{s}}{\text{d}}}{0.25\ \text{kg}\times 1\frac{\text{J}}{\text{kg}}\Big/\text{Gy}}$$

$\dot{D}_{Body\leftarrow kidney} = 2.5 \times 10^{-4}$Gy/day is the initial dose rate to the body from kidneys.

For the K x-rays, mean energy = 0.075 MeV and frequency = 0.127, the energy absorption coefficient (Table 5.3) is 0.027 cm^2/g, and the absorbed fraction is:

$$\phi(0.075\ \text{MeV}) = 1 - e^{-0.027\frac{\text{cm}^2}{\text{g}}\times 3.9\frac{\text{g}}{\text{cm}^2}} = 0.1$$

The initial X-ray dose rate to the body from the kidneys is estimated as

$\dot{D}(\text{X-ray})_{Body\leftarrow kidney} =$

$$\frac{0.45\times 3.7\times 10^{5}\ \text{Bq}\times 1\frac{\text{tps}}{\text{Bq}}\times 0.127\frac{\gamma}{\text{t}}\times 0.075\frac{\text{MeV}}{\gamma}\times 0.1\times 1.6\times 10^{-13}\frac{\text{J}}{\text{MeV}}\times 86400\frac{\text{s}}{\text{d}}}{0.25\ \text{kg}\times 1\frac{\text{J}}{\text{kg}}\Big/\text{Gy}}$$

$\dot{D}(\text{x-ray})_{Body\leftarrow kidney} = 8.77 \times 10^{-6}$ Gy/d

The ^{203}Hg is cleared from the kidney, according to the retention equation, at a rate of 0.0345 per day. The total dose to the body from the ^{203}Hg in the kidney is

$$D_{Body\leftarrow Kidneys} = \frac{D_0}{\lambda_E} = \frac{\left(2.5\times 10^{-4} + 8.8\times 10^{-6}\right)\frac{\text{Gy}}{\text{d}}}{0.0346\text{d}^{-1}} = 7.5 \times 10^{-3}\ \text{Gy}$$

The total dose to the body from both the bodily deposited nuclide and kidney deposited nuclide is:

3.91×10^{-3} Gy + 7.50×10^{-3} Gy = 1.14×10^{-2} Gy = 1.14 rads

Dose to the kidneys

A value of 1 for ϕ is used since it is characteristic radiation (low energy). Assume all the γ's escape from the small volume of the kidneys and consider only the betas and conversion electrons. From Figure 6.13;

	MeV ×	f ×	ϕ	Absorbed Energy
β	0.058	1.00	1	0.058
K_{ce-}	0.1936	0.132	1	0.0256
L_{ce-}	0.2648	0.039	1	0.0103
M_{ce-}	0.2761	0.0117	1	0.0032
			Total	0.097 MeV/t

E_e = 0.097 MeV/t

The retention equation shows that 0.45 of the activity is deposited in the kidneys and that it is cleared from the kidney at a rate of 0.0345 per day. The activity initially deposited in the kidneys is:

$$q_{\text{kidneys}} = 0.45 \times 10\ \mu\text{Ci} = 4.5\ \mu\text{Ci} = 1.665 \times 10^5\ \text{Bq}$$

$$m_{kidneys} = 1.4\ \text{g} = 1.4 \times 10^{-3}\ \text{kg}$$

The dose rate due to an internally deposited radionuclide is given by equation 6.76:

$$\dot{D}_{kidney \leftarrow kidney} = \frac{q\ \text{Bq} \times 1 \frac{\text{tps}}{\text{Bq}} \times E_e \frac{\text{MeV}}{\text{t}} \times 1.6 \times 10^{-13} \frac{\text{J}}{\text{MeV}} \times 8.64 \times 10^4 \frac{\text{s}}{\text{d}}}{m\ \text{kg} \times \frac{1\ \text{J}}{\text{kg}} \Big/ \text{Gy}}$$

$$\dot{D}_{kidney \leftarrow kidney} = \frac{1.665 \times 10^5\ \text{Bq} \times 1\frac{\text{tps}}{\text{Bq}} \times 0.097\frac{\text{MeV}}{\text{t}} \times 1.6 \times 10^{-13}\ \frac{\text{J}}{\text{MeV}} \times 8.64 \times 10^4\ \frac{\text{s}}{\text{d}}}{1.4 \times 10^{-3}\ \text{kg} \times \frac{1\ \text{J}}{\text{kg}} \Big/ \text{Gy}}$$

$\dot{D}_{kidney \leftarrow kidney} = 0.159$ Gy/d is the initial dose rate to the kidneys from nuclide in the kidneys.

Using equation 6.58 to find the dose commitment for the kidneys;

$\lambda_E = 0.0346\ \text{d}^{-1}$ is the term for the kidneys (as given)

$$D_{kidney \leftarrow kidney} = \frac{D_0}{\lambda_E} = \frac{0.159\frac{\text{Gy}}{\text{d}}}{0.0346\frac{1}{\text{d}}} = 4.61\ \text{Gy} = 461\ \text{rad}$$ is the committed dose to the kidneys.

6.10 Iodine is deposited in the thyroid at a rate of 0.139 per hour. If the radioactive half life of ^{123}I is 13 hours, what is the deposition half life? **6.10**

Equation 4.21 is used to solve for the radioactive decay constant:

$T_R = 13$ hours

$$T_B = \frac{0.693}{\lambda_B} = \frac{0.693}{0.139\ \text{hr}^{-1}} = 5\ \text{hr}$$

Putting values into equation 6.54:

$$T_E = \frac{T_R \times T_B}{T_R + T_B} = \frac{13\ \text{hr} \times 5\ \text{hr}}{13\ \text{hr} + 5\ \text{hr}} = 3.6\ \text{hr}$$

6.11

6.11 A patient with cancer of the thyroid has been found to have a thyroid iodine uptake of 50%. How much ^{131}I must be injected to deliver a dose to the thyroid, which weighs 30 g, of 15 grays (1500 rad) in 3 days?
Since no iodine retention time is given for this cancer patient, we will assume the ICRP 28 value and calculate the effective half life using 6.54.

$T_R = 8.05$ d
$T_B = 138$ d (ICRP 28)

$$T_E = \frac{T_R \times T_B}{T_R + T_B} = \frac{8.05 \text{ d} \times 138 \text{ d}}{8.05 \text{ d} + 138 \text{ d}} = 7.6 \text{ d, effective half life } ^{131}\text{I in the body.}$$

Converting to effective elimination constant, using equation 6.52:

$$\lambda_E = \frac{0.693}{T_E} = \frac{0.693}{7.6 \text{ d}} = 0.091 \text{ d}^{-1}$$

Find the initial dose rate (equation 6.57):
$D = 15$ Gy
$\lambda_E = 0.091$ d^{-1}
$t = 3$ days

$$D = \frac{\dot{D}_0}{\lambda_E}\left(1 - e^{-\lambda_E t}\right)$$

$$\dot{D}_0 = \frac{D\lambda_E}{\left(1 - e^{-\lambda_E t}\right)} = \frac{15 \text{ Gy} \times 0.091 \text{d}^{-1}}{\left(1 - \text{e}^{-(0.091)\times 3}\right)} = 5.71 \text{Gy/d is the initial dose rate to the}$$

thyroid

Example problem 6.13 in the text demonstrates how to calculate the average energy ^{131}I imparts per transformation, 0.230 MeV/t.

Using equation 6.47, and knowing that the initial dose rate is 5.71 Gy/d:

$m = 30$ g $= 0.03$ kg thyroid mass (appendix 3)

$$D = \frac{q \text{ Bq} \times 1 \text{tps/Bq} \times E \text{ MeV/t} \times 1.6 \times 10^{-13} \text{J/MeV} \times 8.64 \times 10^4 \text{sec/d}}{m \text{ kg} \times 1 \frac{\text{J}}{\text{kg}} / \text{Gy}}$$

$$5.71\frac{\text{Gy}}{\text{day}} = \frac{q\ \text{Bq} \times \frac{1\text{tps}}{\text{Bq}} \times 0.230\ \frac{\text{MeV}}{\text{t}} \times 1.6 \times 10^{-13}\ \frac{\text{J}}{\text{MeV}} \times 8.64 \times 10^{4}\ \text{sec / day}}{0.03\ \text{kg} \times 1\frac{\text{J}}{\text{kg}} / \text{Gy}}$$

q Bq = 54 × 10^6 Bq = 54 MBq

Since the thyroid uptake is 50% of the activity twice the activity must be administered to deliver the proper radiation dose:

54 × 2 = 108 MBq must be injected to deliver 15 Gy in 3 days.

6.12 The mean concentration of potassium in seawater is 380 mg/kg. What is the dose rate, in milligrays per year and in millirads per year, in the ocean depths due to the dissolved ^{40}K? **6.12**

^{40}K comprises approximately 0.0119% of all potassium (CRC). Please note that the RHH (1970) incorrectly lists 0.118% of all potassium as ^{40}K.

The specific activity of ^{40}K will also be needed:

Use equation 4.31

A_{Ra} = 226
T_{Ra} = 1620 years
A_{K} = 40
T_{K} = 1.26 × 10^9 years

$$\text{SA}_{\text{K-40}} = \frac{A_{Ra}T_{Ra}}{A_K T_K} = \frac{226 \times 1620\ \text{yr}}{40 \times 1.3 \times 10^{9}\ \text{yr}} = 7 \times 10^{-6}\ \text{Ci/g K–40}$$

$$\frac{380\ \text{mg K}}{1\ \text{kg seawater}} \times \frac{1\ \text{g K}}{1000\ \text{mg K}} \times \frac{0.0119\ \text{g}\ ^{40}\text{K}}{100\ \text{g K}} \times \frac{7 \times 10^{-6}\ \text{Ci}}{1\ \text{g}\ ^{40}\text{K}} \times \frac{3.7 \times 10^{10}\ \frac{\text{trans}}{\text{sec}}}{1\ \text{Ci}}$$

= 11.7 (t/s)/kg

$$\frac{11.7\frac{\text{t}}{\text{sec}}}{\text{kg seawater}} \times \frac{3600\ \text{sec}}{\text{hr}} \times \frac{24\ \text{hr}}{\text{day}} \times \frac{365\ \text{day}}{\text{year}} = 3.69 \times 10^{8}\ \text{(t/year)/kg seawater}$$

^{40}K emits the following:
1.46 MeV γ 11% of the time.
0.509 MeV$_{\text{average}}$ β^- is emitted in 89% of the decays.

The average energy therefore is

$$\bar{E} = (0.11 \times 1.46) + (0.89 \times 0.509) = 0.614 \frac{\text{MeV}}{\text{t}}$$

In an infinite medium, the energy emitted = energy absorbed

$$\frac{\frac{3.69 \times 10^{8}\ \text{t/yr}}{\text{kg}} \times \frac{0.614\ \text{MeV}}{\gamma} \times \frac{1.6 \times 10^{-13}\ \text{J}}{\text{MeV}}}{1\frac{\text{J}}{\text{kg}}\Big/\text{Gy}} = 3.6 \times 10^{-5}\ \text{Gy/yr} = 3.6\ \text{mrads/yr}$$

6.13

6.13 Calculate the annual radiation dose to a reference person from the ^{40}K and from the ^{14}C deposited in his body. The specific activity of carbon is 0.255 Bq (6.9 pCi) per gram. Assume in both instances, that the radioisotopes are uniformly distributed throughout the body.

Performing the calculations for potassium first:

In problem 6.12, we calculate the specific activity of ^{40}K to be 7.04×10^{-6} Ci/g (^{40}K)

From appendix 3, table 2, the amount of potassium found in a reference person is 140 grams. The natural abundance of ^{40}K is 0.0119% (Table 4.5). Please note that the RHH (1970) incorrectly lists 0.118% of all potassium as ^{40}K. Calculating the number of transformations of ^{40}K per second in the body:

$$\frac{140 \text{ g K}}{\text{body}} \times \frac{0.0119 \text{ g}^{40}\text{K}}{100 \text{ g K}} \times \frac{7.04 \times 10^{-6}\text{Ci}}{\text{g}^{40}\text{K}} \times \frac{3.7 \times 10^{10} \frac{\text{t}}{\text{sec}}}{\text{Ci}} = 4.3 \times 10^{3} \frac{\text{t}}{\text{sec}} \text{ of } ^{40}\text{K}$$

in body

^{40}K emits the following

$\beta_{average}$ = 0.509 MeV in 89% of all transformations
γ = 1.46 MeV (11% of all transformations)

For uniformly distributed 1.5 MeV gamma, Table 6.8 shows the absorbed fraction to be 0.302.Therefore the total amount of energy absorbed per transformation is:

$$E_e = E_e(\gamma) + E_e(\beta) = (1.46 \text{ MeV} \times 0.302 \times 0.11) + (0.509 \text{ MeV} \times 0.89)$$

$$E_e = 0.502 \text{ MeV/trans}$$

Calculating the dose due to potassium using equation 6.76;

m = 70 kg (appendix 3, table 1)

$q = 4.3 \times 10^{3} \frac{\text{t}}{\text{sec}}$ of ^{40}K

E_e = 0.502 MeV/trans

$$\dot{D} = \frac{q \text{ Bq} \times 1\frac{\text{tps}}{\text{Bq}} \times E_e \frac{\text{MeV}}{\text{trans}} \times 1.6 \times 10^{-13} \frac{\text{J}}{\text{MeV}} \times 8.64 \times 10^{4} \frac{\text{sec}}{\text{day}} \times 365 \frac{\text{days}}{\text{yr}}}{m \text{ kg} \times \frac{1 \text{ J}}{\text{kg}} \Big/ \text{Gy}}$$

$$\dot{D} = \frac{4.3 \times 10^{3} \frac{\text{trans}}{\text{sec}} \times 0.502 \frac{\text{MeV}}{\text{trans}} \times 1.6 \times 10^{-13} \frac{\text{J}}{\text{MeV}} \times 8.64 \times 10^{4} \frac{\text{sec}}{\text{day}} \times 365 \frac{\text{day}}{\text{year}}}{70 \text{ kg} \times \frac{1 \text{ J}}{\text{kg}} \Big/ \text{Gy}}$$

$$\dot{D} = 1.55 \times 10^{-4} \frac{\text{Gy}}{\text{yr}} = 0.155 \frac{\text{mGy}}{\text{yr}} \text{ from the } ^{40}\text{K}$$

Performing the calculations for ^{14}C which is a pure beta emitter where the average beta energy is 0.05 MeV.

From appendix C, the amount of carbon found in a reference person is 16,000 grams. Calculating the number of transformations of ^{14}C per second in the body, using the specific activity given in the problem:

$$q = \frac{16000 \text{ g C}}{\text{body}} \times \frac{0.255 \text{ Bq}}{\text{g C}} \times \frac{1\frac{\text{t}}{\text{sec}}}{1\text{Bq}} = 4080 \frac{\text{t}}{\text{sec}} \text{ of } ^{14}\text{C in body}$$

Calculating the dose due to ^{14}C using equation 6.76;

m = 70 kg (appendix 3, table 1)
q = 4080 Bq of ^{14}C
E_e = 0.05 MeV/trans

$$\dot{D} = \frac{q \text{ Bq} \times 1\frac{\text{tps}}{\text{Bq}} \times E_e \frac{\text{MeV}}{\text{trans}} \times 1.6 \times 10^{-13} \frac{\text{J}}{\text{MeV}} \times 8.64 \times 10^4 \frac{\text{sec}}{\text{day}} \times 365 \frac{\text{d}}{\text{yr}}}{m \text{ kg} \times \frac{1 \text{ J}}{\text{kg}} \Big/ \text{Gy}}$$

$$\dot{D} = \frac{4080 \frac{\text{t}}{\text{sec}} \times 0.05 \frac{\text{MeV}}{\text{trans}} \times 1.6 \times 10^{-13} \frac{\text{J}}{\text{MeV}} \times 8.64 \times 10^4 \frac{\text{sec}}{\text{day}} \times 365 \frac{\text{day}}{\text{year}}}{70 \text{ kg} \times 1\frac{\text{J}}{\text{kg}} \Big/ \text{Gy}}$$

$$\dot{D} = 1.53 \times 10^{-5} \frac{\text{Gy}}{\text{yr}} = 0.0153 \frac{\text{mGy}}{\text{yr}} \text{ from } ^{14}\text{C}$$

Summing the doses from both yields:

$$0.155 \frac{\text{mGy}}{\text{yr}} \text{ from the } ^{40}\text{K} + 0.015 \frac{\text{mGy}}{\text{yr}} \text{ from the } ^{14}\text{C} = 0.17 \frac{\text{mGy}}{\text{yr}}$$

6.14 A thin walled carbon wall ionization chamber, whose volume is 2 cm^3, is filled with standard air at 0°C and 760 torr and is placed inside a tank of water to make a depth dose measurement. A 24 MeV betatron beam produces a current of 0.02 μA in the chamber. What was the absorbed dose rate? **6.14**

According to the Bragg-Gray relationship (equation 6.14)

$$\frac{\text{energy absorbed}}{\text{unit mass}} = \rho_m\, w\, J$$

Mass stopping power ratios for electrons generated by x-rays may be obtained from ICRU 14, Table A.3.

ρ_m = mass stopping power ratio of water for 24 MV X-rays = 1.08

To calculate the number of ion pairs per gram of air:

density of air = 1.293×10^{-3} g/cm^3 (Table 5.2)
1 ion pair = 1.6×10^{-19} coulombs

$$J = \frac{\text{ion pairs}}{\text{gram}_{\text{air}}} = \frac{0.02\,\frac{\mu\text{C}}{\text{sec}} \times \frac{1\text{C}}{1\times 10^{6}\,\mu\text{C}} \times \frac{1\text{ ion pair}}{1.6\times 10^{-19}\,\text{C}}}{2\text{ cm}^3_{\text{air}} \times \frac{1.293\times 10^{-3}\,\text{g}_{\text{air}}}{\text{cm}^3_{\text{air}}}} = 4.8 \times 10^{13}\ \frac{\text{ion pairs}}{\text{gram}_{\text{air}}\cdot\text{sec}}$$

For betas (and electrons), w = 34 electron volts are expended per ion pair in air (Table 5.1).
1.6×10^{-12} erg = 1 eV
1 rad = 100 ergs/gram

Substituting these values into the Bragg-Gray equation and calculating the dose rate, we have

$$\dot{D} = \rho_m \times w\,\frac{\text{eV}}{\text{ip}} \times J\,\frac{\text{ip}}{\text{g}\cdot\text{s}} \times 1.6\times 10^{-12}\,\frac{\text{erg}}{\text{eV}} \times \frac{1\text{ rad}}{100\,\frac{\text{ergs}}{\text{g}}}$$

$$\dot{D} = 1.08 \times 34\,\frac{\text{eV}}{\text{ip}} \times 4.8\times 10^{13}\,\frac{\text{ip}}{\text{g}\cdot\text{s}} \times 1.6\times 10^{-12}\,\frac{\text{erg}}{\text{eV}} \times \frac{1\text{ rad}}{100\,\frac{\text{ergs}}{\text{g}}}$$

$\dot{D}$ = 28.4 rads/s = 284 mGy/s

6.15

6.15 An aluminum ionization chamber containing 10 cm^3 air at 20°C and 760 torr operates under Bragg Gray conditions. After a 1–hour exposure to ^{60}Co gamma rays, 3.6×10^{-9} coulomb of charge is collected. If the relative mass stopping power of Al for the electrons generated by the ^{60}Co gammas is 0.875, what was the dose to the aluminum?

The Bragg Gray rule applies in this problem: $\dfrac{\text{energy absorbed}}{\text{unit mass}} = \rho_m\, w\, J$

$\rho_m = 0.875$
density of air = 1.293×10^{-3} g/cm^3 (Table 5.2)
1 ion pair = 1.6×10^{-19} C
w = 34 eV per ion pair in air (Table 5.1)

Converting the volume of air in the chamber to STP, assuming it is an ideal gas:
Standard Temp = 273 K

$$10\ \text{cm}^3 \times \frac{273\ \text{K}}{293\ \text{K}} = 9.32\ \text{cm}^3 \text{ is the volume in the chamber at STP}$$

$$J = \frac{\text{ion pairs}}{\text{gram}_{\text{air}}} = \frac{3.6 \times 10^{-9}\,\dfrac{\text{C}}{\text{hr}} \times \dfrac{1\ \text{ion pair}}{1.6 \times 10^{-19}\,\text{C}}}{9.32\ \text{cm}^3_{\text{air}} \times \dfrac{1.293 \times 10^{-3}\,\text{g}_{\text{air}}}{\text{cm}^3_{\text{air}}}} = 1.87 \times 10^{12}\ \frac{\text{ion pairs}}{\text{gram}_{\text{air}}}$$

$$w = \frac{34\ \text{eV}}{\text{ion pair}} \times \frac{1.6 \times 10^{-12}\ \text{erg}}{\text{eV}} = 5.44 \times 10^{-11}\ \frac{\text{erg}}{\text{ion pair}}$$

Equation 6.14 gives the Bragg–Gray relationship:

$$D = \rho_{\text{m}} \times w\,\frac{\text{eV}}{\text{ip}} \times J\,\frac{\text{ip}}{\text{g}\cdot\text{s}} \times \frac{1\ \text{rad}}{100\,\dfrac{\text{ergs}}{\text{g}}}$$

$$D = 0.875 \times 5.44 \times 10^{-11}\,\frac{\text{erg}}{\text{ip}} \times 1.87 \times 10^{12}\,\frac{\text{ip}}{\text{g}} \times \frac{1\ \text{rad}}{100\,\dfrac{\text{ergs}}{\text{g}}}$$

$D = 0.889$ rads = 8.9 mGy

6.16 An ion chamber made of 50 grams copper has a 10 cm^3 cavity filled with air at STP. The temperature of the copper rose 0.002 °C after exposure to ^{60}Co gamma rays. If the mass stopping power of Cu is 0.753 relative to air, and if the specific heat of Cu is 0.092 calories per gram per degree C, calculate 6.16
(a) The absorbed dose to the copper,

4.184 J = 1 calorie

$$\frac{0.092 \text{ calories}}{\text{gram}\cdot{}^\circ\text{C}} \times \frac{4.184 \text{ J}}{\text{calorie}} \times 50 \text{ g} \times 0.002^\circ\text{C} = 0.0385 \text{ J deposited in the chamber}$$

$$\frac{0.0385 \text{ J}}{50 \text{ g}} \times \frac{1000 \text{ g}}{\text{kg}} \times \frac{1\text{Gy}}{1\frac{\text{J}}{\text{kg}}} = 0.77 \text{ Gy deposited in chamber}$$

(b) The amount of charge (in coulombs) formed by ionization in the cavity during exposure.

$\rho_m = 0.753$

$$\frac{34 \text{ eV}}{\text{ion pair}} \times \frac{1.6 \times 10^{-19} \text{ J}}{\text{eV}} = 5.44 \times 10^{-18} \frac{\text{J}}{\text{ion pair}}$$

Equation 6.14 gives the Bragg Gray relationship:

$$\dot{D} = \frac{\Delta E_{absorbed}}{\Delta m} = \rho_m \; w \, J$$

$$\dot{D} = \rho_m \times 5.44 \times 10^{-18} \frac{\text{joules}}{\text{ip}} \times J \frac{\text{ip}}{\text{kg}} \times \frac{1 \text{ Gy}}{\text{J}/\text{kg}}$$

Dose determined in part (a) was 0.77 Gy, and the quantity of coulombs is needed, which is a part of the "J" term, so solve for "J"

$$0.77 \text{ Gy} = \rho_m \, w \, J$$

$$0.77 \text{ Gy} = (0.753) \times 5.44 \times 10^{-18} \frac{\text{joule}}{\text{ion pair}} \times J \frac{\text{ip}}{1.293 \times 10^{-5} \text{kg}} \times \frac{1\text{Gy}}{\text{joule}/\text{kg}}$$

$J = 2.43 \times 10^{12}$ ip

Total charge = 2.43×10^{12} ip $\times 1.6 \times 10^{-19}$ C/ip $= 3.9 \times 10^{-7}$ C

6.17

6.17 An aqueous suspension of virus is irradiated by X–rays whose half value layer is 2 mm Cu. If the exposure was 355 C/kg (1.3×10^{6} R), and if the depth of the suspension is 5 mm, what was the absorbed dose, and what was the mean ionization density?

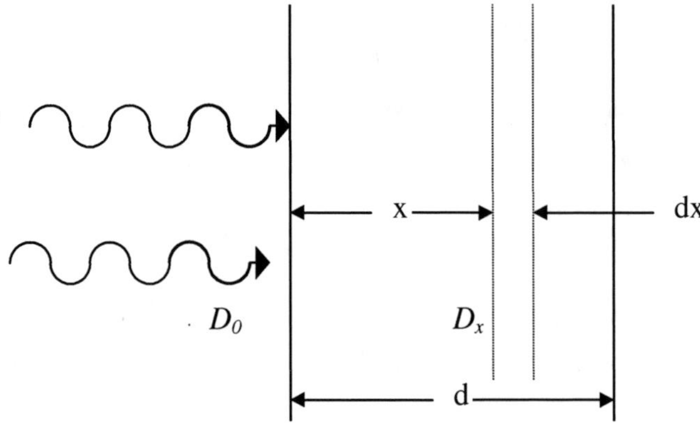

Use equation 5.18B to determine the linear attenuation of the copper;

$t = 2$ mm
$I/I_0 = 0.5$

$\ln I/I_0 = -\mu t$

Rearranging;

$$\mu = \frac{\ln(0.5)}{-2 \text{ mm}} = 0.347 \text{ mm}^{-1} = 3.47 \text{ cm}^{-1}$$ is the linear attenuation of Cu.

Look up in table 5.2 the energy that this attenuation coefficient corresponds to, and it is found that the approximate average energy of the x–rays is 0.112 MeV.

To convert roentgens to rads using equation 6.12,

$\mu_w / \rho_w = 0.0258\ \text{cm}^2/\text{g}$ (Table 5.3 for 0.112 MeV)

$\mu_a / \rho_a = 0.0237\ \text{cm}^2/\text{g}$ (Table 5.3 for 0.112 MeV)

$$\text{rads} = \frac{87.7}{100} \times \frac{\mu_w / \rho_w}{\mu_a / \rho_a}\ \text{roentgen} = \frac{87.7}{100} \times \frac{0.0258}{0.0237}\ \text{R}$$

0.95 rad = 1 R

$$D_0 = 1.3 \times 10^6\ \text{R} = 1.3 \times 10^6\ \text{R} \times \frac{0.95\ \text{rad}}{1\ \text{R}} = 1.24 \times 10^6\ \text{rads}$$

The dose at depth x is

$$D_x = D_0 e^{-\mu x}$$

Let
I = integral dose, gram-rads
A = irradiated area. Since dose is an intensive property, we may use $A = 1\ \text{cm}^2$

ρ_{water} = density of suspension, $1 \frac{\text{g}}{\text{cm}^3}$
μ (0.112 MeV, H_2O) = 0.0258 cm^{-1} (Table 5.3)

The absorbed energy, dI gram-rads, in the thickness dx is:

$$dI = \rho\, A\, D_x dx = \rho\, A\, D_0\, e^{-\mu x}$$

Integrating to find the integral dose through the 5 mm (0.5 cm) of suspension;

$$\int dI = \rho \times (A) \times D_0 \int_0^{0.5} e^{-\mu x} dx$$

$$I = \frac{\rho \times (A) \times D_0}{\mu} \times \left(1 - e^{-\mu x}\right)$$

$$I = \frac{1\frac{\text{g}}{\text{cm}^3} \times 1\ \text{cm}^2 \times 1.24 \times 10^6\ \text{rads}}{0.0258\ \text{cm}^{-1}} \times \left(1 - e^{-0.0258\times(0.5)}\right) = 6.2 \times 10^5\ \text{g·rads}$$

Dividing by the mass of the unit area irradiated:

$$D = \frac{6.2 \times 10^5\ \text{g} \cdot \text{rads}}{0.5\ \text{g}} = 1.24 \times 10^6\ \text{rads} = 1.24 \times 10^4\ \text{Gy}.$$

The number of ion pairs formed per eV in water can be found in "Medical Physics Handbook 15, Fundamentals of Radiation Dosimetry", Second edition, table 2.5, published by Adam Hilger, 1985 as 29.6 eV per ion pair;

$$1.24 \times 10^4\ \text{Gy} \times \frac{1\ \text{J/kg}}{1\ \text{Gy}} \times \frac{\text{eV}}{1.6 \times 10^{-19}\ \text{J}} \times \frac{\text{ion pair}}{29.6\ \text{eV}} \times \frac{\text{kg}}{1000\ \text{g}} = 2.6 \times 10^{18}\ \text{ion pairs/g}$$

6.18

6.18 A child drinks 1 liter of milk per day containing ^{131}I at a mean concentration of 33.3 Bq (900 pCi) per liter over a period of 30 days. Assuming that the child has no other intake of ^{131}I, calculate the dose to the thyroid at the end of the 30 days ingestion period, and the dose commitment.

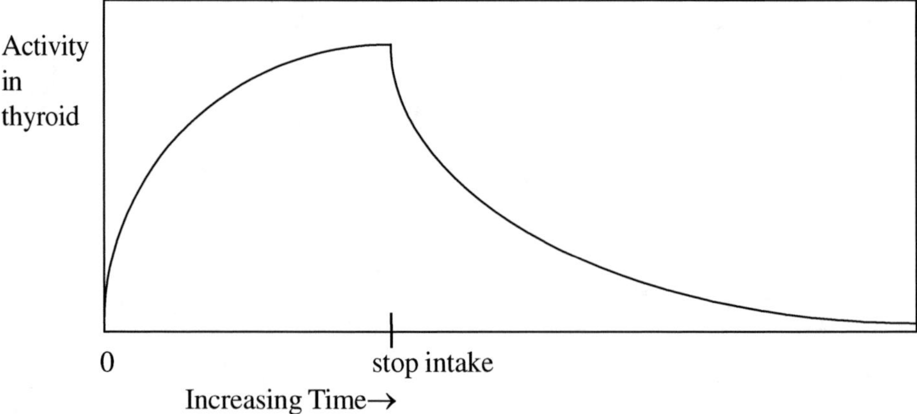

First calculate the effective half life of the I–131 in the body, use equation 6.54:

$T_R = 8.05$ d
$T_B = 138$ d (ICRP 28)

$$T_E = \frac{T_R \times T_B}{T_R + T_B} = \frac{8.05 \text{ d} \times 138 \text{ d}}{8.05 \text{ d} + 138 \text{ d}} = 7.6 \text{ d effective half life of } ^{131}\text{I in body.}$$

Converting to effective elimination constant, using equation 6.52:

$$\lambda_E = \frac{0.693}{T_E} = \frac{0.693}{7.6 \text{ d}} = 0.091 \text{ d}^{-1}$$

The average energy of each ^{131}I beta particle is found (Figure 6.11), and the yield from each decay is also tabulated:

Energy, MeV/t	Yield, *f*
0.0701	0.016
0.0955	0.069
0.1428	0.005
0.1917	0.904
0.2856	0.006

The mean β energy/transformation is:

$$\overline{E}_e(\beta) = \Sigma \overline{E} \times f_{\beta i} = (0.0701 \times 0.016) + (0.0955 \times 0.069) + (0.1428 \times 0.005) + (0.1917 \times 0.904) + (0.2856 \times 0.006)$$

$$\overline{E}_e(\beta) = 0.184 \text{ MeV/t}$$

Calculating the contribution due to the γ, the specific absorbed fraction is found in appendix 4 for an adult. Assume all the ^{131}I is deposited in the thyroid. So for this case, the contribution from the γ is not significant and can be ignored, especially since the child's thyroid is small (~2-5g, ICRP 53).

MeV	*f*	Spec. Abs	MeV/t
0.723	0.016	0.00166	1.92E-05
0.637	0.069	0.00166	7.3E-05
0.503	0.003	0.00166	2.5E-06
0.326	0.002	0.00155	1.01E-06
0.177	0.002	0.00155	5.49E-07
0.365	0.853	0.00155	0.000483
0.284	0.051	0.00155	2.25E-05
0.08	0.051	0.0429	0.000175
0.164	0.006	0.00155	1.53E-06
		Sum	0.000778

The intake is $q = 33.3$ Bq/day, however, only one–third of the iodine is directly deposited in the thyroid (ICRP 30).

$$K = 33.3\frac{\text{Bq}}{\text{d}} \times \frac{1\text{ deposited}}{3\text{ ingested}} = 11.1\frac{\text{Bq}}{\text{d}}$$

Some of the iodine is eliminated daily, so find the concentration in the thyroid at any time:

$$\frac{dq}{dt} = \text{deposition} - \text{disappearance}$$

$$\frac{dq}{dt} = K - \lambda_{eff}\, q$$

Separating the variables, we have

$$\int_0^q \frac{dq}{\left(K - \lambda_{eff}\, q\right)} = \int_0^t dt$$

After integration, and solving for q as a function of t;

$$q(t) = \frac{K}{\lambda}\left(1 - e^{-\lambda t}\right)$$

As $t \to \infty$, q approaches

$$q_{\infty} = \frac{K}{\lambda} = \frac{11.1 \frac{\text{Bq}}{\text{day}}}{0.091 \text{ day}} = 122 \text{ Bq}$$

m = 20 g (for adult, from appendix C), for a child, assume 10% of adult mass (10 CFR 20), 2 g.

Putting values into equation 6.76:

$$\dot{D}_{\infty} = \frac{q_{\infty} \text{ Bq} \times 1\text{tps / Bq} \times E \text{ MeV / t} \times 1.6 \times 10^{-13} \text{J / MeV} \times 8.64 \times 10^{4} \text{sec / d}}{m \text{ kg} \times 1 \frac{\text{J}}{\text{kg}} \text{/ Gy}}$$

$$\dot{D}_{\infty} = \frac{122 \text{ Bq} \times 1\text{tps / Bq} \times 0.184 \text{ MeV / t} \times 1.6 \times 10^{-13} \text{J / MeV} \times 8.64 \times 10^{4} \text{sec / day}}{2 \text{ g} \times \frac{\text{kg}}{1000 \text{ g}} \times 1 \frac{\text{J}}{\text{kg}} \text{/ Gy}}$$

$\dot{D}_{\infty} = 1.55 \times 10^{-4} \frac{\text{Gy}}{\text{day}}$ = 0.155 mGy/d to child's thyroid is the dose rate after an infinite ingestion period at 33 Bq/d.

The total dose at the end of t days of continuous intake is given by

$$D = \int_{0}^{t} \dot{D}(t)dt$$

Since $\dot{D}(t)$ is proportional to $q(t)$, the expression for $\dot{D}(t)$ is analogous to that for $q(t)$.

Therefore the dose rate after t days of intake is:

$$\dot{D}(t) = \dot{D}_\infty\left(1 - e^{-\lambda t}\right)$$

The above equation is integrated with respect to time to find the dose for the 30 day period of intake. The dose rate at an infinite time (the equilibrium dose) is known from the earlier calculation to be 0.155 mGy/day.

$$D = \int_0^t \dot{D}(t)dt$$

$$\dot{D}(t) = \dot{D}_\infty\left(1 - e^{-\lambda t}\right)$$

$$\text{Dose} = \int_0^t \dot{D} \cdot dt = \dot{D}_\infty \int_0^t \left(1 - e^{-\lambda t}\right)dt$$

Integrating yields:

$$D = D_\infty\left[t + \frac{1}{\lambda}\left(e^{-\lambda t} - 1\right)\right]$$

And the accumulated dose at 30 days is:

$\dot{D}_\infty = 0.155$ mGy/day
$\lambda = 0.091\ \text{d}^{-1}$
$t = 30$ d

$$D = 0.155\frac{\text{mGy}}{\text{d}} \times \left[30\ \text{d} + \frac{1}{0.091\text{d}^{-1}} \times \left(\text{e}^{-0.091\times(30)} - 1\right)\right] = 3\ \text{mGy}$$

3 mGy is the accumulated dose at the end of the 30 day period.

The dose commitment is the sum of the dose accumulated during intake, and then during elimination (washout).

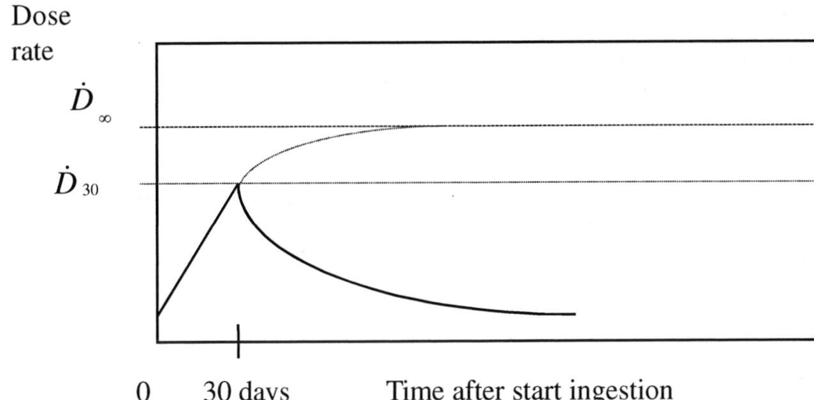

Find the dose rate at t = 30 days

$$\dot{D}_{30} = \dot{D}_\infty (1 - e^{-\lambda t}) = 0.155 \frac{\text{mGy}}{\text{d}} \times \left(1 - \text{e}^{-0.091\times(30)}\right) = 0.145 \ \frac{\text{mGy}}{\text{day}}$$

$$D = \frac{\dot{D}_{30}}{\lambda} = \frac{0.145 \frac{\text{mGy}}{\text{d}}}{0.091 \frac{1}{\text{d}}} = 1.59 \text{ mGy is the dose after ingestion stops.}$$

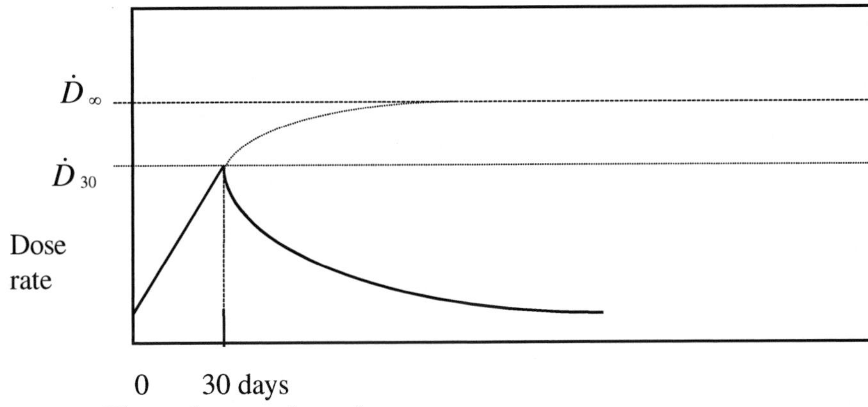

The total dose, from the time intake started to the end of the first 30 days, plus the dose after the intake stopped will be;

3 mGy + 1.6 mGy = 4.6 mGy total dose to the childs thyroid.

6.19

6.19 A patient who weighs 50 kg is given an organic compound tagged with 4 MBq (108 μCi) ^{14}C. On the basis of bioassay measurements, the following whole body retention data were inferred:

Day	0	1	2	3	4	5	6	8	10	12	14
MBq	1	2.94	2.32	1.9	1.6	1.4	1.2	0.9	0.8	0.6	0.5

(a) plot the retention data, and write the equation for the retention curve as a function of time.

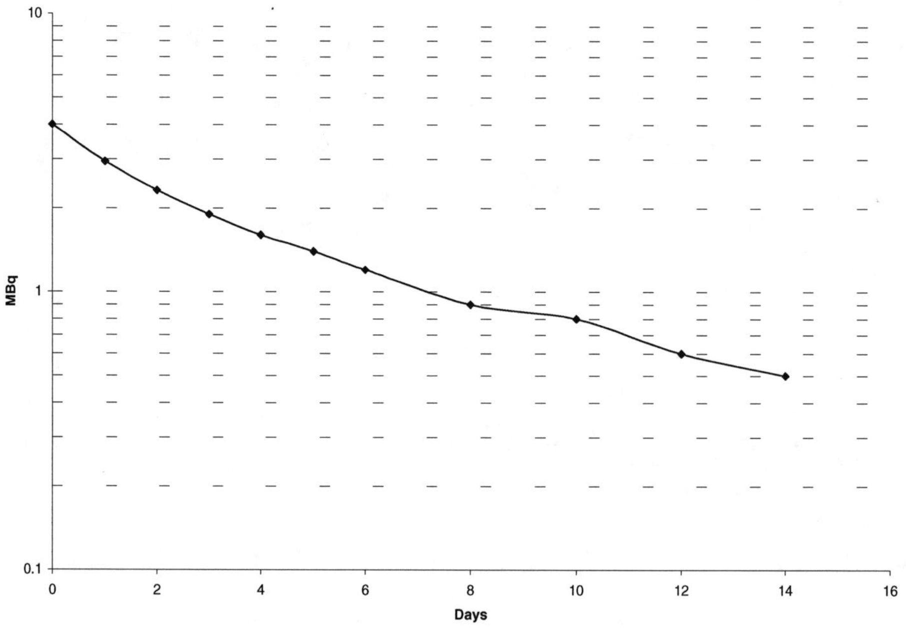

Days are labeled on the x–axis, MBq on the y–axis. The curve appears to have two components to it, a long lived and short lived. To resolve these two components, and determine the equation, draw a line along the long lived portion to the y axis;

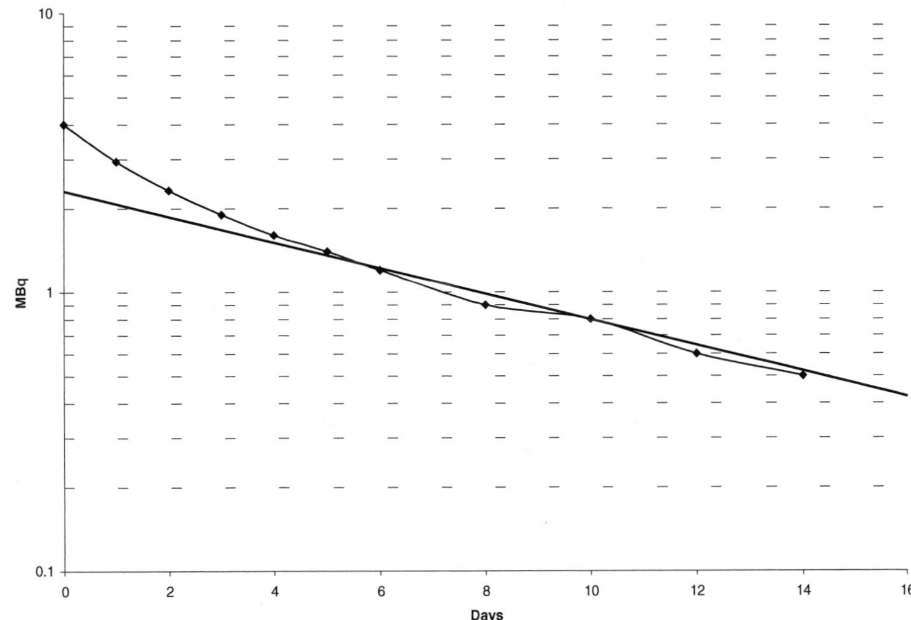

Since the line intercepts the y axis at 2.2 MBq, that is the amount deposited in the long lived compartment. The time for the activity to decrease to one half of the initial activity, to 1.1 MBq, is found from the graph to be 6.5 days. The slope of the line, therefore, is

$$\mu = \frac{0.693}{t_{1/2}} = \frac{0.693}{6.5\ \text{d}} = 0.11\ \text{d}^{-1}$$

and the equation for the long lived component is

$$R\,(t, LL) = 2.2\text{e}^{-0.11t}$$

The short lived component of the curve is found by subtracting the long lived activity from the total activity. Thus, for t = 0, we have

4 MBq – 2.2 MBq = 1.8 MBq

The long lived activity for days 1 - 5 are calculated from the equation for the long lived component, and then are subtracted from the total activity. These differences, which are tabulated and plotted below, fall on a straight line. The half-time for this short lived component is 1.1 days, and the slope is 0.693/1.1 days = 0.63 per day. The equation for the short lived component is therefore $R\ (t, SL) = 1.8e^{-0.63t}$. The equation for the retention curve, which is the sum of the two components is

$$R(t) = 1.8e^{-0.63\,t} + 2.2e^{-0.11\,t}$$

Day	Total	Long lived	Short lived
0	4	2.2	1.8
1	2.94	1.97	0.97
2	2.32	1.77	0.55
3	1.9	1.58	0.32
4	1.6	1.42	0.18
5	1.4	1.27	0.13

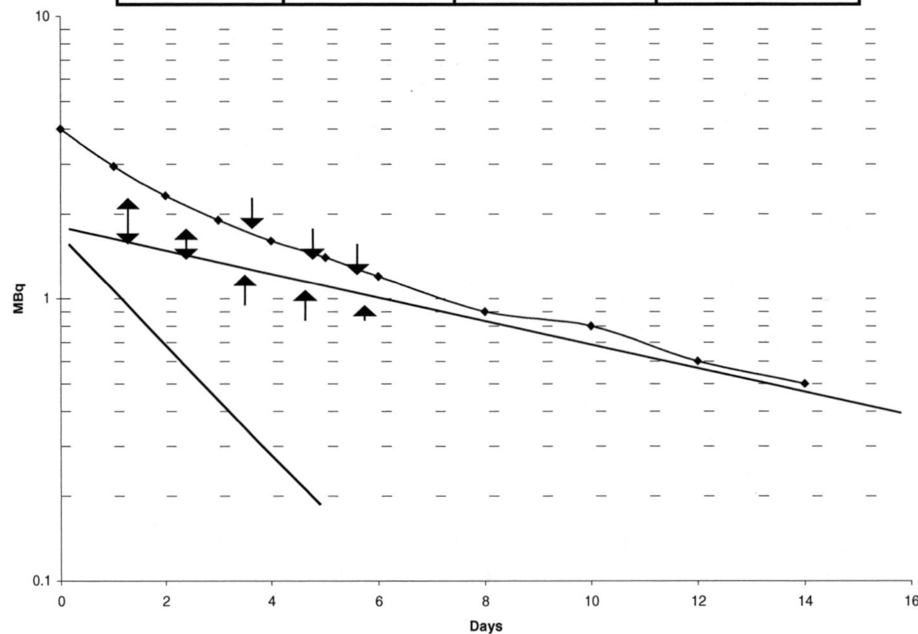

(b) Assuming the ^{14}C to be uniformly distributed throughout the body, calculate the absorbed dose to the patient at day 7 and day 14 after administration of the drug.

$\overline{E}_{avg} = 0.04947$ MeV

$m = 50$ kg

Using equation 6.47 to find the initial dose rate from q Bq:

$$\dot{D} = \frac{q\ \text{Bq} \times \dfrac{1\dfrac{\text{trans}}{\text{sec}}}{\text{Bq}} \times \overline{E}\,\dfrac{\text{MeV}}{\text{trans}} \times 1.6 \times 10^{-13}\,\dfrac{\text{J}}{\text{MeV}} \times 8.64 \times 10^{4}\,\dfrac{\text{sec}}{\text{d}}}{m\ \text{kg} \times \dfrac{1\text{J}}{\text{kg}} \Big/ \text{Gy}}$$

$$\dot{D} = \frac{q\ \text{Bq} \times \dfrac{1\dfrac{\text{trans}}{\text{sec}}}{\text{Bq}} \times 0.04947\,\dfrac{\text{MeV}}{\text{trans}} \times 1.6 \times 10^{-13}\,\dfrac{\text{J}}{\text{MeV}} \times 8.64 \times 10^{4}\,\dfrac{\text{sec}}{\text{d}}}{50\ \text{kg} \times \dfrac{1\text{J}}{\text{kg}} \Big/ \text{Gy}}$$

$$\dot{D} = 1.38 \times 10^{-11} \times q\,\frac{\text{Gy}}{\text{d/Bq}}$$

The sum of the doses from each component gives the total dose. The dose for each component is given by equation 6.57, where $\dot{D}_0$ is the initial dose rate for that component and λ is the clearance rate for that component.

$$D = \frac{\dot{D}_0}{\lambda}\left\{1 - e^{-\lambda t}\right\}$$

$$D = \left[\frac{\dot{D}_{01}}{\lambda_1} \left\{ 1 - e^{-\lambda_1 t} \right\} \right] + \left[\frac{\dot{D}_{02}}{\lambda_2} \left\{ 1 - e^{-\lambda_2 t} \right\} \right]$$

Note equation is split into two lines.

$$D = \left[\frac{\left(1.38 \times 10^{-11} \times 1.8 \times 10^{6}\right) \frac{\text{Gy}}{\text{d}}}{0.63\ \text{d}^{-1}} \times \left\{ 1 - \text{e}^{-0.63 \times (7)} \right\} \right] +$$

$$\left[\frac{\left(1.38 \times 10^{-11} \times 2.2 \times 10^{6}\right) \frac{\text{Gy}}{\text{d}}}{0.11\ \text{d}^{-1}} \left\{ 1 - \text{e}^{-0.11 \times (7)} \right\} \right]$$

$D = 0.19$ mGy is the absorbed dose to the patient after 7 days.

Calculating the dose after 14 days in a similar fashion (Note equation is split into two lines)

$$D = \left[\frac{\left(1.38 \times 10^{-11} \times 1.8 \times 10^{6}\right) \frac{\text{Gy}}{\text{d}}}{0.63\ \text{d}^{-1}} \times \left\{ 1 - \text{e}^{-0.63 \times (14)} \right\} \right] +$$

$$\left[\frac{\left(1.38 \times 10^{-11} \times 2.2 \times 10^{6}\right) \frac{\text{Gy}}{\text{d}}}{0.11\ \text{d}^{-1}} \left\{ 1 - \text{e}^{-0.11 \times (14)} \right\} \right]$$

$D = 0.26$ mGy is the absorbed dose to the patient after 14 days.

(c) What is the dose commitment from this procedure?

$$D = \left[\frac{\left(1.38\times10^{-11}\times1.8\times10^{6}\right)\frac{\text{Gy}}{\text{d}}}{0.63\ \text{d}^{-1}}\right] + \left[\frac{\left(1.38\times10^{-11}\times2.2\times10^{6}\right)\frac{\text{Gy}}{\text{d}}}{0.11\ \text{d}^{-1}}\right]$$

$D = 0.32$ mGy is the dose commitment.

6.20 A 2 MeV electron beam is used to irradiate a sample of plastic whose thickness is 0.5 g/cm^2. If a 250 μamp beam passes through a port 1 cm in diameter to strike the plastic, calculate the absorbed dose rate. **6.20**

First, calculate the range of a 2 MeV electron using equation 5.2;

$E = 2$ MeV

$R = 412E^{1.265-0.0954\times\ln E} = 412\times(2)^{1.265-0.0954\times\ln(2)} = 945.8\,\frac{\text{mg}}{\text{cm}^2}$ is the range of the 2 MeV electron. An approximation is then made that there is a linear relationship between energy and range.

$$\text{Energy deposited} = \frac{\text{range of material}}{\text{range of initial electron}}\times\text{Initial Energy}$$

$\text{Energy deposited} = \dfrac{500\frac{\text{mg}}{\text{cm}^2}}{945.8\frac{\text{mg}}{\text{cm}^2}}\times 2\ \text{MeV} = 1.06\ \text{MeV per electron}$ is the energy deposited in the material using this linear approximation.

Converting the MeV associated with each electron to joules:

250 μA beam (given)

1 A = 1 C/sec

1.6×10^{-19} C/electron (Charge on electron)

$$\frac{1.06\text{ MeV}}{\text{electron}} \times \frac{1.6 \times 10^{-13}\text{ J}}{\text{MeV}} \times \frac{1\text{ electron}}{1.6 \times 10^{-19}\text{ C}} \times 250\ \mu\text{A} \times \frac{1\text{ C / sec}}{1 \times 10^{6}\ \mu\text{A}} = 265\text{ J/sec}$$ is the energy deposited.

Since dose is simply energy deposited per unit mass of material, calculate the mass of the plastic disc:

$d = 1$ cm
$r = 0.5$ cm
Area of plastic = $\pi\, r^2 = \pi \times (0.5)^2 = 0.785\text{ cm}^2$

Calculating the mass:

$$0.785\text{ cm}^2 \times \frac{0.5\text{ g}}{\text{cm}^2} = 0.392\text{ g} = 0.392 \times 10^{-3}\text{ kg}$$

$$\frac{265\dfrac{\text{J}}{\text{sec}}}{0.392 \times 10^{-3}\text{ kg}} \times \frac{1\text{ Gy}}{1\dfrac{\text{J}}{\text{kg}}} = 6.75 \times 10^{5}\text{ Gy/sec}$$

Alternatively, stopping power may also be used to calculate the answer:

$$\text{Stopping power in Lucite} = 1.81\ \frac{\text{MeV}}{\text{g/cm}^2}$$

$$\text{Energy lost in plastic} = 1.81\ \frac{\text{MeV}}{\text{g/cm}^2} \times 0.5\frac{\text{g}}{\text{cm}^2} = 0.905\text{ MeV/e}^-$$

$$\frac{2.5 \times 10^{-4}\ \text{A} \times 1\dfrac{\text{C/s}}{\text{A}} \times \dfrac{1\text{ e}^-}{1.6 \times 10^{-19}\text{ C}} \times 0.905\dfrac{\text{MeV}}{\text{e}^-} \times 1.6 \times 10^{-1}\ \dfrac{\text{J}}{\text{MeV}}}{0.392 \times 10^{-3}\ \text{kg} \times 1\dfrac{\text{J}}{\text{kg}}\Big/\text{Gy}}$$

$= 5.75 \times 10^{5}$ Gy/sec

The different answers are probably due to the fact that range energy equations used in the previous solution are curve fitted experimental equations.

6.21 Calculate the average power density, in watts per kg, of an aqueous solution of ^{60}Co, at a concentration of 10 MBq per liter, in **6.21**

(a) An infinitely large medium,

Cobalt 60 emits a 1.17 MeV and a 1.33 MeV gamma ray with each decay, and a 0.314 MeV (max) energy beta. The average energy of the beta is calculated using the approximation from Chapter 4, by taking one third of the maximum energy:

$$0.314\text{ MeV} \times \frac{1}{3} = 0.1047\text{ MeV (average)}$$

So that the energy that ^{60}Co looses per decay is:
1.17 + 1.33 + 0.1047 = 2.6 MeV

$$\frac{\dfrac{10\text{ MBq}}{\text{L}} \times \dfrac{10^{6}\,\dfrac{\text{trans}}{\text{sec}}}{1\text{ MBq}} \times \dfrac{2.6\text{ MeV}}{\text{trans}} \times \dfrac{1.6\times10^{-13}\text{ J}}{\text{MeV}} \times \dfrac{1\text{ W}}{1\,\dfrac{\text{J}}{\text{sec}}}}{\dfrac{1\text{ kg}}{\text{L (water)}}} = 4.2\times10^{-6}\,\frac{\text{W}}{\text{kg}}$$

(b) a 6 liter spherical tank.

The absorbed energy due to the beta particle is calculated first in the same manner as in part (a);

$$\frac{\dfrac{10\text{ MBq}}{\text{L}} \times \dfrac{10^{6}\,\dfrac{\text{trans}}{\text{sec}}}{1\text{ MBq}} \times \dfrac{0.104\text{ MeV}}{\text{trans}} \times \dfrac{1.6\times10^{-13}\text{ J}}{\text{MeV}} \times \dfrac{1\text{ W}}{1\,\dfrac{\text{J}}{\text{sec}}}}{\dfrac{1\text{ kg}}{\text{L (water)}}} = 1.66\times10^{-7}\,\frac{\text{W}}{\text{kg}}$$

Now calculate the absorbed energy due to the photons, however, some of the photons escape without imparting any energy to the solution. The absorbed fraction of energy is found using table 6.5 and interpolating for a 6 liter (kg) sphere with an average photon energy of 1.25 MeV. A value of ϕ=0.223 is interpolated. So, the average photon energy imparted to the sphere per decay will be:

(1.17MeV + 1.33 MeV) × 0.223 = 0.5575 MeV.

Finding the power density, using the same format as in part (a);

$$\frac{\dfrac{10\text{ MBq}}{\text{L}} \times \dfrac{10^6\,\dfrac{\text{trans}}{\text{sec}}}{1\text{ MBq}} \times \dfrac{0.5575\text{ MeV}}{\text{trans}} \times \dfrac{1.6\times10^{-13}\text{ J}}{\text{MeV}} \times \dfrac{1\text{ W}}{1\dfrac{\text{J}}{\text{sec}}}}{\dfrac{1\text{ kg}}{\text{L (water)}}} = 8.92\times10^{-7}\,\frac{\text{W}}{\text{kg}}$$

Summing the power density from the beta and the gamma–rays;

$8.92\times10^{-7}\,\frac{\text{W}}{\text{kg}} + 1.66\times10^{-7}\,\frac{\text{W}}{\text{kg}} = 1.06\times10^{-6}\,\frac{\text{W}}{\text{kg}}$ is the power density for a 6 liter spherical tank.

6.22

6.22 A 20 liter sealed polyethylene cylinder contains 3700 MBq (100 mCi) ^{137}Cs waste uniformly dispersed in concrete. Neglecting absorption by the cover, estimate the dose rate at the top of the container, and at 1 meter over the top.

$\rho = 2.35\,\frac{\text{g}}{\text{cm}^3}$ (Table 5.2)

$$V_{cylinder} = 20\text{ L}\times\frac{1000\text{ cm}^3}{1\text{ L}} = 2\times10^4\text{ cm}^3$$

$\mu_{concrete} = 0.2\text{ cm}^{-1}$ (Table 5.2)

Energy of ^{137}Cs gamma ray = 0.662 MeV 85% of the time.
The dose rate in an infinite medium can be found first (similar to equation 6.76);

$$\frac{\frac{3.7\times10^{9}\ \text{Bq}}{2\times10^{4}\,\text{cm}^{3}}\times\frac{1\frac{\text{t}}{\text{s}}}{1\ \text{Bq}}\times0.662\frac{\text{MeV}}{\gamma}\times\frac{0.85\ \gamma}{\text{t}}\times1.6\times10^{-6}\frac{\text{erg}}{\text{MeV}}\times3600\frac{\text{s}}{\text{hr}}}{2.35\frac{\text{g}}{\text{cm}^{3}}\times100\frac{\text{ergs}}{\text{g}}\Big/\text{rad}}=2.55\frac{\text{rad}}{\text{hr}}$$

Since the concern is the surface dose rate, half of an infinite medium is a surface, so divide the infinite medium in half to obtain the surface dose rate;

$$2.55\frac{\text{rad}}{\text{hr}}\times0.5=1.27\frac{\text{rad}}{\text{hr}}=12.7\frac{\text{mGy}}{\text{hr}}$$ is the dose rate at the surface.

The dose rate at 1 meter is calculated assuming that the cylinder's diameter is the same as its height:

$d = h$

$$V=\frac{\pi}{4}\times d^{2}\times d$$

$$2\times10^{4}\ \text{cm}^{3}=\frac{\pi}{4}\times d^{2}\times d$$

$d = 29.42$ cm

So the diameter of the 20 liter cylinder is 29.42 cm. Now find the area of the lid:

$$A=\frac{\pi}{4}\times d^{2}=\frac{\pi}{4}\times(29.42\ \text{cm})^{2}=679.8\ \text{cm}^{2}$$

$$C_{V}=\frac{100\ \text{mCi}}{2\times10^{4}\,\text{cm}^{3}}=0.005\frac{\text{mCi}}{\text{cm}^{3}}$$

Absorption coefficient for concrete (Appendix F) and density of concrete (Table 5.2)

$$\mu = 0.029\frac{\text{cm}^2}{\text{g}} = 0.029\frac{\text{cm}^2}{\text{g}} \times 2.35\frac{\text{g}}{\text{cm}^3} = 0.06815\ \text{cm}^{-1}$$

$x = 29.42$ cm height of cylinder

Find the apparent areal concentration of the activity in the 20 liter container by integrating over the volume of the container with respect to height: (equation. 10.14)

$$C_a = \int_0^x C_V e^{-\mu x} dx$$

$$C_a = \frac{C_V}{\mu}\left(1 - e^{-\mu x}\right) = \frac{0.005\frac{\text{mCi}}{\text{cm}^3}}{0.06815\ \text{cm}^{-1}} \times \left(1 - \text{e}^{-0.06815 \times (29.14)}\right) = 0.064\frac{\text{mCi}}{\text{cm}^2}$$

To find the apparent activity on the lid, multiply the surface area of the lid (determined above) by the concentration:

$$0.064\ \frac{\text{mCi}}{\text{cm}^2} \times 679.8\ \text{cm}^2 = 43.16\ \text{mCi}$$

Plane Source Calculation using equation 10.10;

$$\Gamma_{Cs-137} = 0.33\frac{\text{R} \cdot \text{m}^2}{\text{Ci} \cdot \text{hr}} \quad \text{(Table 6.3)}$$

$h = 1$ m
$r = 0.147$ m
$C_a = 0.64$ Ci/m^2

$$\dot{H}_{1\,\text{m}} = \pi \times \Gamma \times C_a \times \ln\left(\frac{r^2 + h^2}{h^2}\right) = \pi \times 0.33\frac{\text{R} \cdot \text{m}^2}{\text{Ci} \cdot \text{hr}} \times 0.64\frac{\text{Ci}}{\text{m}^2} \times \ln\left(\frac{0.147^2 + 1^2}{1^2}\right)$$

$$\dot{H}_{1\,\text{m}} = 0.014\ \text{R/hr} \approx 0.13\ \text{mGy/hr}$$

Alternatively, assuming the apparent activity is approximated by a point source, calculate the dose rate at 1 meter using equation 10.1;

$$\Gamma_{Cs-137} = 0.33\frac{\text{R}\cdot\text{m}^2}{\text{Ci}\cdot\text{hr}} \text{ (Table 6.3)}$$

$s = 1$ m
$n = 43.16$ mCi $= 0.043$ Ci

$$\dot{X} = \frac{n\Gamma}{s^2} = \frac{0.043 \text{ Ci} \times \left(0.33\frac{\text{R}\cdot\text{m}^2}{\text{Ci}\cdot\text{hr}}\right)}{(1 \text{ m})^2} = 0.014\frac{\text{R}}{\text{hr}}$$

Using equation 6.12 to convert to rads;

$$\mu_m/\rho_m = 0.0326 \text{ cm}^2\text{/g (table 5.3)}$$

$$\mu_a/\rho_a = 0.0296 \text{ cm}^2\text{/g (table 5.3)}$$

$$\dot{X} = 0.014\frac{\text{R}}{\text{hr}}$$

$$\text{rads} = \frac{87.7}{100} \times \frac{\mu_m/\rho_m}{\mu_a/\rho_a} \times \text{roentgens} = \frac{87.7}{100} \times \frac{0.0326}{0.0296} \times 0.014\frac{\text{R}}{\text{hr}} = 0.0137\frac{\text{rads}}{\text{hr}}$$

$$\frac{0.0137 \text{ rads}}{\text{hr}} \times \frac{10 \text{ mGy}}{1 \text{ rad}} = 0.14\frac{\text{mGy}}{\text{hr}}$$ is the dose rate at 1 meter from the surface.

Alternative Solution for Surface Dose

Please note that the apparent areal concentration could have also been used to calculate the dose rate on the surface of the lid, rather than assuming an infinite medium. Half of the radiation from the apparent surface activity is assumed to be going up, and half down. The surface dose rate is given by the following equation:

$$\dot{D}=\frac{1}{2}\times\frac{C_a\dfrac{\text{mCi}}{\text{cm}^2}\times\dfrac{3.7\times10^7\,\frac{\text{t}}{\text{s}}}{1\text{ mCi}}\times f\dfrac{\gamma}{\text{t}}\times E\dfrac{\text{MeV}}{\gamma}\times1.6\times10^{-6}\dfrac{\text{erg}}{\text{MeV}}\times\mu_{en_{muscle}}\dfrac{\text{cm}^2}{\text{g}}\times36}{100\dfrac{\text{ergs}}{\text{g}}\Big/\text{rad}}$$

$$\frac{1}{2}\times\frac{0.064\dfrac{\text{mCi}}{\text{cm}^2}\times\dfrac{3.7\times10^7\,\frac{\text{t}}{\text{s}}}{1\text{Ci}}\times0.85\dfrac{\gamma}{\text{t}}\times0.662\dfrac{\text{MeV}}{\gamma}\times1.6\times10^{-6}\dfrac{\text{erg}}{\text{MeV}}\times0.032\dfrac{\text{cm}^2}{\text{g}}\times36}{100\dfrac{\text{ergs}}{\text{g}}\Big/\text{rad}}$$

$=1.22\dfrac{\text{rads}}{\text{hr}}$ is the estimated dose rate on the surface of the container (calculated using the apparent areal concentration)

It can be seen that the 1.22 rads/hr obtained here compares favorably with the 1.27 rads/hr calculated using an infinite medium (within 5% of each other).

6.23

6.23 A nuclear bomb is exploded at an altitude of 200 m. Assuming 10^{18} fissions, in the explosion, 6 fission gammas of 1 MeV each and 2 prompt neutrons of 2 MeV each, estimate the dose from the gammas and from the neutrons at 1500 m from ground zero. Neglect the shielding effect of the air and scattering from the ground.

The distance from the explosion to a point 1500 meters away is:

$$\sqrt{1500^2+200^2}=1513.3\text{ m}$$

Calculating the gamma dose first using equation 6.10;

$$\phi=\frac{10^{18}\text{ fissions}}{4\times\pi\times(1513.3\text{ m})^2}\times\frac{6\,\gamma}{\text{fission}}\times\frac{1\text{ m}^2}{1.0\times10^4\text{cm}^2}=2.08\times10^7\,\frac{\gamma}{\text{cm}^2}$$

$$\mu_m=0.0308\frac{\text{cm}^2}{\text{g}}$$

$$D_\gamma = \frac{\phi \frac{\gamma}{\text{cm}^2} E \frac{\text{MeV}}{\gamma} 1.6 \times 10^{-13} \frac{\text{J}}{\text{MeV}} \mu_m \frac{\text{cm}^2}{\text{g}} \times 10^3 \frac{\text{g}}{\text{kg}}}{\frac{\text{J}/\text{kg}}{\text{Gy}}}$$

$$D_\gamma =$$

$$\frac{2.08 \times 10^7 \frac{\gamma}{\text{cm}^2} \times 1.0 \frac{\text{MeV}}{\gamma} \times 1.6 \times 10^{-13} \frac{\text{J}}{\text{MeV}} \times 0.0308 \frac{\text{cm}^2}{\text{g}} \times 10^3 \times 1}{0.001 \frac{\text{kg}}{\text{cm}^3} \times \frac{\text{J}/\text{kg}}{\text{Gy}}}$$

$= 1 \times 10^{-4}$ Gy γ

Next, calculate the neutron dose. The scattering cross sections for 2 MeV neutrons are approximately the same as for 5 MeV neutrons (cross sections are relatively constant between 1 and 10 MeV). Using the information from example 6.16 and N and f from table 6.12, Synthetic Tissue Composition:

Element	σ cm²/atom	N, atoms/kg	f	$N\sigma f$
O	1.55×10^{-24}	2.69E+25	0.111	4.628
C	1.65×10^{-24}	6.41E+24	0.142	1.502
H	1.50×10^{-24}	5.98E+25	0.5	44.85
N	1.00×10^{-24}	1.49E+24	0.124	0.1848
Na	2.3×10^{-24}	3.93E+22	0.08	0.007231
Cl	2.8×10^{-24}	1.70E+22	0.053	0.002523
			sum	51.17

$$\sum_i N_i \sigma_i f_i = 51.17 \frac{\text{cm}^2}{\text{kg}}$$

$$\phi = \frac{10^{18} \text{ fissions}}{4 \times \pi \times (1513.3 \text{ m})^2} \times \frac{3 \text{ neutrons}}{\text{fission}} \times \frac{1 \text{ m}^2}{1.0 \times 10^4 \text{ cm}^2} = 1.04 \times 10^7 \frac{\text{neutrons}}{\text{cm}^2}$$

Equation 6.103;

$$D = \frac{\phi(E) E \sum_i N_i \sigma_i f_i}{1 \, \mathrm{J/kg} \cdot \mathrm{Gy}}$$

$$D = \frac{1.04 \times 10^7 \, \frac{\text{neutrons}}{\text{cm}^2} \times 2 \text{ MeV} \times 1.6 \times 10^{-13} \, \frac{\text{J}}{\text{MeV}} \times 51.17 \, \frac{\text{cm}^2}{\text{kg}}}{1 \, \mathrm{J/kg} \cdot \mathrm{Gy}} = 1.7 \times 10^{-4} \text{Gy}$$

neutron dose

6.24

6.24 An unmarked, unshielded vial containing 370 MBq (10 mCi) ^{24}Na is left in a hood. A radiochemist not knowing of the presence of the ^{24}Na, spends 8 hours at his bench, which is 2 meters from the ^{24}Na. Based on the ^{24}Na transformation scheme shown in problem 6.5, calculate
(a) the dose rate at 2 meters from the 370 MBq source.

(Equation 10.1)
$A = 10$ mCi
$d = 2$ meters

$$\Gamma = 1.84 \, \frac{\mathrm{R \cdot m^2}}{\mathrm{Ci \cdot hr}} \text{ (table 6.3)}$$

$$\dot{X} = \frac{\Gamma A}{d^2} = \frac{1.84 \frac{\mathrm{R \cdot m^2}}{\mathrm{Ci \cdot hr}} \times 10 \text{ mCi} \times \frac{1 \text{ Ci}}{10^3 \text{ mCi}}}{(2\text{m})^2} = 4.6 \times 10^{-3} \text{ R/hr} = 0.046 \text{ mGy/hr is}$$

the initial dose rate.

(b) The dose commitment from the 8–hour exposure.

^{24}Na decays with a half life of 15 hours. The dose rate therefore is continuously changing. The total dose is therefore;

$$D = \int \dot{D}(t) \cdot dt = \int_0^{8 \text{ hr}} \dot{D}_0 \cdot e^{-\lambda t} dt = \frac{\dot{D}_0}{\lambda}\left(1 - e^{-\lambda t}\right) = \frac{0.046 \frac{\text{mGy}}{\text{hr}}}{\left(\frac{0.693}{15 \text{ hr}}\right)}\left(1 - e^{-\frac{0.693}{15 \text{ hr}} \times 8 \text{ hr}}\right)$$

$D = 0.31$ mGy

6.25 Chlormerodrin tagged either with ^{197}Hg or ^{203}Hg is used diagnostically in studies of renal function. Calculate the dose to the kidneys, for the case of normal uptake, from injection of 3.7 MBq (100μCi) of each of the radioisotopes. Assume very rapid kidney deposition, followed by unusually rapid elimination with a biological half time of 6.5 hours. **6.25**

Calculating ^{197}Hg first:

Table 6.11 gives information on how much Hg will be deposited in the kidneys, and with normal uptake, 35% (0.35) of the injected activity will be deposited in the kidneys.

$A_S(0) = (0.35) \times 3.7 \text{ MBq} = 1.295 \text{ MBq} = 1.3 \times 10^6 \text{ Bq}$

The biological half life is given in the question, so calculating the effective half life for ^{197}Hg using equation 6.54:

$T_R = 65$ hr
$T_B = 6.5$ hours

$$T_E = \frac{T_R T_B}{T_R + T_B} = \frac{65 \text{ hr} \times 6.5 \text{ hr}}{65 \text{ hr} + 6.5 \text{ hr}} = 5.9 \text{ hr}$$

Finding the effective elimination constant by equation 6.52:

$$\lambda_E = \frac{0.693}{T_E} = \frac{0.693}{5.9 \text{ hr}} = 0.117 \text{ hr}^{-1}$$

The cumulated activity is found with equation 6.91;

$$\tilde{A}(\text{kid}) = \frac{A_S(0)}{\lambda_E} = \frac{1.3 \times 10^6 \text{ Bq}}{0.117 \text{ hr}^{-1} \times \dfrac{1 \text{ hr}}{3600 \text{ sec}}} = 4 \times 10^{10} \text{ Bq·sec}$$

Find the value now for S (kidneys←kidneys) from NM/MIRD Pamphlet No. 11, "S," Absorbed Dose per Unit Cumulated Activity for Selected Radionuclides and Organs, Oct. 1975, page 246 and 247 to calculate the dose to the kidneys from the activity deposited in the kidneys;

$$S\,(\text{kidneys}\leftarrow\text{kidneys}) = 5.5 \times 10^{-4}\frac{\text{rad}}{\mu\text{Ci}-\text{hr}}$$

Converting units:

S (kidneys←kidneys) =

$$\frac{5.5\times10^{-4}\text{ rad}}{\mu\text{Ci}\cdot\text{hr}}\times\frac{1\text{ Gy}}{100\text{ rad}}\times\frac{1\ \mu\text{Ci}}{3.7\times10^{4}\text{ Bq}}\times\frac{1\text{ hr}}{3600\text{ sec}}=4.13\times10^{-14}\frac{\text{Gy}}{\text{Bq}\cdot\text{sec}}$$

Now substitute the values in equation 6.97 to find the dose to the kidneys from the activity deposited into the kidneys;

$$D\left(r_k \leftarrow r_h\right) = \tilde{A}_h \times S\left(r_k \leftarrow r_h\right)$$

$$D\,(\text{kidneys}\leftarrow\text{kidneys}) = \tilde{A}_{kidneys} \times S\left(\text{kidneys} \leftarrow \text{kidneys}\right)$$

$$D\,(\text{kidneys}\leftarrow\text{kidneys}) = 4 \times 10^{10}\text{ Bq}\cdot\text{sec} \times \left(4.13\times10^{-14}\frac{\text{Gy}}{\text{Bq}\cdot\text{sec}}\right)$$

D (kidneys←kidneys) = 1.65×10^{-3}Gy is the dose to the kidneys from activity deposited in the kidneys.

Table 6.11 shows that although activity is deposited in the kidneys, it is also deposited in the liver, spleen and whole body in significant quantities. They also contribute dose to the kidneys from the activity deposited in these other places. The spleen will be ignored in this problem since the deposition in it is so small (0.02). Calculating the dose from the liver to the kidneys {S (kidneys←liver)} next:
From table 6.11, 15% (0.15) of the activity deposited into the liver:

$A_S(0) = (0.15) \times 3.7\text{ MBq} = 0.555\text{ MBq} = 5.55 \times 10^5\text{ Bq}$

From Table 6.11, we find the biological half life of Hg in the liver to be 324 hours (13.5 days). Therefore,

$$T_E = \frac{65\text{ h}\times324\text{ h}}{65\text{ h}+324\text{ h}} = 54\text{ h} \text{ and}$$

$$\lambda_E = \frac{0.693}{T_E} = \frac{0.693}{54\ \text{h}} = 0.0128\ \text{h}^{-1}$$

The cumulated activity (equation 6.91) is

$$\tilde{A}(\text{liver}) = \frac{A_{liver}(0)}{\lambda_E} = \frac{5.55 \times 10^5\ \text{Bq}}{0.0128\ \text{h}^{-1} \times \dfrac{1\ \text{h}}{3600\ \text{sec}}} = 1.56 \times 10^{11}\ \text{Bq·sec}$$

To calculate the dose to the kidneys from the activity deposited in the kidneys, first find the value for S(kidneys←liver) from NM/MIRD Pamphlet No. 11, "S," Absorbed Dose per Unit Cumulated Activity for Selected Radionuclides and Organs, Oct. 1975, page 246 and 247.

$$S\ (\text{kidneys} \leftarrow \text{liver}) = 2.7 \times 10^{-6} \frac{\text{rad}}{\mu\text{Ci} \cdot \text{hr}} = 2.03 \times 10^{-16} \frac{\text{Gy}}{\text{Bq} \cdot \text{sec}}$$

Now substitute the values in equation 6.97 to find the dose to the kidneys from the activity deposited into the liver;

$$D\left(r_k \leftarrow r_h\right) = \tilde{A}_h \times S\left(r_k \leftarrow r_h\right)$$

$$D\ (\text{kidneys} \leftarrow \text{liver}) = \tilde{A}_{liver} \times S\left(\text{kidneys} \leftarrow \text{liver}\right)$$

$$D\ (\text{kidneys} \leftarrow \text{liver}) = 1.56 \times 10^{11}\ \text{Bq·sec} \times \left(2.03 \times 10^{-16} \frac{\text{Gy}}{\text{Bq} \cdot \text{sec}}\right) = 3.17 \times 10^{-5}\ \text{Gy}$$

is the dose to the kidneys from the ^{197}Hg in the liver.

Calculating the dose from the total body ^{197}Hg to the kidneys {S (kidneys←body)}:

According to Table 6.11, if 35% + 15% + 2% are deposited in the kidneys, liver, and spleen, then 48% of 3.7 MBq or 1.8×10^6 Bq are distributed throughout the body. The biological half life in the body is given as 240 hours (10 days). The effective half life in the body is

$$T_E = \frac{65\ \text{h} \times 240\ \text{h}}{65\ \text{h} + 240\ \text{h}} = 51\ \text{h} \ \text{ and}$$

$$\lambda_E = \frac{0.693}{T_E} = \frac{0.693}{51\ \text{h}} = 0.0136\ \text{h}^{-1}$$

The cumulated activity in the body is

$$\tilde{A}(\text{body}) = \frac{A_{body}(0)}{\lambda_E} = \frac{1.8 \times 10^6\ \text{Bq}}{0.0136\ \text{hr}^{-1}} = 4.765 \times 10^{11}\ \text{Bq·sec}$$

Find the value now for S(kidneys←body) from NM/MIRD Pamphlet No. 11, "S," Absorbed Dose per Unit Cumulated Activity for Selected Radionuclides and Organs, Oct. 1975, page 246 and 247 to calculate the dose to the kidneys from the activity deposited in the body;

$$S\ (\text{kidneys} \leftarrow \text{body}) = 3.3 \times 10^{-6} \frac{\text{rad}}{\mu\text{Ci} \cdot \text{hr}} = 2.48 \times 10^{-16} \frac{\text{Gy}}{\text{Bq} \cdot \text{sec}}$$

Now substitute the values in equation 6.97 to find the dose to the kidneys from the activity deposited into the body;

$$D\left(r_k \leftarrow r_h\right) = \tilde{A}_h \times S\left(r_k \leftarrow r_h\right)$$

$$D\ (\text{kidneys} \leftarrow \text{body}) = \tilde{A}_{body} \times S\ (\text{kidneys} \leftarrow \text{body})$$

$$D\ (\text{kidneys} \leftarrow \text{body}) = 4.765 \times 10^{11}\ \text{Bq·sec} \times 2.48 \times 10^{-16} \frac{\text{Gy}}{\text{Bq} \cdot \text{sec}}$$

$$D\ (\text{kidneys} \leftarrow \text{body}) = 1.182 \times 10^{-4}\ \text{Gy}$$

Adding the doses together:

1.65×10^{-3} Gy (kidney←kidney) + 3.17×10^{-5} Gy (kidney←liver)+ + 1.18×10^{-4} Gy (kidney←body) = 1.80×10^{-3} Gy to the kidneys

$$1.8 \times 10^{-3}\ \text{Gy} \times \frac{1 \times 10^5\ \text{mrad}}{\text{Gy}} = 180 \text{ mrads to kidneys from the 3.7 MBq } {}^{197}\text{Hg}$$

tagged chlormerodrin.

Since the deposition in other organs is not listed or small, they do not contribute significantly to the dose to the kidneys. Even if the dose from the liver had been omitted the net dose would not have changed significantly.

Now calculate the dose from the same quantity of ^{203}Hg activity to the kidneys using the same format and equations:

Table 6.11 shows that 35% (0.35) of the injected activity will be deposited in the kidneys.

$A_S(0) = (0.35) \times 3.7$ MBq $= 1.295$ MBq $= 1.3 \times 10^6$ Bq

Using the abnormally short biological half life given in the question, the effective half life for ^{203}Hg, using equation 6.54 is:

$T_R = 46.9$ days $= 1125.6$ hr (fig 6.13)
$T_B = 6.5$ hours

$$T_E = \frac{T_R T_B}{T_R + T_B} = \frac{1125.6\ \text{hr} \times 6.5\ \text{hr}}{1125.6\ \text{hr} + 6.5\ \text{hr}} = 6.46\ \text{hr}$$

Finding the effective elimination constant with equation 6.54:

$$\lambda_E = \frac{0.693}{T_E} = \frac{0.693}{6.46\ \text{hr}} = 0.107\ \text{hr}^{-1}$$

Placing values into equation 6.91 to find the cumulated activity;

$$\tilde{A}(\text{kid}) = \frac{A_S(0)}{\lambda_E} = \frac{1.3 \times 10^6\ \text{Bq}}{0.107 \frac{1}{\text{hr}} \times \frac{1\ \text{hr}}{3600\ \text{sec}}} = 4.37 \times 10^{10}\ \text{Bq·sec}$$

Find the value now for S (kidneys←kidneys) from table 6.9 to calculate the dose to the kidneys from the activity deposited in the kidneys;

$$S\text{ (kidneys}\leftarrow\text{kidneys)} = 8.1 \times 10^{-4}\frac{\text{rad}}{\mu\text{Ci}\cdot\text{hr}} = 6.08\times10^{-14}\ \frac{\text{Gy}}{\text{Bq}\cdot\text{sec}}$$

Now substitute these values into equation 6.97 to find the dose to the kidneys from the activity deposited into the kidneys;

$$D\left(r_k \leftarrow r_h\right) = \tilde{A}_h \times S\left(r_k \leftarrow r_h\right)$$

$$D\text{ (kidneys}\leftarrow\text{kidneys)} = \tilde{A}_{\text{kidneys}} \times S\text{ (kidneys}\leftarrow\text{kidneys)}$$

$$D\text{ (kidneys}\leftarrow\text{kidneys)} = 4.37 \times 10^{10}\ \text{Bq}\cdot\text{sec} \times \left(6.08\times10^{-14}\ \frac{\text{Gy}}{\text{Bq}\cdot\text{sec}}\right)$$

$$D\text{ (kidneys}\leftarrow\text{kidneys)} = 2.66 \times 10^{-3}\ \text{Gy} = 266\ \text{mrads}$$

The contributions of the ^{203}Hg activity in the liver and body to the total dose to the kidneys are calculated in the same manner as for ^{197}Hg. For each of these compartments, as well as for the kidneys (whose calculations are detailed above), the numerical values for the parameters were calculated in the same manner as for ^{197}Hg, and are tabulated below

Day	Total	Long lived	Short lived
0	4	2.2	1.8
1	2.94	1.97	0.97
2	2.32	1.77	0.55
3	1.9	1.58	0.32
4	1.6	1.42	0.18
5	1.4	1.27	0.13

The total dose to the kidneys from the 3.7 MBq ^{203}Hg chlormerodrin is the sum of the contributions from each compartment, 3.89×10^{3} Gy, or 389 mrads.

^{197}Hg dose to kidneys = 180 mrads
^{201}Hg dose to kidneys = 389 mrads

6.26 A nuclear medicine procedure used to evaluate pulmanary perfusion uses intravenously injected ^{99m}Tc tagged microspheres that are rapidly taken up by the lungs, where they are temporarily trapped in a small fraction of the capillaries. Absence of radioactivity in a part of the lung means decreased perfusion of that part, and suggests a possible pulmonary embolism. Some 60% of the ^{99m}Tc activity is transferred out of the lung with a biological $T_{1/2}$ of 1.8 hours, and the other 40% has a biological $T_{1/2}$ of 36 hours. **6.26**

(a) What is the mean intrapulmonary residence time of the ^{99m}Tc?

First calculate the effective half life of each compartment using equation 6.54:

Transferred out of the lung (60%)

$T_B = 1.8$ hr
$T_R = 6$ hr

$$T_E = \frac{T_R T_B}{T_R + T_B} = \frac{6 \text{ hr} \times 1.8 \text{ hr}}{6 \text{ hr} + 1.8 \text{ hr}} = 1.385 \text{ hr}$$

Since this is the effective half life of 60%,

1.385 hr × 0.60 = 0.831 hr is the "weighted" effective half life for this compartment.

The "other" 40%;

$T_B = 36$ hr
$T_R = 6$ hr

$$T_E = \frac{T_R T_B}{T_R + T_B} = \frac{6 \text{ hr} \times 36 \text{ hr}}{6 \text{ hr} + 36 \text{ hr}} = 5.143 \text{ hr}$$

Since this is the effective half life of 40%,

5.143 × 0.40 = 2.0572 hr is the "weighted" effective half life for this compartment.

Combining the two "weighted" half times:

0.831 hr + 2.0572 hr = 2.89 hr

However, the mean time is found by equation 4.24:

$$\bar{t} = \frac{1}{\lambda_{eff}} = \frac{1}{0.693/T_E} = \frac{T_E}{0.693} = \frac{2.89\ \text{hr}}{0.693} = 4.16\ \text{hr is the mean intrapulmonary}$$

residence time.

(b) What is the dose to the lung from the intrapulmonary activity per MBq injected?

$$1\ \text{MBq} \times \frac{1\times 10^6\ \text{Bq}}{1\ \text{MBq}} \times \frac{1\times 10^6\ \mu\text{Ci}}{3.7\times 10^{10}\ \text{Bq}} = 27\ \mu\text{Ci}$$

$\tilde{A}$ = activity × mean residence time = 27 μCi × 4.159 hr = 112.3 μCi·hr

From NM/MIRD Pamphlet No. 11, October, 1975, page150, for ^{99m}Tc, or using Table 6.10;

$$S\ (\text{lung}\leftarrow\text{lung}) = 5.2 \times 10^{-5} \frac{\text{rad}}{\mu\text{Ci}\cdot\text{hr}}$$

Using equation 6.97 with the above values:

$$D(\text{lung}\leftarrow\text{lung}) = \tilde{A} \times S(\text{lung}\leftarrow\text{lung})$$

$$D(\text{lung}\leftarrow\text{lung}) = (112.3\ \mu\text{Ci}\cdot\text{hr}) \times 5.2 \times 10^{-5} \frac{\text{rad}}{\mu\text{Ci}\cdot\text{hr}} = 5.84 \times 10^{-3}\ \text{rad}$$

$$D(\text{lung}\leftarrow\text{lung}) = 5.84\ \text{mrad} = 58.4\ \mu\text{Gy}$$

6.27 **6.27** Three mCi ^{99m}Tc labeled sulfur colloid is injected to visualize the liver. 60% of the injectate is deposited in the liver, 30% in the spleen, and 10% in the red bone marrow. Calculate the absorbed dose to:

(a) the liver

The radiological half life , T_R, for ^{99m}Tc = 6 hours. This is very much less than the biological half time in these organs (ICRP 53), therefore, $T_E = T_R$, and

$$\lambda_E = \frac{0.693}{T_E} = \frac{0.693}{6\ \text{h}} = 0.12\ \text{h}^{-1}$$

a. Dose to liver

Since the 3,000 μCi (3 mCi) are injected, and 60% is deposited in the liver, 0.6 × 3000 μCi = 1800 μCi are deposited in the liver.

The radiation dose, in traditional units, is given by equation 6.100

$$D(\text{target}) = \frac{A_0(\text{source})\ \mu\text{Ci}}{\lambda_E\ \text{h}^{-1}} \times S(\text{target} \leftarrow \text{source}) \frac{\text{rad}}{\mu\text{Ci} \cdot \text{hr}}$$

S (liver←liver) $= 4.6 \times 10^{-5} \frac{\text{rad}}{\mu\text{Ci} \cdot \text{hr}}$ for ^{99m}Tc is found in Table 6.10

$$D(\text{liver} \leftarrow \text{liver}) = \frac{0.6 \times 3000\ \mu\text{Ci}}{0.12\ \text{h}^{-1}} \times 4.6 \times 10^{-5} \frac{\text{rad}}{\mu\text{Ci} \cdot \text{hr}} = 0.690\ \text{rad}$$

The spleen's contribution to the liver dose is

$$D(\text{liver} \leftarrow \text{spleen}) = \frac{A_0(\text{spleen})\ \mu\text{Ci}}{\lambda_E\ \text{h}^{-1}} \times S(\text{liver} \leftarrow \text{spleen}) \frac{\text{rad}}{\mu\text{Ci} \cdot \text{hr}}$$

$$D(\text{liver} \leftarrow \text{spleen}) = \frac{0.3 \times 3000\ \mu\text{Ci}}{0.12\ \text{h}^{-1}} \times 9.8 \times 10^{-7} \frac{\text{rad}}{\mu\text{Ci} \cdot \text{hr}} = 7.35 \times 10^{-3}\ \text{rad}$$

The red bone marrow's (RBM) contribution to the liver dose is

$$D(\text{liver} \leftarrow \text{RBM}) = \frac{A_0(\text{RBM})\ \mu\text{Ci}}{\lambda_E\ \text{h}^{-1}} \times S(\text{liver} \leftarrow \text{RBM}) \frac{\text{rad}}{\mu\text{Ci} \cdot \text{hr}}$$

$$D(\text{liver} \leftarrow \text{RBM}) = \frac{0.1 \times 3000\ \mu\text{Ci}}{0.12\ \text{h}^{-1}} \times 9.2 \times 10^{-7} \frac{\text{rad}}{\mu\text{Ci} \cdot \text{hr}} = 2.3 \times 10^{-3}\ \text{rad}$$

D (Liver) = 0.690 + 0.0074 + 0.0023 = 0.7 rad

The dose to the spleen and to the RBM is calculated in a similar manner, using the parameter values and the results tabulated below:

Liver as target (liver←source)

Source	Activity, μCi	λ_E, h^{-1}	$S\ \frac{rad}{\mu Ci \cdot h}$	Dose, rad
Liver	1800	0.12	4.6×10^{-5}	0.6900
spleen	900	0.12	9.8×10^{-7}	0.0074
RBM	300	0.12	9.2×10^{-7}	0.0023
			Dose(liver)	0.7

(b)

Spleen as target (spleen←source)

Source	Activity, μCi	λ_E, h^{-1}	$S\ \frac{rad}{\mu Ci \cdot h}$	Dose, rad
Liver	1800	0.12	9.2×10^{-7}	0.0138
spleen	900	0.12	3.3×10^{-4}	2.4750
RBM	300	0.12	9.2×10^{-7}	0.0023
			Dose(spleen)	2.5

(c)

RBM as target (RBM←source)

Source	Activity, μCi	λ_E, h^{-1}	$S\ \frac{rad}{\mu Ci \cdot h}$	Dose, rad
Liver	1800	0.12	1.6×10^{-6}	0.0240
spleen	900	0.12	1.7×10^{-6}	0.0128
RBM	300	0.12	3.1×10^{-5}	0.0775
			Dose(spleen)	0.1

6.28

6.28 A patient is treated for Graves disease with 111 MBq (3 mCi) I-131. Uptake studies with a tracer dose of I-125 showed a thyroid uptake of 60% and a biological $T_{1/2}$ = 2 days. Assuming a very rapid thyroid uptake, calculate the dose to the thyroid from this treatment.

First calculate the effective half life using equation 6.54:

$T_B = 2$ d
$T_R = 8.05$ d

$$T_E = \frac{T_R T_B}{T_R + T_B} = \frac{8.05\text{ d} \times 2\text{ d}}{8.05\text{ d} + 2\text{ d}} = 1.6\text{ d} = 38.45\text{ hr}$$

Find the effective clearance constant for the thyroid with equation 4.21;

$$\lambda_{eff} = \frac{0.693}{T} = \frac{0.693}{38.45\text{ hr}} = 1.8 \times 10^{-2}\text{ hr}^{-1}$$

Equation 6.91 is used to find $\tilde{A}$;

$$\tilde{A} = \frac{\text{activity} \times \text{fraction depos.}}{\lambda} = \frac{\left(3\text{ mCi} \times \frac{1 \times 10^3\,\mu\text{Ci}}{1\text{ mCi}}\right) \times 0.6}{1.8 \times 10^{-2}\text{ hr}^{-1}} = 1 \times 10^5\ \mu\text{Ci·hr}$$

$$S\text{ (thyroid}\leftarrow\text{thyroid)} = 2.2 \times 10^{-2}\ \frac{\text{rad}}{\mu\text{Ci} \cdot \text{hr}}\ \text{(From MIRD pamphlet 11)}$$

Putting values into equation 6.97;

$$D\text{ (thyroid}\leftarrow\text{thyroid)} = \tilde{A} \times S\text{ (thyroid}\leftarrow\text{thyroid)}$$

$$D\text{ (thyroid}\leftarrow\text{thyroid)} = 1 \times 10^5\mu\text{Ci·hr} \times \left(2.2 \times 10^{-2}\ \frac{\text{rad}}{\mu\text{Ci} \cdot \text{hr}}\right) = 2200\text{ rads} = 22\text{ Gy}$$

is the dose to the thyroid.

An alternative method is to calculate the initial dose rate, $\dot{D}_0$, using the effective energy deposited in the thyroid as calculated in Chapter 6, 0.227 MeV per transformation for ^{131}I, and the mass of the thyroid, 20 grams, and a 60% deposition:

$$\dot{D} = \frac{\frac{60}{100} \times 111\text{ MBq} \times \frac{1 \times 10^6\text{ t}}{\text{sec}} \times \frac{0.227\text{ Mev}}{\text{t}} \times \frac{1.6 \times 10^{-13}\text{ J}}{\text{MeV}} \times \frac{3600\text{ sec}}{\text{hr}}}{20\text{ g} \times \frac{1\text{ kg}}{1000\text{ g}} \times \frac{1\text{ J}/\text{kg}}{\text{Gy}}} = 0.44\ \frac{\text{Gy}}{\text{hr}}$$

The total dose is then found using the effective elimination constant calculated earlier:

$$D = \frac{\dot{D}}{\lambda_{eff}} = \frac{0.44 \frac{\text{Gy}}{\text{hr}}}{1.8 \times 10^{-2}\ \text{hr}^{-1}} = 24\ \text{Gy}$$

This is close to the value calculated more formally of 22 Gy.

6.29

6.29 A well insulated water sample is irradiated with gamma rays at a rate of 10 Gy (1000 rads) per hour. What is the rate of temperature rise in the water, °C/hr.

$$1\frac{\text{Gy}}{\text{hr}} = \frac{1\ \text{J}/\text{kg}}{\text{hr}} \text{ by definition.}$$

The specific heat of water is 1°C/10^3cal/kg

$$10\ \text{Gy} \times \frac{\frac{1\ \text{J}/\text{kg}}{\text{hr}}}{\text{Gy}} \times \frac{1\ \text{cal}}{4.186\ \text{J}} \times \frac{1^\circ\ \text{C}}{1 \times 10^3\ \text{cal}/\text{kg}} = 2.4 \times 10^{-3}\ \frac{^\circ\text{C}}{\text{hr}}$$

6.30

6.30 A laboratory worker who weighs 70 kg was accidentally exposed for several hours in an atmosphere containing tritiated water vapor. Urine analysis for tritium were made for 7 weeks, starting 1 day after exposure, and the following data were obtained on a 24 h urine samples:

Day	1	2	3	5	7	10	14	21	28	35	42	49
Bq	524	485	450	402	342	293	227	147	94	60	40	26

According to reference man, 47% of the daily water output is via the urine. Assuming that the tritium is uniformly distributed throughout the body's water,

(a) plot the data and write the equation for the clearance curve,

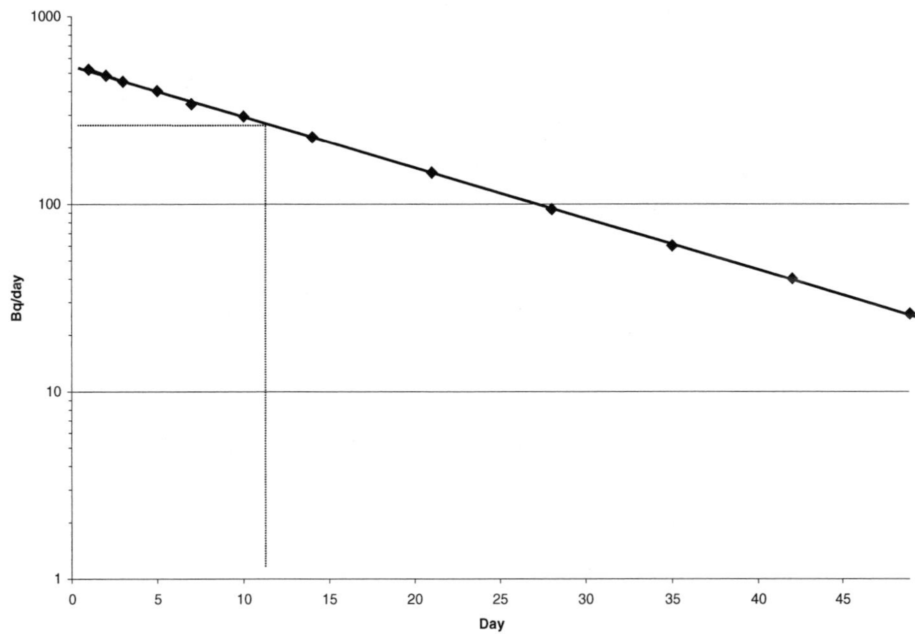

The clearance curve, when plotted on semi-log paper, forms a straight line. Therefore, the equation of the curve is

$$A\,(t) = A_0\, e^{-\lambda t}$$

By extrapolating the line to $t = 0$, A_0 is found to be 555 Bq/day. The clearance half time is found from the graph to be 10.8 days. The slope of the curve, λ, is

$$\lambda = \frac{0.693}{T_{1/2}} = \frac{0.693}{10.8\ \text{d}} = 0.064\ \text{d}^{-1}$$

The equation for the clearance curve is

$$\dot{A}(t) = 555e^{-0.064t}\ \text{Bq / day}$$

(b) calculate the worker's dose commitment from this accidental exposure.

To calculate the dose commitment from this accidental exposure from basic principles with equation 6.47, where $\overline{E}\,(^3\text{H}) = 5.7 \times 10^{-3}$ MeV/transformation:

Since 47 % of the daily water output is via the urine, the total extrapolated initial daily water output is

$$\dot{A}_0 = \frac{555\text{ Bq}}{0.47} = 1181\text{ Bq/day}.$$

The total amount of ^{3}H that was absorbed is equal to the total excreted, which is given by the area under the clearance curve.

$$A = \int_0^\infty \dot{A}(t)dt = \dot{A}_0 \int_0^\infty e^{-\lambda t}dt = \frac{\dot{A}_0}{\lambda} = \frac{1181\frac{\text{Bq}}{\text{d}}}{0.064\text{ d}^{-1}} = 1.85 \times 10^4\text{ Bq}$$

The initial dose rate due to this ^{3}H activity is

$$\dot{D}_0 = \frac{q\text{ Bq} \times \frac{1\text{ t}}{\text{sec}}\Big/\text{Bq} \times \overline{E}\frac{\text{MeV}}{\text{t}} \times \frac{1.6 \times 10^{-13}\text{ J}}{\text{MeV}} \times \frac{86400\text{ sec}}{\text{day}}}{m\text{ kg} \times 1\text{ J}\Big/\text{kg}\Big/\text{Gy}} = \frac{\text{Gy}}{\text{day}}$$

$$\dot{D}_0 = \frac{1.85 \times 10^4\text{ Bq} \times \frac{1\text{ t}}{\text{sec}}\Big/\text{Bq} \times \frac{5.7 \times 10^{-3}\text{ Mev}}{\text{t}} \times \frac{1.6 \times 10^{-13}\text{ J}}{\text{MeV}} \times \frac{86400\text{ sec}}{\text{day}}}{70\text{ kg} \times 1\text{ J}\Big/\text{kg}\Big/\text{Gy}}$$

$$\dot{D}_0 = 2.1 \times 10^{-8}\ \frac{\text{Gy}}{\text{day}}$$

Now find the dose commitment using equation 6.58:

$\dot{D}_0 = 2.1 \times 10^{-8}$ Gy/day

$\lambda_E = 0.064\text{ d}^{-1}$ (see part a)

$$D = \frac{\dot{D}_0}{\lambda_E} = \frac{2.1 \times 10^{-8}\frac{\text{Gy}}{\text{d}}}{0.064\text{ d}^{-1}} = 3.4 \times 10^{-7}\text{ Gy} = 0.034\text{ mrad}$$

Solutions for Chapter 9

HEALTH PHYSICS INSTRUMENTATION

9.1 If a certain counting standard has a mean activity of 400 cpm, **9.1**
(a) What is the probability of observing exactly 400 counts in one minute?

Find the standard deviation of 400 counts in one minute. Since we can approximate this using the Poisson distribution, equation 9.36 is used:

$\bar{n} = 400$

$\sigma = \sqrt{\bar{n}} = \sqrt{400} = 20$

Use equation 9.31 to obtain the probability of exactly 400 counts in one minute.

$\bar{n} = 400$
$\sigma = 20$

$$p(n) = \frac{1}{\sigma\sqrt{2\pi}} e^{-(n-\bar{n})^2/2\sigma^2} = p(400) = \frac{1}{20 \times \sqrt{2\pi}} e^{-(400-400)^2/2(20)^2} = 0.02$$

(b) What is the probability of measuring 390 - 410 counts in 1 minute?

Calculate the number of standard deviations away 410 is from the mean, using equation 9.49;

$\bar{n} = 400$
$\sigma = 20$ (from part a)

$t = \dfrac{n-\bar{n}}{\sigma} = \dfrac{410-400}{20} = 0.5$ is the number of standard deviations from the mean.

Look this number up in a table of values, the area under the normal distribution curve from the mean to 0.5 standard deviations away is 0.1915.

Calculating t for 390,

$$t = \frac{390 - 400}{20} = -0.5$$

Since the normal curve is symmetric, the area is the same, 0.1915. The probability of a count between 390 and 410 is given by the area under the normal curve between -0.5σ and $+0.5\sigma = 0.38$

9.2

9.2 A sample counted 560 counts in 10 min., while the background counted 390 counts in 15 minutes.

(a) What is the standard deviation of the gross and background counting rates?

$n_g = 560$
$t_g = 10$

Equation 9.37 gives us the solution:

$$r \pm \sigma_r = \frac{n}{t} \pm \frac{\sqrt{n}}{t}$$

$$r_g \pm \sigma_g = \frac{560}{10} \pm \frac{\sqrt{560}}{10} = 56 \pm 2.37 \text{ cpm for the sample gross count rate}$$

Background is calculated the same way, using equation 9.37:

$n_b = 390$
$t_b = 15$

$$r_b \pm \sigma_b = \frac{n}{t} \pm \frac{\sqrt{n}}{t}$$

$$r_b \pm \sigma_b = \frac{390}{15} \pm \frac{\sqrt{390}}{15} = 26 \pm 1.32 \text{ cpm for the background count rate}$$

(b) What is the standard deviation of the net counting rate?

Using equation 9.43 and the results from part (a);

$$\sigma_n = \sqrt{\sigma_g^2 + \sigma_b^2} = \sqrt{(2.37)^2 + (1.32)^2} = 2.71 \text{ cpm}$$

(c) What are the 90% and 99% confidence limits for the net counting rate?

Using the information from part (a), the net counting rate is:

$r_g - r_b = 56 - 26 = 30$ cpm

The confidence limits are found by multiplying the standard deviation of the net counting rate, as found in part (b), by the number of standard deviations associated with the 90% confidence level. The 90% confidence level is associated with 1.645 standard deviations (as found in chapter 9), giving:

$r_n \pm 1.645\sigma$

$30 \pm 1.645 \times (2.7)$

30 ± 4.44

34.44 to 25.56 cpm is the 90% confidence interval

For the 99% confidence limits, 2.575 standard deviations are required;

$r_n \pm 2.575\sigma$

$30 \pm 2.575 \times (2.7)$

30 ± 7

37 to 23 cpm is the 99% confidence level

9.3 A 10 min sample count yielded 1,000 counts. A 10 min background measurement gave 250 counts. Assuming negligible radioactive decay of the sample during the counting period, what is the sample net count rate and its 95% confidence interval? **9.3**

$n_g = 1000$ counts
$t_g = 10$ min
$n_b = 250$ counts

$t_b = 10$ min

$$r_g = \frac{1000 \text{ counts}}{10 \text{ min}} = 100 \text{ cpm}$$

$$r_b = \frac{250 \text{ counts}}{10 \text{ min}} = 25 \text{ cpm}$$

$$r_n = r_g - r_b = 100 \text{ cpm} - 25 \text{ cpm} = 75 \text{ cpm}$$

Using equation 9.43 to find the standard deviation of the net counts;

$$\sigma_n = \sqrt{\frac{r_g}{t_g} + \frac{r_b}{t_b}} = \sqrt{\frac{100}{10} + \frac{25}{10}} = 3.5$$

Chapter 9 gives the number of standard deviations that the 95% confidence interval must cover as 1.96σ, so, the solution would be;

$$r_n \pm 1.96\sigma$$

substituting in values,

$$75 \pm (1.96 \times 3.5) \text{ cpm}$$

$$75 \pm 6.9 \text{ cpm}$$

9.4

9.4 A 10 minute sample count was 756 and a 40 min background was 600 counts.
(a) What is the net count rate and its standard deviation?

$n_g = 756$ counts
$t_g = 10$ min
$n_b = 600$ counts
$t_b = 40$ min

$$r_g = \frac{756 \text{ counts}}{10 \text{ min}} = 75.6 \text{ cpm}$$

$$r_b = \frac{600 \text{ counts}}{40 \text{ min}} = 15 \text{ cpm}$$

$r_n = r_g - r_b = 75.6 \text{ cpm} - 15 \text{ cpm} = 60.6 \text{ cpm}$

Using equation 9.43 to find the standard deviation of the net count rate;

$$\sigma_n = \sqrt{\frac{r_g}{t_g} + \frac{r_b}{t_b}} = \sqrt{\frac{75.6}{10} + \frac{15}{40}} = 2.8 \text{ cpm}$$

60.6 ± 2.8 cpm

(b) What is the precision of the measurement, expressed as %?

The precision of this measurement expressed as percent is defined as the standard deviation divided by the net count rate times 100,

$$\text{precision} = \frac{\sigma_n}{r_n} 100 = \frac{2.8}{60.6} \times 100 = 4.65\%$$

9.5 A background counting rate of 30 cpm was determined by a 60 min count. A sample that was counted for 5 min gave a gross count of 170. **9.5**
(a) At the 90% confidence level, is there activity in the sample?

$t_b = 60$
$n_g = 170$
$t_g = 5$
$r_g = 170/5 = 34$ cpm
$r_b = 30$ cpm

$r_1 = M_1 = 34$

$r_2 = M_2 = 30$

Using equation 9.49

$$t = \frac{M_1 - M_2}{\sqrt{\frac{r_1}{t_1} + \frac{r_2}{t_1}}} = \frac{34 - 30}{\sqrt{\frac{34}{60} + \frac{30}{5}}} = 1.47$$

$t = 1.47$ standard deviations difference between the two means. A one tail test must be used for this problem since the question is asking only whether the sample is *greater* than background. For a 1 tailed test, the critical value for t (90%) = 1.28. Since we found $t = 1.47$, we conclude that activity is present at the 90% confidence level.

(b) Is there activity in the sample at the 95% confidence level?

Since t (the number of standard deviations) was calculated in part (a) as 1.47, and the critical value for t (95%) = 1.645 for a 1 tailed test, we conclude that there is not activity present at the 95% confidence level.

9.6

9.6 As a test of the operation of a certain counter, two measurements were made on the same long–lived sample. The first gave 10,210 counts in 10 minutes, and the second gave 4995 in 5 minutes. Is the counter operating satisfactorily?

$n_1 = 10210$
$t_1 = 10$
$n_2 = 4995$
$t_2 = 5$

$$r_1 = M_1 = \frac{10210}{10} = 1021\text{cpm}$$

$$r_2 = M_2 = \frac{4995}{5} = 999\text{cpm}$$

Using equation 9.49

$$t = \frac{|M_1 - M_2|}{\sqrt{\frac{r_1}{t_1} + \frac{r_2}{t_2}}} = \frac{|1021 - 999|}{\sqrt{\frac{1021}{10} + \frac{999}{5}}} = 1.27$$

A two tail test is used for this problem since we are only looking for differences between the two measurements. The critical value for t (90%) for a 2 tailed test is 1.645. Since the measurements show that $t = 1.27$, we conclude that there is no difference between the two means, and that yes, the counter is operating properly.

9.7 A 1 minute count shows a gross activity of 35 counts. If the background is 1560 in 60 min, how long must the sample be counted in order to be within ±10% of the true activity at the 95% confidence level? **9.7**

$t_g = 1$
$r_g = 35$ cpm
$n_b = 1560$
$t_b = 60$

$$r_b = \frac{n_b}{t_b} = \frac{1560}{60} = 26 \text{ cpm}$$

Find the net counting rate:

$r_g - r_b = 35 - 26 = 9$ cpm

The estimated true counting rate is 9 cpm. If it is desired to be within 10% of 9 cpm, the estimate must be within 0.1 × (9 cpm) = 0.9 cpm
To find the net standard deviation associated with 0.9 cpm at 95% confidence interval:
1.96 standard deviations are associated with a 95% confidence level (Chapter 9).

$0.9 = 1.96\sigma$

$\sigma = 0.459$

Now use equation 9.43 to solve for the time the sample should be counted (t_g):

$$\sigma_n = \sqrt{\frac{r_g}{t_g} + \frac{r_b}{t_b}}$$

$$0.459 = \sqrt{\frac{35}{t_g} + \frac{26}{60}}$$ $t_g = -160$ Since the solution is negative, it is not possible to obtain the stated accuracy and precision in the problem, unless the background counting time is increased.

9.8

9.8 A sample that had been counted for 15 min showed a counting rate of 32 cpm. The background, counted for 10 min, was 15 cpm.

(a) What is the net counting rate, at the 95% confidence limit?

$r_g = 32$ cpm
$t_g = 15$ min
$r_b = 15$ cpm
$t_b = 10$ min

$r_{net} = r_g - r_b = 32 - 15 = 17$ cpm is the net count rate

Use equation 9.43 to find the standard deviation associated with the net count rate:

$$\sigma_n = \sqrt{\frac{r_g}{t_g} + \frac{r_b}{t_b}} = \sqrt{\frac{32}{15} + \frac{15}{10}} = 1.91\text{cpm}$$

Chapter 9 gives the 95% confidence level as 1.96 standard deviations, so the result is:

$r_n \pm 1.96\,\sigma$

$17 \pm 1.96 \times (1.91)$

17 ± 3.7 cpm

(b) What is the coefficient of variation (relative error at ± 1 standard deviation) of the net counting rate?

Use equation 9.39b and data from part (a);

$n = 17$
$\sigma = 3.7$

$$\%\text{ relative probable error} = 100 \times \frac{\sigma}{n} = 100 \times \frac{1.91}{17} = 11\ \%$$

9.9

9.9 A sample has an estimated gross counting rate of 35 cpm (based on a 2 minute count). The background, determined by a 1 hour count, is 10 counts per minute. How long should the sample be counted if we want to be 95% certain that the net counting rate is within ± 5% of the true net counting rate?

$r_g = 35$ cpm
$t_g = 2$ min
$r_b = 10$ cpm
$t_b = 60$ min

Estimate the net count rate first:

$$r_{net} = r_g - r_b = 35 - 10 = 25 \text{ cpm}$$

The estimated true net counting rate is 25 cpm. If it is desired to be within 5% of 25 cpm, the estimate must be within 0.05(25cpm) = 1.25 cpm

To find the net standard deviation associated with 1.25 cpm at 95% confidence interval: 1.645 standard deviations are associated with a 95% confidence level for a one tail test. A one tail test is used since we wish to see whether the sample is greater than the background.

$1.25 = 1.645\sigma$
$\sigma = 0.76$

Now use equation 9.43 to solve for the time the sample should be counted (t_g):

$$\sigma_n = \sqrt{\frac{r_g}{t_g} + \frac{r_b}{t_b}}$$

$$0.76 = \sqrt{\frac{35}{t_g} + \frac{10}{60}}$$

$t_g = 85$ minutes.

9.10 (a) The gross 1 minute count on a sample was 100, and the background, counted during 1 minute was 50 counts. What was the net counting rate at the 90% confidence level? **9.10**

$r_g = 100$ cpm
$t_g = 1$ min
$r_b = 50$

$t_b = 1$ min

$r_{net} = r_g - r_b = 100 - 50 = 50$ cpm

Use equation 9.43 to find the standard deviation associated with the net count rate:

$$\sigma_n = \sqrt{\frac{r_g}{t_g} + \frac{r_b}{t_b}} = \sqrt{\frac{100}{1} + \frac{50}{1}} = 12.25$$

The number of standard deviations associated with 90% is 1.645 (from chapter 9)

$r_n \pm 1.645\sigma_n = 50 \pm (1.645) \times 12.25 = 50 \pm 20$ cpm

9.10(b) If the sample and background were each counted for 10 minutes, and gave counting rates of 100 and 50 cpm respectively, what was the net counting rate at the 95% confidence interval?

$r_g = 100$ cpm
$t_g = 10$ min
$r_b = 50$
$t_b = 10$ min

$r_{net} = r_g - r_b = 100 - 50 = 50$ cpm

Use equation 9.43 to find the standard deviation associated with the net count rate:

$$\sigma_n = \sqrt{\frac{r_g}{t_g} + \frac{r_b}{t_b}} = \sqrt{\frac{100}{10} + \frac{50}{10}} = 3.87$$

The number of standard deviations associated with 95% is 1.96 (from chapter 9)

$r_n \pm 1.96\sigma_n = 50 \pm (1.96) \times 3.87 = 50 \pm 8$ cpm

9.11

9.11 A shielded low background counter has an average counting rate of 2 cpm. What is the probability that a 1 min counting period will record?

(a) 2 counts, (b) 4 counts, (c) 0 counts.

Use equation 9.34

$\bar{n} = 2$
$n = 2$

$$p(n) = \frac{(\bar{n})^n e^{-\bar{n}}}{n!} = p(2) = \frac{2^2 e^{-2}}{2!} = 0.271$$

(b) 4 counts,

$\bar{n} = 2$
$n = 4$

$$p(n) = \frac{(\bar{n})^n e^{-\bar{n}}}{n!} = p(4) = \frac{2^4 e^{-2}}{4!} = 0.09$$

(c) 0 counts,

$\bar{n} = 2$
$n = 0$

$$p(n) = \frac{(\bar{n})^n e^{-\bar{n}}}{n!} = p(0) = \frac{2^0 e^{-2}}{0!} = 0.135$$

9.12 A sample of river water was taken near the waste discharge pipe of an isotope laboratory, and another sample was taken upstream of the discharge point. Each sample was counted for 10 min, and gave 225 and 210 cpm, respectively. At the 99% confidence level, is the downstream water more radioactive than the water upstream? **9.12**

$t_g = 10$
$t_b = 10$
$r_g = 225$ cpm
$r_b = 210$ cpm

$r_1 = M_1 = 225$
$r_2 = M_2 = 210$

Using equation 9.49 without absolute values, because there is a reason for the ordering of the values,

$$t = \frac{M_1 - M_2}{\sqrt{\frac{r_1}{t_1} + \frac{r_2}{t_1}}} = \frac{225 - 210}{\sqrt{\frac{225}{10} + \frac{210}{10}}} = 2.27$$

$t = 2.27$ standard deviations difference between the two means. A one tail test is used since we are only checking to determine whether the activity downstream is greater than upstream t (99%, 1 tail) = 2.327. Since the measurement $t < 2.327$, the downstream water is not more radioactive than the upstream.

9.13

9.13 A certain counting standard has a true mean counting rate of 50 cpm. (a) What is the probability of observing exactly 50 counts in 1 minute?

Find the standard deviation of 50 counts in one minute. Since we can describe the distribution of count rates by the Poisson distribution, equation 9.36 is used:

$$\sigma = \sqrt{\bar{n}} = \sqrt{50} = 7.07$$

Since the mean, 50>30, we can use either the Poisson distribution, equation 9.34, or the normal distribution, equation 9.31 to obtain the probability of exactly 50 counts in one minute. Assuming the normal distribution we have:

$\bar{n} = 50$
$\sigma = 7.07$

$$p(n) = \frac{1}{\sigma\sqrt{2\pi}} e^{-(n-\bar{n})^2/2\sigma^2} = p(50) = \frac{1}{7.07\sqrt{2\pi}} e^{-(50-50)^2/2(7.07)^2} = 0.056$$

(b) What is the probability of measuring 43–57 counts in 1 min?

43 - 57 = mean $\pm$ 1σ

Since 68% of the area under the normal curve is included between $\pm$ 1σ, then, the probability of measuring 43-57 counts is 0.68.

(c) What is the probability of finding more than 57 counts in 1 min?

Since 50% of the area of a normal probability curve lies above 50 counts (the mean), and 57 counts is one standard deviation from the mean (34% of the area), the remaining area would be 50% – 34%=16%.
The probability of obtaining greater than 57 counts is 0.16.

9.14 A counting system has a background of 360 counts during a 20 minute counting period. What is the lower limit of detection with this system for counting times of **9.14**
(a) 2 min.

$n_b = 360$ counts
$t_b = 20$ min

$$r_b = \frac{360 \text{ counts}}{20 \text{ min}} = 18 \text{ cpm}$$

$t_s = 2$ min

Equation 9.53 is used;

$$\text{LLD} = \frac{3.29\sqrt{r_b t_s\left(1+\frac{t_s}{t_b}\right)}+3}{t_s} = \frac{3.29\times\sqrt{\left(18\frac{\text{counts}}{\text{min}}\right)\times 2\text{ min}\times\left(1+\frac{2\text{ min}}{20\text{ min}}\right)}+3}{2\text{ min}}$$

LLD = 12 cpm

(b) $t_s = 20$ minutes

$$\text{LLD} = \frac{3.29\times\sqrt{\left(18\frac{\text{counts}}{\text{min}}\right)\times 20\text{ min}\times\left(1+\frac{20\text{ min}}{20\text{ min}}\right)}+3}{20\text{ min}} = 4.6\text{ cpm}$$

(c) $t_s = 200$ min.

$$\text{LLD} = \frac{3.29\times\sqrt{\left(18\frac{\text{counts}}{\text{min}}\right)\times 200\text{ min}\times\left(1+\frac{200\text{ min}}{20\text{ min}}\right)}+3}{200\text{ min}}$$

LLD = 3.3 cpm

9.15

9.15 To determine possible low level contamination, smears are counted for 10 minutes at an overall counting efficiency of 10%. The smear is considered positive if its activity exceeds the MDA. If the blank gives 400 counts in 10 minutes, what is the MDA for this counting system.

Equation 9.54 is used;

$k = 10\% = 0.1$ counting efficiency
$t_b = 10$ min
$n_b = 400$

$$\text{MDA} = \frac{4.66\sqrt{n_b}+3}{kt} = \frac{4.66 \times \sqrt{400}+3}{0.1 \times (10)} = 96.2 \text{ dpm}$$

$$\text{MDA} = \frac{96.2 \text{ d}}{\text{min}} \times \frac{1 \text{ min}}{60 \text{ sec}} \times \frac{1 \text{ Bq}}{1\text{d}/\text{sec}} = 1.6 \text{ Bq}$$

9.16

9.16 A blank in an alpha counter records 28 counts in 2 hours. Calculate the lower limit of detection for a 1 hour and a 2 hour sample count.

Calculating for 1 hour;

$n_b = 28$ counts
$t_b = 2 \text{ hr} = 120 \text{ min.}$

$$r_b = \frac{28 \text{ counts}}{120 \text{ min}} = 0.23 \text{ cpm}$$

$t_s = 1 \text{ hr} = 60 \text{ min}$

Equation 9.53 is used;

$$\text{LLD} = \frac{3.29\sqrt{r_b t_s\left(1+\frac{t_s}{t_b}\right)}+3}{t_s} = \frac{3.29 \times \sqrt{\left(14\frac{\text{counts}}{\text{hr}}\right) \times 1 \text{ hr} \times \left(1+\frac{1 \text{ hr}}{2 \text{ hr}}\right)}+3}{1 \text{ hr} \times \frac{60 \text{ min}}{\text{hr}}}$$

LLD = 0.30 cpm above background

For $t_s = 2$ hours, we can use either equation 9.53, as above

$$\text{LLD} = \frac{3.29 \times \sqrt{\left(14\,\frac{\text{counts}}{\text{hr}}\right) \times 2\text{ hr} \times \left(1 + \frac{2\text{ hr}}{2\text{ hr}}\right)} + 3}{2\text{ hr} \times \frac{60\text{ min}}{\text{hr}}}$$

LLD = 0.23 cpm above background

or, since $t_s = t_b$, we can use equation 9.50

$$\text{LLD} = \frac{4.66\sigma_b + 3}{t_s} = \frac{4.66\sqrt{n} + 3}{t_s}$$

$$\text{LLD} = \frac{4.66\sqrt{28} + 3}{120\text{ min}} = 0.23\text{ cpm above background}$$

9.17 A counting standard was counted for 5 minutes before an experiment, and gave mean count rate of 5965 cpm. After the experiment, the standard was counted again, and gave 6070 cpm during a 2 minute check. Was the counting system operating as expected? **9.17**

Use the two tail test (since we are only looking for a difference between the two counts) to determine if there is a difference between the two counts, equation 9.49:

$M_1 = 5965$ cpm
$M_2 = 6070$ cpm
$r_1 = 5965$ cpm
$r_2 = 6070$ cpm
$t_1 = 5$ min
$t_2 = 2$ min

$$t = \frac{|M_1 - M_2|}{\sqrt{\frac{r_1}{t_1} + \frac{r_2}{t_2}}} = \frac{|5965 - 6070|}{\sqrt{\frac{5965}{5} + \frac{6070}{2}}} = 1.615$$

"t" is less than 1.96, so there is no difference between the two count rates at the 95% confidence level.

Yes, the counter is operating properly.

9.18

9.18 An unsealed air wall ionization chamber whose volume is 275 cm^3 is calibrated at an atmospheric pressure of 760 torr and a temperature of 20°C. A measurement is made at an altitude of 7000 ft (2120 m), where the pressure is 589 torr and the temperature is 25°C. The meter reading was 10 mR/hr (2.58 μC/kg/hr). What is the corrected exposure rate?

The air is less dense at measurement, due to lower pressure and higher temperature, than at calibration. When corrected for pressure and temperature, we have

$$\dot{X}(\text{corrected}) = 10\frac{\text{mR}}{\text{h}} \times \frac{760}{589} \times \frac{273+25}{273+20} = 13.1\frac{\text{mR}}{\text{h}}$$

9.19

9.19 A 0.0025 μCi (92.5 Bq) ^{14}C source is placed into an air filled current ionization chamber whose detection efficiency is 40%. The ionization current produces a 10 mV drop when it flows through a 10^{12} ohm load resistor. What is the mean energy of the ^{14}C beta particles?

Basic electricity equation;

$V = 10$ mV $= 0.01$ V
$R = 10^{12}$ ohm

$$I = \frac{V}{R} = \frac{0.01\text{ V}}{10^{12}\text{ ohm}} = 1 \times 10^{-14}\text{ A}$$

Table 5.1 gives the average energy lost by beta particles in air as 33.7 eV per electron produced by ionization.

$$1\times10^{-14}\text{ A}\times\frac{1\text{C}/\text{sec}}{1\text{ A}}\times\frac{\text{electron}}{1.6\times10^{-19}\text{C}}\times\frac{100\text{ e}^{-}\text{ produced}}{40\text{ e}^{-}\text{ detected}}\times\frac{33.7\text{ eV}}{\text{electron}} = 5.3\times10^{6}\frac{\text{eV}}{\text{sec}}$$

$$92.5\text{ Bq} = 92.5\frac{\text{t}}{\text{sec}}$$

$$\frac{5.3\times10^{6}\text{eV}}{\text{sec}}\times\frac{\text{sec}}{92.5\text{ t}} = 57\times10^{3}\text{ eV} = 57\text{ keV is the mean energy.}$$

9.20 A survey meter whose time constant is 6 sec is used to measure the scattered radiation from an x–ray machine. After a 0.2 second exposure time, the meter read 10 mR (258 μC/kg)/hr. What was the actual exposure rate? **9.20**

Meter reading, $\dot{X} = 10$ mR
$t = 0.2$ sec
$RC = 6$ sec

If the measurement time, t, is small relative to the time constant, RC, then the actual exposure rate, $\dot{X}_0$, is related to the meter reading, $\dot{X}$ by

$$\dot{X} = \dot{X}_0(1 - e^{-t/RC})$$

$$\dot{X}_0 = \frac{\dot{X}}{(1-e^{-t/RC})} = \frac{10\frac{\text{mR}}{\text{hr}}}{(1-e^{-0.2\text{sec}/6\text{sec}})} = 305\frac{\text{mR}}{\text{hr}}$$

9.21 What is the gamma threshold energy for a Cerenkov counter whose index of refraction is 1.6? **9.21**

Using equation 9.7 to find the energy of the electron that produces the Cerenkov radiation:

$n = 1.6$

$$E = 0.51\left(\frac{1}{\sqrt{1-\frac{1}{n^2}}} - 1\right) = 0.51 \times \left(\frac{1}{\sqrt{1-\frac{1}{1.6^2}}} - 1\right) = 0.143 \text{ MeV}$$

So a 0.143 MeV electron would produce the desired effect. What energy γ ray would produce a 0.143 MeV Compton electron when back scattered 180° (a 180° back scattered electron would have the most energy that could be transferred by a γ ray to an electron) ?

$$E_{\text{compton(e)}} = E(\gamma)_{\text{initial}} - E(\gamma)_{\text{scattered}} = 0.143 \text{ MeV}$$

Solve for the scattered photon energy next, $E(\gamma)_{\text{initial}} - 0.143 \text{ MeV} = E(\gamma)_{\text{scattered}}$

Replace E′ in equation 5.31A with the above term for the scattered photon;

$$E' = \frac{E}{1 + \left(\frac{E}{m_0 c^2}\right)(1 - \cos\theta)}$$

$$E - 0.143 \text{ MeV} = \frac{E}{1 + \left(\frac{E}{m_0 c^2}\right)(1 - \cos\theta)}$$

$\theta = 180°$
$m_0 c^2 = 0.511$ MeV (energy equivalence of an electron)

$$E - 0.143 \text{ MeV} = \frac{E}{1 + \left(\frac{E}{0.511 \text{ MeV}}\right) \times (1 - \cos[180])}$$

$E = 0.275$ MeV is the threshold gamma ray energy (Note you will need to use the quadratic equation to solve for E)

9.22 **9.22** An ionization chamber has a window thickness of 2 mg/cm^2. If a 0.01 μCi (370 Bq) ^{210}Po source is located 1 cm in front of the window, so that the counting geometry is 25%, calculate the saturation ionization current.

Equation 9.10 is used to solve for the current:

$$I = \frac{N \frac{\text{particles}}{\text{sec}} \times \overline{E} \frac{\text{eV}}{\text{particle}} \times 1.6 \times 10^{-19} \frac{\text{C}}{\text{ion}}}{w \frac{\text{eV}}{\text{ion}}} = \text{current in amps}$$

The energy of the ^{210}Po α will be degraded by traveling through the air and the window.
First, calculate the range of the 5.3 MeV α in air, using equation 5.14:

$E = 5.3$ MeV
R cm = 1.24E MeV – 2.62 = 1.24 × (5.3 MeV) –2.62 = 3.95 cm range in air.

Convert the range of the α into aerial density units (mg/cm^2):

$$R = 1.293\ \frac{\text{mg}}{\text{cm}^3} \times 3.95\ \text{cm} = 5.1\ \text{mg/cm}^2$$

The range is reduced by passing through the 1 cm of air, so convert the 1 cm air to aerial density units by multiplying by the density of air:

$$\rho_{air} = 1.293 \times 10^{-3}\ \text{g/cm}^3 = 1.293\ \text{mg/cm}^3$$

$$1\ \text{cm} \times \frac{1.293 \times 10^{-3}\,\text{g}}{\text{cm}^3} \times \frac{1000\ \text{mg}}{\text{g}} = 1.293\ \text{mg/cm}^2$$

Since the window is given as 2 mg/cm^2 thick, it is already in aerial density units, it is now possible to sum the two materials that the α must pass through, the air and the window:

1.293 mg/cm^2(air)+ 2 mg/cm^2(window) = 3.293 mg/cm^2

Using a ratio of the range of the α in air (5.1 mg/cm^2 as calculated above), calculate the energy of the α after passing through 3.293 mg/cm^2 of materials:

$$\frac{5.1\frac{\text{mg}}{\text{cm}^2} - 3.293\frac{\text{mg}}{\text{cm}^2}}{5.1\frac{\text{mg}}{\text{cm}^2}} \times 5.3\ \text{MeV} = 1.88\ \text{MeV}$$ is the energy of the α after passing through the air and window

N = 370 α per second from ^{210}Po (given) × 0.25 (only 25% efficient) = 92.5 α/sec
w = 35.5 eV/ion (based on information in Chapter 9)

Substituting to find the current:

$$I = \frac{92.5\frac{\text{particles}}{\text{sec}} \times 1.88\frac{\text{MeV}}{\text{particle}} \times 1.6 \times 10^{-19}\frac{\text{C}}{\text{ion}}}{35.5\frac{\text{eV}}{\text{ion}} \times \frac{1\ \text{MeV}}{10^6\,\text{eV}}} = 7.8 \times 10^{-13}\ \text{C/sec}$$

$I = 7.8 \times 10^{-13}$ A

9.23

9.23 An air wall, air–filled ionization chamber, whose volume is 100 cm^3, gives a saturation current of 10^{-12} A when placed in an X–ray field. If the temperature was 27 °C, and the atmospheric pressure was 740 mm Hg, what was the radiation exposure rate?

3×10^9 sC = 1 C
1 statcoulomb/cm^3 = 1 roentgen

$$\frac{1\times 10^{-12}\,\text{A}}{100\ \text{cm}^3} \times \frac{1\frac{\text{C}}{\text{sec}}}{1\ \text{A}} \times \frac{3\times 10^{9}\,\text{sC}}{\text{C}} \times \frac{3600\ \text{sec}}{1\ \text{hr}} = \frac{10.8\ \text{sC / hr}}{100\ \text{cm}^3}$$

Note that roentgens are measured at a standard temperature of 273 K and 760 mm, so the exposure rate must be temperature corrected:

27 °C = 300 K

Convert statcoulombs per cm^3 into roentgens by correcting for temperature and pressure. Both the temperature and pressure, in this case, act to decrease the number of molecules with which the radiation can interact. Therefore both temperature and pressure correction factors must be greater than one.

$$\frac{10.8\ \text{sC / hr}}{100\ \text{cm}^3} \times \frac{1\ \text{R}}{1\frac{\text{sC}}{\text{cm}^3}} \times \frac{760\ \text{mm}}{740\ \text{mm}} \times \frac{300\ \text{K}}{273\ \text{K}} = 0.122\ \text{R/hr or } 122\ \text{mR/hr}$$

9.24

9.24 (a) What value resistor, to be placed in series with the ion chamber, in problem 23, is required to generate a voltage drop of 10 mV?

For DC circuits:
$V = 10$ mV = 10×10^{-3} V
$I = 1 \times 10^{-12}$ A

$$R = \frac{V}{I} = \frac{10\times 10^{-3}\,\text{V}}{1\times 10^{-12}\,\text{A}} = 1 \times 10^{10} \text{ ohms is the value of resistor required.}$$

(b) If the capacity of the chamber is 250 μμF, what is the time constant of the detector circuit?

As explained in Chapter 9, the product RC is the time constant, τ. The resistance was calculated in part (a):

$R = 1 \times 10^{10}$ ohms
$C = 250\ \mu\mu F = 250 \times 10^{-12}$ F

$\tau = RC = 1 \times 10^{10}$ ohms $\times\ 250 \times 10^{-12}$ F $= 2.5$ sec

(c) How much time is required before the meter will read 99% of the saturation current?

$RC = 2.5$ sec (from part b)

I is the saturation current

$V = IR$

Using equation 9.9:

$V = IR\ (1 - e^{t/RC})$

where V is the voltage at some time t, and IR is the saturation current times resistance of the circuit, or V_0.

$V = V_0\ (1 - e^{t/RC})$

$$\frac{V}{V_0} = (1 - e^{t/RC})$$

To find when 99% of the saturation voltage is reached, $\dfrac{V}{V_0} = 0.99$,

$0.99 = (1 - e^{t/RC})$

substituting in the values,

$0.99 = (1 - e^{t/2.5\ \mathrm{sec}})$

$t = 11.5$ sec

9.25 **9.25** A pocket dosimeter has a capacitance of 5 μμF and a sensitive volume of 1.5 cm^3. What is the charging voltage if it is to be used in the range 0 - 200 mR (0 - 51.5 μC/kg) and the voltage across the dosimeter should be one–half the charging voltage when the dosimeter reads 200 mR?

$C = 5\ \mu\mu\text{F} = 5 \times 10^{-12}\ \text{F}$

density of air = $1.293 \times 10^{-6}\ \text{kg/cm}^3$ (Table 5.2)

$$Q = \frac{51.5\mu\text{C}}{\text{kg}_{\text{air}}} \times \frac{1.293 \times 10^{-6}\,\text{kg}_{\text{air}}}{\text{cm}^3_{\text{air}}} \times 1.5\ \text{cm}^3 \times \frac{1\ \text{C}}{1 \times 10^6\,\mu\text{C}} = 9.988 \times 10^{-11}\ \text{C}$$

Use equation 2.66

$\Delta V = \frac{Q}{C} = \frac{9.988 \times 10^{-11}\,\text{C}}{5 \times 10^{-12}\,\text{F}}$ =20 Volts for the difference in charge, from full to half charge.

Therefore the charging voltage = $2 \times \Delta V$ = 40 volts

9.26 **9.26** A Geiger tube has a capacitance of 25 μμF. The time required to collect all the positive ions is 221×10^{-6} sec. In order to produce sharp output pulses, it is desired to limit the time constant of the detector to 50 μsec.
(a) What is the value of the series resistor?

$\tau = 50\ \mu\text{sec} = 50 \times 10^{-6}\ \text{sec}$

$C = 25\ \mu\mu\text{F} = 25 \times 10^{-12}\text{F}$

As explained in Chapter 9, the product *RC* is the time constant, τ.

$\tau = RC$

$R = \frac{\tau}{C} = \frac{50 \times 10^{-6}\,\text{sec}}{25 \times 10^{-12}\,\text{F}}$ = $2 \times 10^6\ \Omega$ (ohms) is the value of the series resistor

(b) If 10^8 ion pairs are formed per Geiger pulse, what is the upper limit of the output voltage pulse?

First, find Q:

$$Q = \frac{10^8 \text{ions}}{\text{pulse}} \times \frac{1.6 \times 10^{-19}\,\text{C}}{\text{ion}} = 1.6 \times 10^{-11}\ \text{C}$$

$C = 25\ \mu\mu\text{F} = 25 \times 10^{-12}\text{F}$ (given in question)

Use equation 9.1:

$$V = \frac{Q}{C} = \frac{1.6 \times 10^{-11}\,\text{C}}{25 \times 10^{-12}\,\text{F}} = 0.64\ \text{V is the maximum output voltage.}$$

9.27 A Geiger counter has a resolving time of 250 μsec. What fraction of counts is lost due to the counter's dead time if the observed counting rate is 30,000 cpm? 9.27
Using equation 9.5, where:

$R_0 = 30{,}000$ cpm

$$\tau = 250\ \mu\text{sec} = 250\mu\ \text{sec} \times \frac{1\ \text{sec}}{10^6\ \mu\ \text{sec}} \times \frac{1\ \text{min}}{60\ \text{sec}} = 4.17 \times 10^{-6}\ \text{min}$$

$$R_t = \frac{R_0}{1 - R_0\tau} = \frac{30000}{1 - (30000) \times 4.17 \times 10^{-6}} = 34{,}286\ \text{cpm}$$

Finding the fraction of counts lost:

$$1 - \frac{30000}{34286} = 0.125$$

12.5% of the counts are lost.

9.28 The fact that the gas multiplication in a proportional counter is very much less than that in a Geiger counter means that a pulse amplifier for use with a proportional counter must have a lower input sensitivity than one used with a 9.28

Geiger counter. Calculate the input sensitivity for an amplifier to be used with a 2 in. dia. hemispherical windowless gas-flow proportional counter whose capacitance is 20 μμF and which is operated to give a gas amplification of 5×10^3. Assume that the output pulse is "clipped" to one–half its maximum height.

Use equation 9.1:

$$C = 20\ \mu\mu F = 20 \times 10^{-12}\ F$$

$$Q = \frac{5 \times 10^3 \text{ ion pairs}}{\text{event}} \times \frac{1.6 \times 10^{-19}\ C}{\text{ion pair}} = 8 \times 10^{-16}\ C$$

$$V = \frac{Q}{C} = \frac{8 \times 10^{-16}\ C}{20 \times 10^{-12}\ F} = 4 \times 10^{-5}\ V$$

Since the pulse is "clipped" by 50% ,

$$4 \times 10^{-5}\ V \times 50\% = 2 \times 10^{-5}\ V$$

9.29 **9.29** What is the sensitivity of a thermal neutron detector whose volume is 50 cm^3, and is filled with 96% enriched BF_3 to a total pressure of 70 cm Hg? (Assume the temperature is 293 K).

Use the Ideal gas law to find the number of moles of BF_3 gas in the detector:

$$P = 70 \text{ cm Hg} \times \frac{1 \text{ atm}}{76 \text{ cm Hg}} = 0.921 \text{ atm}$$

$$V = 50\ cm^3 \times \frac{1\ L}{1000\ cm^3} = 0.05\ L$$

$$R = 0.082\ \frac{L \cdot atm}{mole \cdot K}$$

$$T = 293\ K$$

Substituting in the values:

$$\frac{PV}{RT} = n = \frac{0.921\ atm \times 0.05\ L}{0.082 \frac{L \cdot atm}{mole \cdot K} \times 293\ K} = 1.92 \times 10^{-3} \text{ moles gas}$$

Calculate the number of atoms of ^{10}B in the detector, since the thermal neutron cross section for absorption for the other atoms in the gas is orders of magnitude smaller:

$$N = 1.92 \times 10^{-3}\,\text{moles gas} \times \frac{0.96\ \text{moles}\ ^{10}\text{B}}{1\ \text{mole gas}} \times \frac{6.02 \times 10^{23}\,\text{atoms}\ ^{10}\text{B}}{1\ \text{mole}\ ^{10}\text{B}}$$

$N = 1.1 \times 10^{21}$ atoms ^{10}B gas

The cross section for thermal neutron absorption for ^{10}B can be found in Chapter 9 as:

$\sigma = 4010\ \text{b} = 4010 \times 10^{24}\ \text{cm}^2/\text{atom}$

Sensitivity is defined by equation 9.18,

$$\text{Sensitivity} = \frac{CR}{\phi}$$

and is calculated with equation 9.17

$$\frac{N\sigma_0}{1.128} = \frac{CR}{\phi}$$

Substituting:

$$\text{Sensitivity} = \frac{N\sigma}{1.128} = \frac{1.1 \times 10^{21}\ \text{atoms} \times 4010 \times 10^{-24}\ \dfrac{\text{cm}^2}{\text{atom}}}{1.128}$$

$$\text{Sensitivity} = 3.95\ \text{cps}\Big/\frac{\text{neutron}}{\text{cm}^2 \cdot \text{sec}}$$

9.30 If the BF_3 tube of problem 29 is used as a current ionization chamber, what saturation current would result from a thermal flux of 10^9 neutrons per cm^2/sec ? **9.30**

Calculate the amount of energy released by the thermal neutrons per neutron reaction:

$$^{10}_{5}\text{B} + ^{1}_{0}\text{n} \rightarrow ^{7}_{3}\text{Li}^{+3} + ^{4}_{2}\text{He}^{+2} + \text{energy}$$

$M\,(^{10}\text{B}) + m\,(\text{n}) = M\,(^{7}\text{Li}) + M\,(^{4}\text{He}) + Q$

The nuclear masses of each isotope is used in this mass energy balance equation.

10.016114 (B-10) + 1.008982 (neutron) = 7.018185 (Li-7) + 4.003873 (He-4)

$Q = 11.025096 - 11.022058 = 3.038 \times 10^{-3}$ AMU/reaction

931 MeV = 1 AMU

$$3.038 \times 10^{-3}\ \text{AMU} \times \frac{931\ \text{MeV}}{\text{AMU}} = 2.83\ \text{MeV/reaction}$$

^{7}Li emits a 0.48 MeV capture gamma 6% of the time, which is assumed to escape the chamber, so the average kinetic energy released per neutron capture is::

$2.83\ \text{MeV} \times 0.94 = 2.66$

$(2.83 - 0.48) \times 0.06 = 0.141$

0.141 + 2.66 = 2.8 MeV average kinetic energy imparted by each thermal neutron reaction. This energy will be expended in producing ions in the BF_3 gas at a rate of 1 ion pair per 35.6 eV.

From problem 9.29:

$N = 1.1 \times 10^{21}$ atoms
$\phi = 10^{9}$ neutrons/cm^{2}/sec
$\sigma_0 = 4010$ barns $= 4010 \times 10^{-24}$ cm^{2}

Equation 9.17 is used to find the neutron reaction rate, *RR*, in the detector:

$$RR = \frac{N\sigma_0}{1.128}\phi = \frac{1.1\times 10^{21}\,\text{atoms} \times 4010 \times 10^{-24}\,\text{cm}^2}{1.128} \times 10^{9}\,\frac{\text{neutrons}}{\text{cm}^2\ /\ \text{sec}}$$

$RR = 3.91 \times 10^{9}$ reactions/sec

Equation 9.10

$$I = \frac{RR\,\frac{\text{reactions}}{\text{sec}} \times \overline{E}\,\frac{\text{eV}}{\text{reaction}} \times 1.6\times10^{-19}\,\frac{\text{C}}{\text{ion}}}{w(\text{eV / ion})} \times 1\ \text{A}\Big/\frac{\text{C}}{\text{s}}$$

$$I = \frac{3.91\times10^{9}\,\frac{\text{reations}}{\text{sec}} \times 2.8\times10^{6}\,\frac{\text{eV}}{\text{reaction}} \times 1.6\times10^{-19}\,\frac{\text{C}}{\text{ion}} \times 1\,\frac{\text{A}}{\text{C/s}}}{35.6\,\frac{\text{eV}}{\text{ion}}}$$

9.31 How long would it take for the sensitivity of the BF_3 detector of problem 30 to decrease by 10%? **9.31**

From problem 9.29:

1.1×10^{21} atoms ^{10}B
3.91×10^{9} neutron interactions/sec

For the sensitivity to decrease by 10%, the number of ^{10}B atoms must decrease by 10%, that is
1.1×10^{21} atoms $\times\ 0.1 = 1.1 \times 10^{20}$ atoms ^{10}B must be consumed by neutron captures.

At the reaction rate of 3.91×10^{9} reactions/second, the time to produce 1.1×10^{20} reactions is

$$T = \frac{1.1\times10^{20}\ \text{reactios}}{3.91\times10^{9}\ \text{reactions / sec}} = 2.8\times10^{10}\ \text{sec}$$

$$T = 2.8\times10^{10}\ \text{sec} \times \frac{1\ \text{hr}}{3600\ \text{sec}} \times \frac{1\ \text{d}}{24\ \text{hr}} \times \frac{1\ \text{yr}}{365\ \text{d}} = 892\ \text{yr}$$

9.32 What is the sensitivity for 1 MeV and for 10 MeV neutrons (amps per neutron per cm^2/second) of an ion chamber that is filled with CH_4 gas to a pressure of 760 mm Hg, if its volume is 500 cm^3 ? **9.32**

Calculate the number of H atoms in the ion chamber:

$P = 760$ mm Hg = 1 atm
$V = 500\ cm^3 = 0.5$ L
$T = 20$ °C = 293 K

$$R = 0.082\ \frac{L \cdot atm}{mole \cdot K}$$

$$n = \frac{PV}{RT} = \frac{0.5\ L \times 1\ atm}{0.082 \frac{L \cdot atm}{mole \cdot K} \times 293\ K} = 0.0208 \text{ moles } CH_4 \text{ in the ion chamber}$$

Since CH_4 has 4 atoms of hydrogen per molecule,

$1.25 \times 10^{22} \times 4 = 5.02 \times 10^{22}$ hydrogen atoms are in the chamber.

Find the neutron capture cross section for each of the energies. Carbon is not considered important in this problem since it is not as effective at transferring energy due to its comparatively smaller cross section. We cannot use equation 5.53 to determine the cross section at energies higher than 1000 eV (see pages 157, 380), since capture energies tend to become flat at very high energies. The cross section can be found in the "Barn Book", 1955 or from Brookhaven National Laboratories database.

$\sigma_{1\ MeV\ H} = 4.5$ b $= 4.5 \times 10^{-24} cm^2$/atom

An average of 50% of a neutron's energy is lost in each collision with H, and assuming that each neutron only collides once with a hydrogen atom. We may assume that only one collision occurs is because the mean free path of a neutron is significantly larger than the chamber:

$$MFP = \frac{1}{4.5 \times 10^{-24} \frac{cm^2}{atom\ H} \cdot \frac{5.02 \times 10^{22}\ atoms}{500\ cm^3\ chamber}} = 2213\ cm$$

Using equation 9.17 to determine the number of neutrons per second reacting (Note that the beams are monoenergetic, so a correction for the most probable energy is not required):

$RR = \phi N \sigma_0$

$$\frac{RR}{\phi} = 5.02 \times 10^{22}\,\text{atom} \times 4.5 \times 10^{-24}\,\frac{\text{cm}^2}{\text{atom}}$$

$$\frac{RR}{\phi} = 0.226 \; \frac{\text{reactions}}{\text{sec}} \bigg/ \frac{\text{neutron}}{\text{cm}^2 \cdot \text{sec}}$$

$w = 28.2$ eV/ion pair in CH_4 (Attix)

$\overline{E} = 1\text{ MeV} = 1 \times 10^6\text{ eV}$

Using equation 9.9 and accounting for only 50% of the neutron's energy being transferred, the current is,

$$I = 0.5 \times \frac{RR\,\frac{\text{reactions}}{\text{sec}}\,\overline{E}\,\frac{\text{eV}}{\text{reactions}}\,1.6 \times 10^{-19}\,\frac{\text{C}}{\text{ion}} \times 1\,\frac{\text{A}}{\text{C/sec}}}{w\,\frac{\text{eV}}{\text{ion}}}$$

$$I = \frac{0.226\;\frac{\text{reactions}}{\text{sec}} \bigg/ \frac{\text{neutrons}}{\text{cm}^2 \cdot \text{sec}} \times 0.5 \times 10^6\,\frac{\text{eV}}{\text{reaction}} \times 1.6 \times 10^{-19}\,\frac{\text{C}}{\text{ion}} \times \frac{1\text{ A}}{\text{C / sec}}}{28.2\,\frac{\text{eV}}{\text{ion}}}$$

I (amps) $= 6.4 \times 10^{-16}$ amp per neutron per cm^2

For 10 MeV neutrons, a similar calculation is performed:

$\sigma_{10\text{ MeV H}} = 1\text{ b} = 1 \times 10^{-24}\text{ cm}^2/\text{atom} \times 4\text{ atoms }{}^1\text{H} = 4 \times 10^{-24}\text{ cm}^2/\text{ atom}$

Using equation 9.17 to determine the number of neutrons per second reacting (Note that the beams are monoenergetic, so a correction for the most probable energy is not required):

$$\frac{CR}{\phi} = 5.02 \times 10^{22}\,\text{atom} \times 1 \times 10^{-24}\,\frac{\text{cm}^2}{\text{atom}} = 0.0502\ \frac{\frac{\text{reactions}}{\text{s}}}{\frac{\text{neutron}}{\text{cm}^2 \cdot \text{s}}}$$

w =28.2 eV/ion pair CH_4

Using equation 9.9 multiplied by 50% (as explained earlier):

$$I = 0.5 \times \frac{RR\dfrac{\text{reactions}}{\text{s}}\,\overline{E}\,\dfrac{\text{eV}}{\text{reaction}}\,1.6 \times 10^{-19}\,\dfrac{\text{C}}{\text{ion}} \times \dfrac{1\ \text{A}}{\text{C/s}}}{w(\text{eV / ion})}$$

$$I = \frac{0.0502\ \dfrac{\frac{\text{reactions}}{\text{s}}}{\frac{\text{neutrons}}{\text{cm}^2 \cdot \text{s}}} \times 5 \times 10^6\,\dfrac{\text{eV}}{\text{reaction}} \times 1.6 \times 10^{-19}\,\dfrac{\text{C}}{\text{ion}} \times \dfrac{1\text{A}}{\text{C/s}}}{28.2\,\dfrac{\text{eV}}{\text{ion}}}$$

I =1.4 × 10^{-15} amp per neutron per cm^2 per second for 10 MeV neutrons

9.33

9.33 A 1000 MBq (27 mCi) ^{60}Co source is lost. At what distance can the lost source be detected with a survey meter whose sensitivity is 0.013 μC/kg per hour (0.05 mR/hr) above background?

$\dot{X}$ = 0.05 mR/hr = 0.05 × 10^{-3} R/hr
A = 27 mCi = 27 × 10^{-3} Ci
I (amps) =1.4 × 10^{-15} amps per neutron per cm^2 per second for 10 MeV neutrons
$\Gamma = 1.32\ \dfrac{\text{R} \cdot \text{m}^2}{\text{Ci} \cdot \text{hr}}$ (table 6.3)

Equation 10.1:

$$\dot{X} = \frac{\Gamma A}{d^2}$$

$$d = \sqrt{\frac{\Gamma A}{\dot{X}}} = \sqrt{\frac{1.32\dfrac{\text{R}-\text{m}^2}{\text{Ci}-\text{hr}} \times 27 \times 10^{-3}\,\text{Ci}}{0.05 \times 10^{-3}\,\text{R / hr}}} = 26.7 \text{ meters}$$

9.34 The thermal neutron flux from a moderated ^{252}Cf neutron calibration source is determined by irradiating a gold foil 1cm diameter × 0.013 cm thick for a period of 7 days at a distance of 100 cm from the source. The foil was counted immediately after the end of the irradiation period, and found to have an activity of 100Bq (2.7 nCi).). What was the thermal flux at the point where the foil was irradiated? The activation cross section for gold is 98.5 barns. **9.34**

Volume of the gold foil:

$$r = \frac{1 \text{ cm}}{2} = 0.5 \text{ cm}$$

$t = 0.013$ cm

$$V = \pi r^2 t = \pi \times 0.5^2 \times 0.013 = 0.0102 \text{ cm}^3$$

$\rho = 19.32$ g/cm^3

Calculating the number of atoms of gold in the foil:

$$0.0102 \text{ cm}^3 \times \frac{19.32 \text{ g}}{\text{cm}^3} \times \frac{1 \text{ mole}}{197 \text{ g}} \times \frac{6.02 \times 10^{23} \text{ atoms}}{\text{mole}} = 6.03 \times 10^{20} \text{ atoms in foil}$$

Use equation 5.59:

$\lambda N = 100$ sec^{-1}
$\sigma = 98.5$ barns $= 98.5 \times 10^{-24}$ cm^2/atom
$n = 6.02 \times 10^{20}$ atoms in the foil
$t = 7$ days

$$\lambda = \frac{\ln(2)}{t_{1/2}} = \frac{0.693}{2.698 \text{ days}} = 0.257 \text{ d}^{-1}$$

$$\lambda N = \phi \sigma n \left(1 - e^{-\lambda t}\right)$$

$$100 \text{ sec}^{-1} = \phi \times 98.5 \times 10^{-24} \frac{\text{cm}^2}{\text{atom}} \times 6.03 \times 10^{20} \text{atoms in foil} \times \left(1 - e^{-0.257 \times 7}\right)$$

$\phi = 2 \times 10^3$ neutrons/cm^2/sec at the 100 cm irradiation point

9.35

9.35 A thermal neutron counter 1 cm diameter × 10 cm long is filled with BF_3 gas at atmospheric pressure and 20°C. What is the counting rate when the counter is in a thermal neutron flux (E_{mp} = 0.025 eV) of 1000 neutrons per square cm per second?

The fluorine atomic cross section for thermal neutrons (E_{mp} = 0.025 eV) is so small (0.01 barns) compared to the cross section for boron (753 barns) that only boron will be considered for this problem (cross sections from NRHH). Calculate the number of moles of gas in the counter, using the ideal gas law:

$P = 1$ atm

$$V_{cyl} = (\text{length} \times (\text{diameter})^2 \times \frac{\pi}{4} = 10\text{ cm} \times 1^2\text{ cm}^2 \times 0.785 = 7.85\text{ cm}^3$$

$$V_{cyl} = 7.85\text{ cm}^3 \times \frac{1\text{ L}}{1000\text{ cm}^3} = 7.85 \times 10^{-3}\text{ L}$$

$$R = 0.082\ \frac{\text{L}\cdot\text{atm}}{\text{mole}\cdot\text{K}}$$

$$T = 20°\text{C} = 293\text{ K}$$

$$n = \frac{PV}{RT} = \frac{1\text{ atm} \times 7.85 \times 10^{-3}\text{L}}{0.082\frac{\text{L}\cdot\text{atm}}{\text{mole}\cdot\text{K}} \times 293\text{ K}} = 3.26 \times 10^{-4}\text{ moles gas in the counter}$$

Converting moles gas into atoms of boron in the counter:

$$N = 3.26{\times}10^{-4}\text{ mole} \times \frac{6.02 \times 10^{23}\text{ molecules}}{\text{mol}} \times \frac{1\text{ atom B}}{\text{molecule}} = 1.96 \times 10^{20}$$

ϕ = 1000 neutrons/cm^2/ sec

σ = 753 b for thermal neutrons for boron

Since thermal neutrons are used, equation 9.17 is used to find the number of counts per second;

$$CR = \frac{N\phi\sigma_0}{1.128} = \frac{1.96\times 10^{20}\,\text{atoms B}\times\dfrac{1000\text{ neutrons}}{\text{cm}^2/\text{sec}}\times\dfrac{753\text{ b}}{\text{atom B}}\times\dfrac{1\times 10^{-24}\,\text{cm}^2}{1\text{ b}}}{1.128}$$

$CR = 132$ cps

Solutions for Chapter 10

EXTERNAL RADIATION PROTECTION

10.1 A Po-Be neutron source emits 10^7 neutrons per second, of average energy 4 MeV. The source is to be stored in a paraffin shield of sufficient thickness to reduce the fast flux at the surface to 10 neutrons per cm^2/sec. Consider paraffin to be essentially CH_2 (for the purpose of this problem) and to have a density of 0.89 g/cm^3. **10.1**

(a) What is the minimum thickness of the paraffin shield?

The unshielded fast flux at a distance equal to the shield thickness is

$$\phi \frac{\text{n}}{\text{cm}^2 \cdot \text{sec}} = \frac{S\ {}^{\text{n}}\!/\!_{\text{sec}}}{4\pi[t\ \text{cm}]^2}$$

With a shielding thickness t and a buildup factor B, ϕ at the shield's surface is

$$\phi = \frac{BS}{4\pi t^2} e^{-\mu t}$$

The attenuation coefficient, μ, for fast neutrons from a Po-Be source is 0.126 cm^{-1} (RHH), and B for thick (20 cm) hydrogenous shields is 5. Substituting these values into the shielding equation gives

$$10 \frac{\text{n}}{\text{cm}^2 \cdot \text{sec}} = \frac{5 \times 10^7\ {}^{\text{n}}\!/\!_{\text{sec}}}{4\pi[t\ \text{cm}]^2} e^{-0.126t}$$

This equation is most easily solved by assuming a value for t, and then calculating the resulting ϕ . This process is repeated until the value for t is found that gives the desired ϕ. By this method of iteration,

t = 44 cm results in ϕ = 8 n/cm^2/sec, which is close to the desired maximum of 10.

(b) If the slowing down length is 6 cm, the thermal diffusion length is 3 cm, and the diffusion coefficient is 0.381 cm, what will be the thermal neutron leakage at the surface of the field?

The thermal neutron leakage is given by equation 5.51:

$$\phi = \frac{Se^{-R/L}}{4\pi RD}$$

Where

$S = 10^7$ n/sec
$R = 44$ cm
$D = 0.381$ cm
$L = 3$ cm

Substituting these values into the equation, we have

$$\phi_{th} = \frac{10^7 \frac{\text{n}}{\text{sec}}}{4 \times \pi \times 44 \text{ cm} \times 0.381 \text{ cm}} e^{-\frac{44 \text{ cm}}{3 \text{ cm}}}$$

$$\phi_{th} = 0.08 \frac{\text{n}}{\text{cm}^2\text{sec}}$$

(c) What is the gamma ray dose rate, due to the hydrogen capture gammas, at the surface of the shield?

The capture of a thermal neutron by a hydrogen atom results in the emission of a 2.26 MeV gamma ray (example 10.11). The paraffin, therefore , acts as a distributed source of gamma radiation. The surface dose rate due to the hydrogen capture gammas in the paraffin shield is calculated with equation 10.37: This equation treats the hydrogen capture gammas as if the paraffin shield contained a uniformly distributed gamma emitter.

$$\dot{D} = \frac{1}{2} C\Gamma \frac{4\pi}{\mu}\left(1 - e^{-\mu r}\right)$$

The concentration C of the gamma emitter is equal to the difference between the source emission rate, S, and the neutron escape rate from the surface, divided by the volume of the shield

$$C = \frac{S - 4\pi r^2\left(\phi_{\text{fast}} + \phi_{\text{thermal}}\right)}{\frac{4}{3}\pi r^3}$$

$$C = \frac{10^7 \frac{\text{n}}{\text{s}} - 4\pi(44\text{ cm})^2(8 + 0.08)\frac{\text{n}}{\text{cm}^2 \cdot \text{s}}}{\frac{4}{3}\pi(44)^3} = 27.5 \frac{\gamma/\text{sec}}{\text{cm}^3} = 27.5 \frac{\text{"Bq"}}{\text{cm}^3}$$

$C = 27.5 \times 10^{-6}$ "MBq"/cm^3

Γ is calculated using equation 6.5 and 6.17

$$\Gamma = 3.69 \times 10^{-9} \sum f_i E_i \frac{(\text{C/kg})\text{m}^2}{\text{MBq} \cdot \text{h}} \times 34 \frac{\text{Gy}}{\text{C/kg}}$$

$$\Gamma = 3.69 \times 10^{-9} \times 2.26\text{ MeV} \frac{(\text{C/kg})\text{m}^2}{\text{MBq} \cdot \text{h}} \times 10^4 \frac{\text{cm}^2}{\text{m}^2} \times 34 \frac{\text{Gy}}{\text{C/kg}}$$

$$\Gamma = 2.8 \times 10^{-3} \frac{\text{Gy} \cdot \text{cm}^2}{\text{MBq} \cdot \text{h}} = 2.8 \frac{\text{mGy} \cdot \text{cm}^2}{\text{MBq} \cdot \text{h}}$$

The energy absorption coefficient for paraffin for 2.26 MeV gammas is calculated by interpolating between 2 and 3 MeV data for water (Table 5.3): μ_{en}(2.26 MeV, H_2O) = 0.0252 cm^2/g. Since $H_2C \cong H_2O$ for gamma energy absorption, we calculate the linear energy absorption coefficient for paraffin with μ_m for water.

$\mu_l = \mu_m \times \rho$

$\mu_l = 0.252$ cm^2/g $\times$ 0.89 g/cm^3 = 0.022 cm^{-1}

Inserting these values into the dose rate equation, we have

$$\dot{D} = \frac{1}{2} C\Gamma \frac{4\pi}{\mu}\left(1 - e^{-\mu r}\right)$$

$$\dot{D} = \frac{1}{2} \times \frac{27.5 \times 10^{-6}\ \text{MBq}}{\text{cm}^3} \times \frac{2.8\ \text{mGy} \cdot \text{cm}^2}{\text{hr} \cdot \text{MBq}} \times \frac{4 \times \pi}{0.022\text{cm}^{-1}}\left(1 - \text{e}^{-0.022 \times (44)}\right)$$

$$\dot{D} = 0.014 \frac{\text{mGy}}{\text{hr}} = 1.4 \frac{\text{mrads}}{\text{hr}}$$

10.2

10.2 An x-ray therapy machine operates at 250 kVp and 20 mA. At a target to skin distance of 100 cm, the exposure rate is 20 R/min. The workload is 10,000 mA min/week. The x–ray tube is constrained to point vertically downward. At a distance of 4 m from the target is an uncontrolled waiting room. Calculate the thickness of lead to be added to the wall if the total thickness of the wall (which is made of hollow tile and plaster, density 2.35 g/cm^3) is 2 in.

Since the primary beam is directed downward, the wall shields only scattered and leakage radiation. We calculate the shielding requirement separately for each of these. If they differ by < 1 TVL, the thicker one is adequate. IF they differ by < 1 TVL, then we add 1 HVL to the thicker barrier.

The scattered radiation attenuation requirement is calculated with equation 10.23:

$$K_{ux} = \frac{P}{aWT}\left(d_{sca}\right)^2\left(d_{\sec}\right)^2 \frac{400}{F}$$

where

P = 0.002 R (uncontrolled area)
W = 10,000 mA min/week @ 1 meter
a = ratio of scattered intensity, at 1 m and 90° scatter, to primary intensity = 0.0019 (from table 10.3)
T = Occupancy Factor = 1 (table 10.1)
d_{sca} = 1 m
d_{sec} = 4 m
F = area (assumed in this case) of beam in scattering plane = 400 cm^2

Substituting these values into the equation, we find the attenuation factor to be

$K_{ux} = 1.68 \times 10^{-3}$ R/mA·min ≅ 1 meter.

Use figure 10.14 on the 250 kVp curve to locate the required thickness of lead, which is 4.5 mm.

The leakage radiation from a therapy housing ≤ 500 kV = 1 R/hr at 1 meter. The required attenuation factor to give an average exposure of *P* R/wk at a distance of *d* meters from a tube whose beam current is *I* mA, is given by equation 10.29:

$$B_{\text{LX}} = \frac{P \times d^2 \times 60I}{WT}$$

Substituting the respective values into the equation, we have

$B_{\text{LX}} = 3.84 \times 10^{-3}$

The number of HVL's required to attain this value is:

$$3.84 \times 10^{-3} = \frac{1}{2^n}$$

$n = 8$

One HVL (Pb, 250 kV) = 0.88 mm (Table 10.2), therefore,
the required thickness = 8 HVL × 0.88 mm/HVL = 7.04 mm Pb

The difference between the barrier thickness for leakage and for scattered radiation is

$\Delta t = 7.04 \text{ mm} - 4.5 \text{ mm} = 2.54 \text{ mm}$

Since 1 TVL = 2.9 mm Pb (Table 10.2) > 2.54 mm, we add 1 HVL to the greater thickness inaccordance with NCRP49. The total required thickness is

$t = 7.04 \text{ mm} + 0.88 \text{ mm} = 7.92 \text{ mm Pb} = 9$ HVL's

The wall thickness is 2" (5.08 cm) plaster. Since the plaster has the same density as concrete, we may use the HVL of concrete to find the wall equivalent

$$T(\text{wall}) = \frac{5.08\ \text{cm}}{2.8\,\text{cm/HVL}} = 1.81\ \text{HVL}$$

The additional lead requirement is

$$T\ (\text{Pb}) = 9\ \text{HVL} - 1.8\ \text{HVL} = 7.2\ \text{HVL}$$

$$T\ (\text{Pb}) = 7.2\ \text{HVL} \times 0.88\ \text{mm/HVL} = 6.3\ \text{mm Pb}$$

From Table 10.5, we find that 6.35 mm, or one quarter inch lead sheet which is commercially available.

10.3 **10.3** A 7.4×10^{13} Bq (2000 Ci) ^{60}Co teletherapy unit is to be installed in an existing concrete room in the basement of a hospital so that the source is 4 m from the north and west walls - which are 30 in. thick. Beyond the north wall is a fully occupied control room. Beyond the west wall is a parking lot. The useful beam is to be directed toward the north wall for a maximum of 5 hr per week. The useful beam is to be directed at the west wall 1 hr per week. Considering only the radiation from the primary beam, how much additional shielding, if any, is required for each of the walls?

Control Room P = 100 mrems/wk

30"(0.76 m)

Public Parking Lot
P = 2 mrems/wk

5 hr/wk 4.76 m

30"(0.76 m) 1 hr/wk

4 m

Consider the ^{60}Co to be a point source. Use equation 10.1 to determine the exposure rate unshielded at the boundary:

$$d = 4\ \text{m} + 0.76\ \text{m} = 4.76\ \text{m}$$

$$\Gamma_{\text{Co}-60} = 1.32 \frac{\text{R} \cdot \text{m}^2}{\text{Ci} \cdot \text{hr}} \quad \text{(table 6.3)}$$

$A = 2000$ Ci

$$\dot{X} = \frac{A\Gamma}{d^2} = \frac{2000\text{Ci} \times \left(1.32\,\frac{\text{R}\cdot\text{m}^2}{\text{Ci}\cdot\text{hr}}\right)}{(4.76\text{ m})^2} = 116.5\text{ R/hr}$$

$\frac{116.4\text{ R}}{\text{hr}} \times \frac{5\text{ hr}}{\text{wk}}$ = 582 R/wk (Directed to control room wall 5 hrs/wk as stated in problem)

According to p.434, 5000 mrem/50 weeks a year, 0.1 R/wk is allowed. Also according to NCRP 49, page 6, the maximum permissible occupational exposure (controlled room) is 0.1 R/wk. Assume 100% occupancy for the control room.

The broad beam HVL for ^{60}Co photons of concrete in Table 10.2 is used to calculate the broad beam attenuation coefficient;

$$\mu = \frac{0.693}{\text{HVL}} = \frac{0.693}{6.2\text{ cm}} = 0.112\text{ cm}^{-1}$$

Since the attenuation coefficient is for broad beam geometry, no buildup factor is required.

Calculate the shielding required under conditions of broad beam geometry, the thickness required for the north wall (control room) with equation 5.19;

$I = I_0 e^{-\mu t}$

$\mu = 0.112\text{ cm}^{-1}$
I_0 = 582 R/wk = 582×10^3 mR/wk (as calculated above)
I = 100 mR/wk

$$t = \frac{\ln\left(\frac{I}{I_0}\right)}{-\mu} = \frac{\ln\left(\frac{100\,\frac{\text{mR}}{\text{wk}}}{582\times10^3\,\frac{\text{mR}}{\text{wk}}}\right)}{-0.112\text{ cm}^{-1}}$$ = 77.4 cm concrete needed for the north wall.

Since we need 77.4 cm, and 76 cm is installed, 1.4 cm of concrete is needed for the control room.

$$\# \text{HVL} = \frac{\text{thickness}}{\text{HVL}} = \frac{1.4 \text{ cm concrete}}{6.2 \text{ cm concrete HVL}} = 0.225 \text{ HVL required (Table 10.2)}$$

0.225 HVL of lead is 3.1 mm thick for ^{60}Co photons (Table 10.2). The next available commercial lead thickness (Table 10.5) is 1/8" sheet, which must be added to the control room wall shielding.

For the parking lot; The maximum permissible dose for uncontrolled areas (parking lot), is 100 mrem/year (2 mrem/wk), according to 10CFR20.1301.a.1. NCRP Report 102 indicates a limit of 2 mrem/wk as well for the general public. An occupancy factor of 1/4 from table 10.1 is also applied, so that the maximum exposure in the parking lot must not exceed:

$2\frac{\text{mrem}}{\text{wk}} \times \frac{4}{1}(\text{Occupancy factor}) = 8\frac{\text{mrem}}{\text{wk}}$ limit thus applies to the parking lot wall.

Calculate the shielding required under conditions of broad beam geometry, the thickness required for the parking lot with equation 5.19;

$$I = I_0 e^{-\mu t}$$

$\mu = 0.112 \text{ cm}^{-1}$ (from first part)

$I_0 = 116.5\frac{\text{R}}{\text{hr}} \times \frac{1\text{hr}}{\text{wk}} = 116.5\frac{\text{R}}{\text{wk}} = 116.5 \times 10^3 \frac{\text{mR}}{\text{wk}}$ (one hour towards this wall, as stated in problem)

$I = 8$ mrem/wk

$$t = \frac{\ln\left(\frac{I}{I_0}\right)}{-\mu} = \frac{\ln\left(\frac{8\frac{\text{mrem}}{\text{wk}}}{116.4 \times 10^3 \frac{\text{mrem}}{\text{wk}}}\right)}{-0.112 \text{ cm}^{-1}}$$ = 85.6 cm concrete needed for the parking lot.

Since 76 cm is present, 85.6 cm – 76 cm = 9.6 cm concrete needed.

$$\# \text{HVL} = \frac{\text{thickness}}{\text{HVL}} = \frac{9.6 \text{ cm concrete}}{6.2 \text{ cm concrete HVL}} = 1.55 \text{ HVL needed}$$

1.55 × 12 mm (Pb HVL) = 18.5 mm Pb needed. The nearest commercially available lead sheet is 1" thick.

10.4 A radiochemist wants to carry a small vial containing 2×10^9 Bq (50 mCi) ^{60}Co solution from one hood to another. If the estimated carrying time is 3 min, what would be the minimum length of the tongs used to carry the vial in order that his dose not exceed 60 μGy (6 mrad) during the operation? **10.4**

By definition, 6 mrads gamma radiation = 6 mrems. For radiation safety purposes, 6 mR = 6 mrems. Therefore, 6 mrads gamma = 6 mR. According to equation 10.1

$$\dot{H} = \frac{\Gamma \dfrac{\text{R} \cdot \text{m}^2}{\text{Ci} \cdot \text{hr}} \times A \text{ Ci}}{(d \text{ m})^2} \times w_R$$

For a 3 minute exposure time, the radiation exposure rate is

6 mrems = $\dot{H}$ mrems/hr × 3/60 hr

$\dot{H}$ = 120 mrems/hr = 0.12 rem/hr

Substituting

$\dot{H}$ = 0.12 rem/hr

$\Gamma_{\text{Co-60}} = 1.32 \dfrac{\text{R} \cdot \text{m}^2}{\text{Ci} \cdot \text{hr}}$ (Table 6.3)

A = 0.05 Ci (50 mCi)

into the equation above, and solving for d, we find

$$d = \sqrt{\frac{1.32 \dfrac{\text{R} \cdot \text{m}^2}{\text{Ci} \cdot \text{hr}} \times 0.05 \text{ Ci} \times 1 \dfrac{\text{rem}}{\text{R}}}{0.12 \dfrac{\text{rem}}{\text{hr}}}} = 0.74 \text{ m} = 74 \text{ cm}$$

10.5

10.5 A viewing window for use with an isotope that emits 1-MeV gamma rays is to be made from a saturated aqueous solution of KI in a rectangular battery jar. What will be the attenuation factor, assuming conditions of good geometry, if the solution thickness is 10 cm, and if the glass walls are equivalent in their attenuation property to 1 mm lead? A saturated solution of KI may be made by adding 30 g KI to 21 mL water to give 30 mL solution at 25 °C. Total attenuation cross sections for 1 MeV gamma rays for the elements in the solution are:

The attenuation factor is calculated from equation 5.19:

$$I/I_0 = e^{-\mu t}$$

The linear attenuation of the KI solution is calculated with the aid of equation 5.23

$$\mu_1 = \Sigma N_i \sigma_i,$$

where N_i is the concentration of the ith atom or molecule per cc, and σ_i is its cross section. For the components of the solution, we have:

K (A = 39.100) = 4 barns
H (A = 1) = 0.2 barns
I (A= 126.91) = 12 barns
O (A = 16) = 1.7 barns
KI (MW = 166.01) = 16 barns
H_2O (MW = 18) = 2.1 barns

The concentrations, N_i, are

$$\text{KI:}\ \frac{30\ \text{g}}{166.01\ \ \text{g/mol} \times 30\ \text{cm}^3} = 6.02 \times 10^{-3}\ \frac{\text{mol KI}}{\text{cm}^3}$$

$$\text{H}_2\text{O:}\ \frac{21\ \text{g}}{18\ \ \text{g/mol} \times 30\ \text{cm}^3} = 3.89 \times 10^{-2}\ \frac{\text{mol H}_2\text{O}}{\text{cm}^3}$$

Since there are 6.02×10^{23} molecule/mole and 10^{-24} cm^2/b

$$\mu_1\ (\text{solution}) = 6.02\times10^{23}\times10^{-24}(6.02\times10^{-3}\times16+3.89\times10^{-2}\times2.1) = 0.107\ \text{cm}^{-1}$$

$$\mu_1\ (\text{Pb, 1 MeV}) = 0.771\ \text{cm}^{-1}\ (\text{Table 5.2})$$

$$\frac{I}{I_0} = e^{-0.107\ \text{cm}^{-1} \times 10\ \text{cm}} \times e^{-0.771\ \text{cm}^{-1} \times 0.1\ \text{cm}} = 0.32$$

10.6 Lead foil consists of an alloy containing 87% Pb and 12% Sn, 1% Cu. Its specific gravity is 10.4. If the mass attenuation coefficients for these three elements are 3.50, 1.17, and 0.325 cm²/g respectively, for X-rays whose wavelength is 0.098 angstroms **10.6**

(a) calculate the mass and linear absorption coefficients for lead foil,

Mass;

$\mu_{mass}\ \Sigma f_i\, \mu_i$

Element	fraction present, f	Attenuation coef., μ	$f_i \times \mu_i$
Pb	0.87	3.5	3.045
Sn	0.12	1.17	0.1404
Cu	0.01	0.325	0.00325
		Sum	**3.19 cm²/g**

μ (linear) = $\rho\Sigma f_i\, \mu_i = \rho\Sigma f_i\, \mu$ (mass)

$$\mu\ (\text{linear}) = 10.4\frac{\text{g}}{\text{cm}^3} \times 3.19\frac{\text{cm}^2}{g} = 33.2\ \text{cm}^{-1}$$

(b) What thickness of lead foil would be required to attenuate the intensity of ^{57}Co gamma rays E(gamma) = 0.123 MeV, by a factor of 25?

Equation 5.19;

$I/I_0 = e^{-\mu t}$

$\mu = 33.16\ \text{cm}^{-1}$
$I/I_0 = 1/25 = 0.04$

$$t = \frac{\ln\left(\frac{I}{I_0}\right)}{-\mu} = \frac{\ln(0.04)}{-33.12\ \text{cm}^{-1}} = 0.097\ \text{cm}$$

10.7

10.7 A hypodermic syringe that will be used in an experiment in which ^{90}Sr solution will be injected has a glass barrel whose wall is 1.5 mm thick. If the density of the glass is 2.5 g/cm^3, how many mm thick must we make a Lucite sleeve that will fit around the syringe if no beta particles are to come through the Lucite? The density of Lucite is 1.2 g/cm^3.

Strontium 90, which emits a 0.55 MeV beta, decays to ^{90}Y, which emits a 2.27 MeV beta (RHH). The shield must therefore be designated to stop the 2.27 MeV beta. Using equation 5.2 to find the range of the beta:

$$R = 412(E \text{ MeV})^{1.265 - 0.0954 \ln(E)}$$

$R = 412 \times (2.27)^{1.265 - 0.0954 \ln(2.27)} = 1090$ mg/cm^2 =1.09 g/cm^2 is the density thickness required.

Already there is glass shielding present, whose density thickness is:

$$0.15 \text{ cm} \times \frac{2.5\text{g}}{\text{cm}^3} = 0.375 \text{ g/cm}^2$$

Calculating the amount of additional shielding required:

1.09 g/cm^2 – 0.357 g/cm^2 = 0.715 g/cm^2 needed.

Lucite is 1.2 g/cm^3, so calculating the additional thickness required:

$$\frac{0.715 \text{ g}}{\text{cm}^2} \times \frac{\text{cm}^3}{1.2 \text{ g}} \times \frac{10 \text{ mm}}{1 \text{ cm}} = 6 \text{ mm Lucite}$$

10.8

10.8 A room in which a 7.4×10^{13} Bq (2000 Ci) ^{137}Cs source will be exposed has the following layout. Calculate the thickness t of concrete so that the exposure rate at the outside surface of the wall does not exceed 0.64 μC/kg (2.5 mR) per hour.

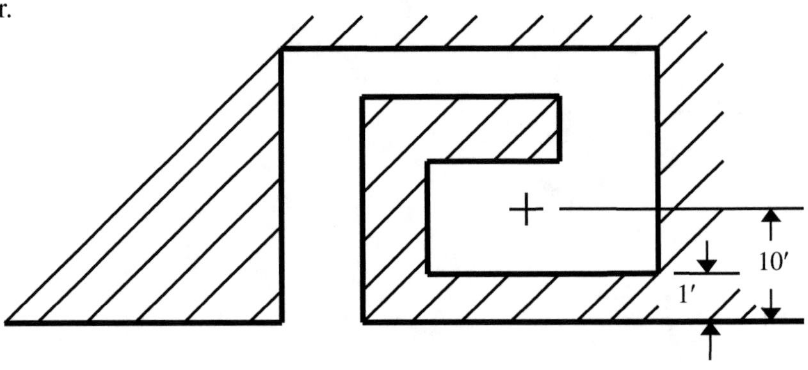

Consider the ^{137}Cs to be a point source. Use equation 10.1 to determine the exposure rate unshielded at the boundary:

$d = 10\text{ ft} = 3.048\text{ m}$

$\Gamma_{\text{Cs-137}} = 0.33\dfrac{\text{R}\cdot\text{m}^2}{\text{Ci}\cdot\text{hr}}$ (table 6.3)

$A = 2000\text{ Ci}$

$$\dot{X} = \frac{A\Gamma}{d^2} = \frac{2000\text{Ci}\times\left(0.33\dfrac{\text{R}\cdot\text{m}^2}{\text{Ci}\cdot\text{hr}}\right)}{(3.048\text{ m})^2} = 71\text{ R/hr is the exposure rate unshielded.}$$

The desired exposure rate is:

$$\frac{2.5\text{ mR}}{\text{hr}}\times\frac{1\text{ R}}{1000\text{ mR}} = 0.0025\text{ R/hr}$$

Determine the required attenuation;

$$\text{Required fraction attenuation} = \frac{0.0025\dfrac{\text{R}}{\text{hr}}}{71\dfrac{\text{R}}{\text{hr}}} = 3.5\times10^{-5}$$

The broad beam HVL of concrete for ^{137}Cs is listed as 4.8 cm (Table 10.2). The number of HVL's needed to reduce the transmitted radiation by this factor is

$$\frac{1}{2^n} = 3.5\times10^{-5}$$

$$n = \frac{-\log\left(3.5\times10^{-5}\right)}{\log\ 2} = 14.8$$

Therefore, the required thickness = 14.8 HVL's × 4.8 cm/HVL = 71 cm = 28 in.

Alternatively, if the broad beam attenuation data for the nuclide of concern are not available, the following procedure may be utilized.

Calculate the shielding required under conditions of "good" or collimated geometry first, to obtain an estimate of the minimum thickness required with equation 5.19;

$$I/I_0 = e^{-\mu t}$$

and then recalculated using a buildup factor, B, equation 10.17

$$I/I_0 = Be^{-\mu t}$$

μ= 0.184 cm^{-1} (table 5.2)
I_0 =71 R/hr
I = 0.0025 R/hr

$$t = \frac{\ln\left(\frac{I}{I_0}\right)}{-\mu} = \frac{\ln\left(\frac{0.0025 \text{ R/hr}}{71 \text{ R/hr}}\right)}{-0.184 \text{ cm}^{-1}}$$ =55.7 cm concrete needed under conditions of "good" geometry.

Now estimate the required thickness when the buildup factor is included by adding one Half Value Layer (HVL) to the value for thickness under conditions of "good" (collimated) geometry. The HVL for concrete is calculated

$$\text{HVL} = \frac{0.693}{\mu} = \frac{0.693}{0.184 \text{ cm}^{-1}} = 3.8 \text{ cm}$$

55.7 + 3.8 = 59.5 cm as a first estimate of the thickness required.

The number of relaxation lengths, μt, for this thickness will be:

μt = 59.5 × (0.184) = 11 relaxation lengths.
In the absence of specific data for B, B may be estimated as

$$B \cong 1 + \mu t$$

Recalculating the exposure rate using equation 10.17,
$\mu t = 11$
$t = 59.5$ cm,
$B = 1 + 11 = 12$
$I_0 = 71$ R/hr

$$I = BI_0 e^{-\mu t} = 12 \times \left(71 \frac{\text{R}}{\text{hr}}\right) \times \text{e}^{-11} = 0.0142 \frac{\text{R}}{\text{hr}}$$

This is approximately six times higher than the required 0.0025 R/hr. Add 3 more HVL's,

59.5 + 3(3.8) = 71 cm as a second estimate of the thickness required.

The number of relaxation lengths, μt, for this thickness is:

$\mu t = 71 \times (0.184) = 13$ relaxation lengths.

$B = 1 + \mu t = 14$

Recalculating the exposure rate using equation 10.17,
$\mu t = 13$
$t = 71$ cm,
$B = 14$
$I_0 = 71$ R/hr

$$I = BI_0 e^{-\mu t} = 14 \times \left(71 \frac{\text{R}}{\text{hr}}\right) \times \text{e}^{-13} = 0.0023 \frac{\text{R}}{\text{hr}}$$

Thus, the shield is 71 cm or 28 inches concrete, which is the same value that was calculated using the broad beam HVL's in Table 10.2 or NCRP 49.

10.9 What minimum density thickness must a pair of gloves have to protect the hands from ^{32}P radiation? **10.9**

Maximum β energy for ^{32}P is 1.708 MeV

Input this into equation 5.2 to find the maximum range of the β;

$$R = 412(E\ \text{MeV})^{1.265-0.0954\times\ln(E\ \text{MeV})} = 412 \times (1.708\ \text{MeV})^{1.265-0.0954\times\ln(1.708\ \text{MeV})} = 789\frac{\text{mg}}{\text{cm}^2}$$

10.10

10.10 When a radium source containing 50 mg Ra encapsulated in 0.5 mm thick Pt is placed into a Pb storage container, the measured exposure rate at a distance of 1 m from the source is 5.41 μC/kg (21 mR) per hour. If this same container is used for storing ^{137}Cs, how many MBq may be kept in it for a period of 4 h without exceeding an exposure of 10.3 μC/kg (40 mR) at a distance of 50 cm from the source?

$$\dot{X} = \frac{A\Gamma}{d^2}$$

$d = 1$ m

$$\Gamma_{\text{Ra}-226} = 0.825\frac{\text{R}\cdot\text{m}^2}{\text{Ci}\cdot\text{hr}}\ \text{(table 6.3)}$$

$$A = 50\ \text{mg Ra} \times \frac{1\ \text{g}}{1000\ \text{mg}} \times \frac{1\ \text{Ci}}{1\ \text{g Ra}} = 50 \times 10^{-3}\text{Ci}$$

$$\dot{X} = \frac{A\Gamma}{d^2} = \frac{50 \times 10^{-3}\text{Ci} \times \left(0.825\frac{\text{R}\cdot\text{m}^2}{\text{Ci}\cdot\text{hr}}\right)}{(1\ \text{m})^2} = 0.041\ \text{R/hr} = 41\ \text{mR/hr is the exposure}$$

rate unshielded.

$I_0 = 41$ mR/hr

The reduction in intensity due to the lead shield is

$$\frac{I}{I_0} = \frac{21\frac{\text{mR}}{\text{hr}}}{41\frac{\text{mR}}{\text{hr}}} = 0.5$$

Thus, one half value layer (HVL) for Ra is provided by the shielding. Since broad beam geometry is involved, find the HVL for radium broad beam geometry in Table 10.2 as 1.66 cm of Pb. Thus, 1.66 cm of Pb is the thickness of the lead in the shield.

We want the shielded ^{137}Cs exposure rate to be 40 mR/4 hr = 10 mR/hr at 0.5 m. The unshielded gamma ray intensity of the stored ^{137}Cs is calculated with equation 5.19, using the broad beam HVL from Table 10.2 (or NCRP 49) to determine the broad beam attenuation coefficient of the lead storage container.

$$\mu = \frac{0.693}{\text{HVL}} = \frac{0.693}{0.65 \text{ cm}} = 1.066 \text{ cm}^{-1}$$

Substituting into the attenuation equation, we have

$$10 \frac{\text{mR}}{\text{hr}} = I_0 e^{-1.066 \text{ cm}^{-1} \times 1.66 \text{ cm}}$$

$I_0 = 58.7$ mR/hr

Use equation 10.1 to determine the activity;
$d = 0.5$ m

$$\Gamma_{\text{Cs-137}} = 330 \frac{\text{mR} \cdot \text{m}^2}{\text{Ci} \cdot \text{hr}} \quad \text{(table 6.3)}$$

$A = ?$
$\dot{X} = 58.7$ mR/hr

$$\dot{X} = \frac{A\Gamma}{d^2}$$

Solving for A (activity);

$$A = \frac{\dot{X}d^2}{\Gamma} = \frac{58.7 \times (0.5)^2}{330 \frac{\text{mR} \cdot \text{m}^2}{\text{Ci} \cdot \text{hr}}} = 0.043 \text{ Ci}$$

$$A = 0.043 \text{ Ci} \times \frac{3.7 \times 10^4 \text{ MBq}}{\text{Ci}} = 1.6 \times 10^3 \text{ MBq}$$

10.11 What is the maximum working time in a mixed radiation field consisting of 6 mC/kg (20 mR) per hour gamma, 40 μGy (4 mrad) per hour fast neutrons, and 50μGy (5 mrad) per hour thermal neutrons, if a maximum dose equivalent of 3 mSv (300 mrem) has been specified for the job? **10.11**

Since this problem involves legal units (rad, rem), for regulatory purposes, let 1 R = 1 rem.

The quality factors for converting rads to rems can be found in Table 7.8 and in 10 CFR 20, Table 20.1004(b).1, (1994).

$Q_{gamma} = 1$
$Q_{fast\ n} = 10$
$Q_{thermal\ n} = 2$

Multiplying the quality factor times each type of radiation to obtain rems:

$20 \text{ mrads/hr} \times Q_{gamma} = 20 \times 1 = 20 \text{ mrems/hr}$
$4 \text{ mrads/hr} \times Q_{fast\ n} = 4 \times 10 = 40 \text{ mrems/hr}$
$5 \text{ mrads/hr} \times Q_{thermal\ n} = 5 \times 2 = \underline{10 \text{ mrems/hr}}$
Total = 70 mrems/hr

Since only 300 mrems are allowed,

$$300 \text{ mrems} \times \frac{1 \text{ hr}}{70 \text{ mrems}} = 4.29 \text{ hours stay time allowed, or 4 hours 17 minutes}$$

10.12

10.12 Maintenance work must be done on a piece of equipment that is 2 meters from an internally contaminated (with ^{137}Cs) valve. The exposure rate at 30 cm from the valve is 500 R/hr (0.13 C/kg–hr). If 4 hours is the estimated repair time, what thickness of lead shielding is required to limit the dose equivalent of the maintenance persons to 1 mSv (100 millirems)?

Determine the exposure rate at 2 meters without shielding (equation 9.20):

$I_1 = 500$ R/hr
$d_1 = 30 \text{ cm} = 0.30$ m
$d_2 = 2$ m

$$I_2 = \frac{I_1 d_1^2}{d_2^2} = \frac{500 \times (0.3^2)}{2^2} = 11.25 \text{ R/hr}$$

1 R of exposure = 1 rem of dose equivalent gamma rays for radiation safety purposes.

Since the repairs should only take 4 hours, and the maximum dose allowed is 100 mrem, the required dose rate after shielding is:

$$\frac{100 \text{ mrems}}{4 \text{ hours}} \times \frac{1 \text{ rem}}{1000 \text{ mrems}} = 0.025 \text{ rem/hr}$$

Use Table 10.2 to find the HVL for Cs-137 as 0.65 cm under conditions of broad beam geometry. Calculate the broad beam attenuation coefficient;

$$\mu = \frac{0.693}{\text{HVL}} = \frac{0.693}{0.65 \text{ cm}} = 1.07 \text{ cm}^{-1}$$

Equation 5.19 gives the shielding thickness:

$I_0 = 11.25$ rem/hr

$I = 0.025$ rem/hr
$\mu = 1.07 \text{ cm}^{-1}$

$I = I_0 e^{-\mu t}$

$0.025 = 11.25 \times e^{-1.07 \times (t)}$

$t = 5.7$ cm

An alternative solution which could be utilized if broad beam attenuation curves are not available but generalized curves of build up factors, such as figures 10.9 and 10.10 in the textbook are available.

Equation 5.19 gives an estimate for the shielding thickness under conditions of "good" geometry:

$I_0 = 11.25$ rem/hr
$I = 0.025$ rem/hr
$\mu = 1.34 \text{ cm}^{-1}$ (Table 5.2, for 0.661 MeV gamma and Pb)
HVL = $0.693/1.34 \text{ cm}^{-1} = 0.52$ cm

$I = I_0 e^{-\mu t}$

$0.025 = 11.25 \times e^{-1.34 \times (t)}$

$t = 4.56$ cm

Since the shield must be thicker than this to allow for buildup, add one half value layer (HVL) to give 4.56 + 0.52 = 5.08 cm.

Now, find in Fig. 10.9 that for 0.66 MeV gamma in Pb, for

$\mu t = 1.34 \text{ cm}^{-1} \times 5.08 \text{ cm} = 6.8$, $B = 2$.

Using this increased thickness, with $B = 2$, in equation 10.17

$I = I_0 B e^{-\mu t}$

and solving for I, we find
$I = 11.25 \times 2 \times e^{-6.8} = 0.025$,

which is the desired value. Thus, a Pb shield 5.08 cm (2 in.) thick is satisfactory. This calculated thickness is in good agreement with the 4.56 cm thickness previously calculated.

10.13

10.13 Calculate the exposure rate from a 100,000 MBq (2.7 Ci) ^{60}Co "point" source, at a distance of 1.25 meters, if the source is shielded with 10 cm Pb?

Equation 10.1 is used to first obtain the exposure rate without shielding:

$\Gamma_{\text{Co-60}} = 1.32 \text{ (R–m}^2\text{)/(Ci–hr)}$ From Table 6.3
$A = 2.7$ Ci
$d = 1.25$ m

$$\dot{X} = \frac{\Gamma A}{d^2} = \frac{1.32 \times 2.7}{(1.25)^2}$$ = 2.28 R/hr is the exposure rate unshielded.

Next, calculate the shielded exposure rate, and account for the buildup factor by using the broad beam HVL (Table 10.2) to calculate the broad beam attenuation coefficient.

$$\mu_{\text{broad beam}} = \frac{0.693}{HVL} = \frac{0.693}{1.2 \text{ cm Pb}} = 0.578 \text{ cm}^{-1}$$

$$I = BI_0 e^{-\mu t} = 2.28 e^{-0.578 \times 10} = 7 \times 10^{-3} \text{ R/hr} = 7 \text{ mR/hr}$$

10.14 A stainless steel bolt came loose from a reactor vessel. It is planned to pick up the bolt with a remotely operated set of tongs and transport it for inspection and study. The bolt had been in a mean thermal neutron flux of 2×10^{12} n/cm^2·sec for a period of 900 days, and will be picked up 21 days after reactor shut–down. Calculate the gamma ray dose rate at a distance of 1 meter from the bolt if the bolt weighs 200 grams and has the following composition by weight: **10.14**

Fe	80%
Ni	19%
Mn	0.5%
C	0.5%

Check the NRHH to find which isotopes are produced and which are significant and to obtain their cross sections for activation. In this alloy, the activated ^{56}Mn and ^{54}Ni have very short half lives, and thus will have decayed away in 21 days. Carbon is not activated (^{14}C emits only betas) and ^{55}Fe emits no gammas. Iron 59, $T_{1/2}$ = 44.6 days, which is produced by ^{58}Fe (n,γ)^{59}Fe is the only gamma emitter; it emits a 1.1 MeV gamma in 56% and 1.29 MeV gamma in 44% of all its decays. The isotopic abundance of ^{58}Fe is 0.31% and its activation cross section is 1.28 barns (NRHH). Since the ^{59}Fe half life is 44.6 days, saturation activity, equation 5.59, is attained:

$$A(\text{sat}) = \lambda N = \phi \sigma n$$

n, the number of target ^{58}Fe atoms, is calculated

$$n = 200\text{ g} \times \frac{80\text{ g Fe}}{100\text{ g}} \times \frac{0.31\,^{58}\text{Fe}}{100\text{ g Fe}} \times \frac{1\text{ mole}\,^{58}\text{Fe}}{58\text{ g}\,^{58}\text{Fe}} \times \frac{6.02 \times 10^{23}\text{ atoms}\,^{58}\text{Fe}}{1\text{ mole}\,^{58}\text{Fe}}$$

atoms

Substituting these values into the activity equation:

$$A(\text{sat}) = \frac{2 \times 10^{12}\text{ n}}{\text{cm}^2 \cdot \text{sec}} \times 1.28 \times 10^{-24}\text{ cm}^2 \times 5.15 \times 10^{21}\text{ atoms} = 1.32 \times 10^{10}\text{dps}$$

$A(\text{sat}) = 1.32 \times 10^{10}$ dps $= 1.32 \times 10^{10}$ Bq $= 1.32 \times 10^{4}$ MBq

After 21 days, the activity is

$$A = 1.32 \times 10^4 \text{ MBq } e^{-\frac{0.693}{44.6 \text{ d}} \times 21 \text{ d}}$$

$$A = 9.525 \times 10^3 \text{ MBq}$$

The dose rate at one meter from this activity is calculated with equation 10.1.

$$\dot{H} = \frac{\Gamma A}{d^2}$$

$$\Gamma = 3.65 \times 10^{-9} \sum f_i E_i \frac{\text{C/kg} \cdot \text{m}^2}{\text{MBq}} \times 34 \frac{\text{Sv}}{\text{C/kg}}$$

$$\Gamma = 3.65 \times 10^{-9} (0.561 \times 1.1 + 0.44 \times 1.29) \times 34 = 1.4 \times 10^{-7} \frac{\text{Sv} \cdot \text{m}^2}{\text{MBq}}$$

$$H = \frac{1.4 \times 10^{-7} \frac{\text{Sv} \cdot \text{m}^2}{\text{MBq} \cdot \text{h}} \times 9.525 \times 10^3 \text{ MBq}}{(1 \text{ m})^2}$$

$$H = 1.4 \times 10^{-3} \text{ Sv} = 1.4 \text{ mSv}$$

10.15

10.15 A circular area 1 meter in diameter is accidentally contaminated with 10 MBq (270 μCi) ^{131}I. What is the maximum dose equivalent rate at a distance of 1 meter above the contaminated area?

The dose rate at a height of 1 meter is the sum of the gamma and beta dose rates. The gamma dose rate is calculated with equation 10.10:

$$\dot{H} = 34(\pi)\Gamma(C_a)\ln\left(\frac{R^2 + h^2}{h^2}\right)$$

The area contaminated is:
$A = \pi R^2 = \pi \times (0.5\text{m})^2 = 0.785 \text{ m}^2$
$R = 0.5$ m (radius of the circular area)
$h = 1$ m (height above circular area)

$$C_a = \frac{10 \text{ MBq}}{0.785 \text{ m}^2} = 12.73 \frac{\text{MBq}}{\text{m}^2}$$

$$\Gamma_{\text{I-131}} = 1.53 \times 10^{-9} \frac{\text{X} \cdot \text{m}^2}{\text{MBq} \cdot \text{hr}} \text{ (Table 6.3)}$$

Using equation 10.10;

$$\dot{H} = 34 \times \pi \times 1.53 \times 10^{-9} \frac{\text{X} \cdot \text{m}^2}{\text{MBq} \cdot \text{hr}} \times \left(12.73 \frac{\text{MBq}}{\text{m}^2}\right) \times \ln\left(\frac{(0.5 \text{ m})^2 + (1 \text{ m})^2}{(1)^2}\right)$$

$\dot{H} = 0.46 \times 10^{-6}$ Sv/hr = 0.46 μSv/hr is the photon dose.

The beta dose is calculated next. Iodine emits 5 groups of betas. The mean value of the maximum energies of these, $\overline{E}_{max} = 0.595$ MeV, and the average energy of all these betas is $\overline{E} = 0.195$ MeV/transformation. The dose rate to the skin at a distance d above the contaminated area is given by equation 6.31a.

$$\dot{D}_b = C_a \times 1.3 \times 10^3 \times \overline{E} \times e^{-\mu_a d} \times e^{-\mu_t 0.007} \times \mu_t \text{ mrads/h}$$

where

$\mu_a = 16 (E_m - 0.036)^{-1.4} = 16 (0.585 - 0.036)^{-1.4} = 37.04 \text{ cm}^2/\text{g}$ (Equation 6.20)

$\mu_t = 18.6 (E_m - 0.036)^{-1.37} = 18.6 (0.585 - 0.036)^{-1.37} = 42.3 \text{ cm}^2/\text{g}$ (Equation 6.21)

Substituting $C_a = \dfrac{270 \ \mu\text{Ci}}{\pi \left(\dfrac{100 \text{ cm}}{2}\right)^2}$, $\overline{E} = 0.195$ MeV/transformation, and

$d = 100 \text{ cm} \times 1.293 \times 10^{-3} \text{ g/cm}^3 = 0.1293 \text{ g/cm}^2$, and the respective values for μ_a and μ_t, we have

$$\dot{D}_b = \frac{270 \ \mu\text{Ci}}{\pi \left(\frac{100 \text{ cm}}{2}\right)^2} \times 1.3 \times 10^3 \times 0.195 \text{ MeV} \times e^{-37.04 \times 0.129} \times e^{-42.3 \times 0.007} \times 42.3$$

$\dot{D}_b = 2.3$ mrad/hr = 23 μSv/hr

The total dose rate is 23 + 0.46 = 24 μSv/hr

10.16

10.16 Design a spherical lead storage container that will attenuate the radiation dose rate from 5×10^{10} Bq (1.35 Ci) ^{24}Na to 100 μGy/hr (10 mrad/hr) at a distance of 1 meter from the source. (The source is physically small enough to be considered a "point.")

Sodium 24 emits 2 photons per transformation:

(1) 2.75 MeV gamma

$\mu(\text{Pb}) = 0.476\ \text{cm}^{-1}$ (Table 5.2)
$\text{HVL} = 0.693/0.476\ \text{cm}^{-1} = 1.5\ \text{cm}$

(2) 1.37 MeV gamma

$\mu(\text{Pb}) = 0.621\ \text{cm}^{-1}$ (Table 5.2)
$\text{HVL} = 0.693/0.621\ \text{cm}^{-1} = 1.12\ \text{cm}$

$$\Gamma\left({}^{24}\text{Na}\right) = 12.8 \times 10^{-9}\ \frac{\text{C/kg} \cdot \text{m}^2}{\text{MBq} \cdot \text{h}} \times 34 \frac{\text{Gy}}{\text{C/kg}}$$

$$\Gamma\left({}^{24}\text{Na}\right) = 4.4 \times 10^{-7}\ \frac{\text{Gy} \cdot \text{m}^2}{\text{MBq} \cdot \text{h}}\ \text{(Table 6.3)}$$

Dose rate at 1 meter,

$$\dot{D}(1\ \text{m}) = 4.4 \times 10^{-7}\ \frac{\text{Gy} \cdot \text{m}^2}{\text{MBq} \cdot \text{h}} \times 5 \times 10^4\ \text{MBq} \times 10^6\ \frac{\mu\text{Gy}}{\text{Gy}}$$

$$\dot{D}(1\ \text{m}) = 2.2 \times 10^4\ \frac{\mu\text{Gy}}{\text{h}}$$

The required attenuation:

$$\frac{I}{I_0} = \frac{100\ \mu\text{Gy/h}}{2.2 \times 10^4\ \mu\text{Gy/h}} = 4.6 \times 10^{-3}$$

The number of HVL's to attain this attenuation

$$\frac{I}{I_0} = 4.6 \times 10^{-3} = \frac{1}{2^n}$$

$n = 7.8 = 8$ HVL's

Each of the two gammas contribute to the shielded dose rate, but the lead shield will attenuate the 1.37 MeV gamma much more than the 2.75 MeV gamma. Let us first consider the attenuation only of the 2.75 MeV gamma by 8 HVL's plus 1 HVL to account for the 1.37 MeV gamma and for buildup. The estimated shield thickness thus is

$t = 9$ HVL × 1.5 cm/HVL = 13.5 cm..

The buildup factor, B, for the 2.75 MeV gamma is

B (Pb, $\mu t = 0.476\ \text{cm}^{-1} \times 13.5\ \text{cm} = 6.4$) = 3 (Fig. 10.9)

The unshielded dose rate at 1 meter due to the 2.75 MeV gamma is (equation 6.17 and 6.5)

$$\dot{D}_0(2.75\ \text{MeV}) = (3.65 \times 10^{-9} \times 2.75)\frac{\text{C/kg} \cdot \text{m}^2}{\text{MBq} \cdot \text{h}} \times 5 \times 10^4\ \text{MBq} \times 34\frac{\text{Gy}}{\text{C/kg}}$$

$$\dot{D}_0(2.75\ \text{MeV}) = 1.7 \times 10^{-2}\ \frac{\text{Gy}}{\text{h}}$$

and the shielded dose rate is

$$\dot{D} = \dot{D}_0 B e^{-\mu t} = 1.7 \times 10^{-2}\ \frac{\text{Gy}}{\text{h}} \times 3 \times e^{-6.4}$$

$$\dot{D} = 8.5 \times 10^{-5}\ \frac{\text{Gy}}{\text{h}} = 85\frac{\mu\text{Gy}}{\text{h}}$$

For the 1.37 MeV gamma, the unshielded dose rate at 1 meter is

$$\dot{D}_0(1.37\ \text{MeV}) = (3.65 \times 10^{-9} \times 1.37)\frac{\text{C/kg} \cdot \text{m}^2}{\text{MBq} \cdot \text{h}} \times 5 \times 10^4\ \text{MBq} \times 34\frac{\text{Gy}}{\text{C/kg}}$$

$$\dot{D}_0(1.37\ \text{MeV}) = 0.85 \times 10^{-2}\ \frac{\text{Gy}}{\text{h}}$$

and the shielded dose rate, with a value of

B (Pb, $\mu t = 0.621\ \text{cm}^{-1} \times 13.5\ \text{cm} = 8.4$) = 3.8 is

$$\dot{D} = \dot{D}_0 B e^{-\mu t} = 0.85 \times 10^{-2}\ \frac{\text{Gy}}{\text{h}} \times 3.8 \times e^{-8.4}$$

$$\dot{D} = 7.3 \times 10^{-6}\ \frac{\text{Gy}}{\text{h}} = 7\ \frac{\mu\text{Gy}}{\text{h}}$$

The total dose rate at 1 meter with 13.5 cm of lead shielding is

$\dot{D}$ = 85 + 7 = 92 μGy/h, which is compatible with the 100 μGy/h requirement.

10.17

10.17 What thickness of standard concrete is needed to reduce the intensity of a collimated beam of 10 MeV X-rays from 10^4 mW/cm^2 to an intensity corresponding to 2.5×10^{-3} centisieverts per hour?

The exposure rate is measured in mW/cm^2 because the roentgen and C/kg are defined only for x-rays or gammas whose energy is less than 3 MeV.

Calculate the flux required to obtain $10^4\ \frac{\text{mW}}{\text{cm}^2}$;

$$\frac{10\ \text{MeV}}{\gamma} \times \frac{\phi_0}{\text{cm}^2 \cdot \text{sec}} \times \frac{1.6 \times 10^{-13}\ \text{J}}{\text{MeV}} \times \frac{1\ \text{W}}{1\ \text{J}/\text{sec}} \times \frac{10^3\ \text{mW}}{\text{W}} = 10^4\ \frac{\text{mW}}{\text{cm}^2}$$

Incident flux, $\phi_0 = 6.25 \times 10^{12}\ \frac{\text{photons}}{\text{cm}^2 \cdot \text{sec}}$

Now calculate the flux required to produce 2.5×10^{-3} cSv/hr in tissue (equation 6.10). The absorption coefficient in tissue is utilized since the units are Sv. The energy absorption coefficient for tissue is 0.0154 cm^2/g (Table 5.3).

$$2.5\times10^{-3}\frac{\text{cSv}}{\text{hr}}=\frac{\phi\dfrac{\gamma}{\text{cm}^2\cdot\text{sec}}\times\dfrac{10\text{ MeV}}{\gamma}\times\dfrac{1.6\times10^{-13}\text{ J}}{\text{MeV}}\times0.0154\dfrac{\text{cm}^2}{\text{g}}}{\left(0.001\dfrac{\text{J/g}}{\text{Gy}}\right)\times\dfrac{1\text{ Gy}}{100\text{ cSv}}}$$

Solving the above equation for photon flux;

$\phi = 1 \times 10^6$

The required attenuation factor is

$$\frac{I}{I_0}=\frac{1\times10^6}{6.25\times10^{12}}=1.6\times10^{-7}$$

The number of HVL's to attain this attenuation is

$$\frac{1}{2^n}=1.6\times10^{-7}$$

n = 22.6 HVL's

The broad beam HVL of concrete for 10 MeV photons is listed in Table 10.2 as 11.9 cm. The required thickness therefore is

t = 22.6 HVL's × 11.9 cm/HVL = 269 cm

10.18 A Ra-Be neutron source emits about 1.2×10^7 fast neutrons (average energy = 4 MeV) per gram Ra. What fraction of the dose equivalent from an unshielded source is due to the neutrons? **10.18**

Find the exposure from the Ra gamma rays first:

A = 1 g Ra = 1 Ci Ra (to yield 1.2×10^7 fast neutrons)

$$\Gamma_{\text{Ra-226}}=0.825\frac{\text{R}\cdot\text{m}^2}{\text{Ci}\cdot\text{hr}}\text{ (table 6.3)}$$

The unshielded gamma ray exposure rate at the distance of 1 meter from 1 gram of Ra is 0.825 R/hr.

For radiation safety purposes, 1 R = 1 rem = 0.01 Sv, so no conversion factors are applied.
The gamma dose rate is 0.825 rem/hr = 8.25 mSv/hr.

Now calculate the neutron flux at one meter unshielded. Assume the neutrons are isotropically distributed over a spherical area whose radius is 100 cm (1 m). Using 1 Ci Ra, 1.2×10^7 fast neutrons are produced per second. Dividing this by the spherical area at one meter will yield the neutron flux at one meter,

$$\frac{1.2 \times 10^7 \text{ n/sec}}{4\pi(100 \text{ cm})^2} = 95.5 \frac{\text{n}}{\text{cm}^2 \cdot \text{sec}}$$

From Table 9.5 it is found that for a 40 hour exposure to 4 MeV neutrons

$$9.2 \frac{\text{n}}{\text{cm}^2 \cdot \text{sec}} = 1 \frac{\text{mSv}}{\text{wk}}$$

Using this information and the calculated neutron flux above, ratio the two values to find the neutron dose rate from the Ra-Be neutrons

$$\frac{95.5 \dfrac{\text{n}}{\text{cm}^2 \cdot \text{sec}}}{\dot{D}_n} = \frac{9.2 \dfrac{\text{n}}{\text{cm}^2 \cdot \text{sec}}}{1 \dfrac{\text{mSv}}{\text{wk}}}$$

$$\dot{D}_n = 10.38 \frac{\text{mSv}}{\text{wk}}$$

Now calculate the fraction of dose equivalent due to the neutrons:

$$f = \frac{\dot{D}_n}{\dot{D}_n + \dot{D}_\gamma} = \frac{10.38 \dfrac{\text{mSv}}{\text{wk}}}{\left(8.25 \dfrac{\text{mSv}}{\text{hr}} \times \dfrac{40 \text{ h}}{\text{wk}}\right) + \left(10.38 \dfrac{\text{mSv}}{\text{wk}}\right)}$$

$$f = 0.03 = 3\%$$

10.19 Transport regulations for shipping a radioactive package specify a maximum surface dose rate equivalent of 2 mSv/hr (200 mrem/hr) and a maximum of 0.1 mSv/hr (10 mrem/hr) at 1 meter from the surface. If aqueous ^{137}Cs waste is to be mixed with cement for disposal, what is the maximum specific activity of the concrete if it is to be cast in 20 liter cylindrical polyethylene containers 30 cm diameter for shipment to the waste burial site? **10.19**

1 R = 1 rem for radiation safety purposes. The top surface of the cylindrical container approximates a plane source. The dose rate would be found using equation 10.11. In this case, solve equation 10.11 for C_a;

$$\dot{H} = \pi \times \Gamma \frac{\text{R} \cdot \text{m}^2}{\text{Ci} \cdot \text{hr}} \times C_a \frac{\text{Ci}}{\text{m}^2} \times \ln \frac{r^2 + h^2}{h^2}$$

r = 15 cm = 0.15 m
h = 1 m

$$\Gamma_{Cs-137} = 0.33 \frac{\text{R} \cdot \text{m}^2}{\text{Ci} \cdot \text{hr}} \quad \text{(Table 6.3)}$$

$\dot{H}$ = 10 mrems/hr = 0.01 rem/hr

Substitute in the values;

$$0.01 \frac{\text{rem}}{\text{hr}} = \pi \times 0.33 \frac{\text{R} \cdot \text{m}^2}{\text{Ci} \cdot \text{hr}} \times C_a \frac{\text{Ci}}{\text{m}^2} \times \ln \frac{(0.15\ \text{m})^2 + (1\ \text{m})^2}{(1\ \text{m})^2}$$

$C_a \frac{\text{Ci}}{\text{m}^2} = 0.434 \frac{\text{Ci}}{\text{m}^2} = 0.0438 \frac{\text{mCi}}{\text{cm}^2}$ which is the apparent areal concentration of activity of the top of the cylindrical container.

Use equation 10.14 to find the volumetric concentration that results in this areal concentration at the container top:

$$C_v = \frac{C_a \mu}{\left(1 - e^{-\mu t}\right)}$$

$$\mu = 0.0290 \frac{\text{cm}^2}{\text{g}} \times 2.35 \frac{\text{g}}{\text{cm}^3} = 0.068\ \text{cm}^{-1} \text{(Appendix E, Table 5.2)}$$

$$C_a = 0.0438 \frac{\text{mCi}}{\text{cm}^2}$$

$$t = \frac{2 \times 10^4 \text{ cm}^3}{\pi (15 \text{ cm})^2} = 28.3 \text{ cm (height of container)}$$

Substituting these values into the equation above, we find

$C_v = 3.5 \times 10^{-3} \dfrac{\text{mCi}}{\text{cm}^3} = 3.5 \dfrac{\mu\text{Ci}}{\text{cm}^3}$ is the concentration of ^{137}Cs which will produce a dose rate of 10 mrems/h at a distance of 1 meter above the surface of the container.

Now check the surface dose rate when a ^{137}Cs concentration of $3.5 \times 10^{-3} \dfrac{\text{mCi}}{\text{cm}^3}$ is used. The surface dose rate must not exceed 200 mrems/h. To calculate the surface dose rate, we will assume that the concrete cylinder is infinitely thick, and use equation 6.44a.

$$\dot{D} = 1.1 \times 10^3 \times C_v \sum f_i E_i$$

where
$E_{\text{Cs-137}}$ = 0.661 MeV/gamma
$f_{\text{Cs-137}}$ = 0.85 gamma/transformation

C_v = concentration, μCi/g

and density of concrete = 2.35 g/cm^3

$$\dot{D} = 1.1 \times 10^3 \times \frac{3.5\, \mu\text{Ci}/\text{cm}^3}{2.35\, \text{g}/\text{cm}^3} \times 0.85 \times 0.661 = 920 \frac{\text{mrems}}{\text{hr}}$$

Since this is too high, we must reduce C_v to

$$\frac{200}{920} \times 3.5 \frac{\mu\text{Ci}}{\text{cm}^3} = 0.76 \frac{\mu\text{Ci}}{\text{cm}^3}$$

The maximum activity that can be mixed into the 20 L concrete slug for disposal is

$$A = 0.76 \frac{\mu\text{Ci}}{\text{cm}^3} \times 2 \times 10^4 \text{ cm}^3 = 15.2 \times 10^3\, \mu\text{Ci} = 562 \text{ MBq}$$

10.20 A technician's job in a radiopharmaceutical laboratory involves simultaneous handling of 5000 MBq (135 mCi) ^{125}I, 4000 MBq (108 mCi) ^{198}Au and 2000 MBq (54 mCi) ^{24}Na for 1 hour per day, 5 days per week for an indefinitely long time. Her average dose equivalent during the other 7 hours will be 0.01 mSv (1 millirem). Her body will be 75 cm from the sources while she works with them, and manipulators will be provided so that her hands will not be exposed inside the shield. **10.20**

(a) What is the source strength for each of the sources?

Traditional units will be used to solve this problem because the regulations of the USNRC are written in traditional units. The source strength for each radioisotope is calculated with the specific gamma ray constant given in Table 6.3. Since we are dealing with gamma radiation, 1 mR = 1 mrem.

Isotope	$\Gamma \frac{\text{mrem}\cdot\text{m}^2}{\text{mCi}\cdot\text{hr}}$	A, mCi	Source Strength $\frac{\text{mrem}\cdot\text{m}^2}{\text{hr}}$	$\dot{H} = \frac{\text{SS}}{(0.75\text{ m})^2}$
^{125}I	0.07	135	9.45	16.8 mrems/hr
^{198}Au	0.23	108	24.8	44.1 mrems/hr
^{24}Na	1.84	54	99.4	176.7 mrems/hr

(b) What thickness of lead shielding is required if her weekly dose equivalent is to be within ALARA guidelines, that is, at 1/10 of the maximum permissible dose?

The USNRC's annual dose limit is 5000 mrems, which is reduced by ALARA policy to 500 mrems. For a nominal 250 day work year, the operational hourly limit is 2 mrems/day. If the technician receives 1 mrem during 7 hours, she is limited to 1 mrem while working with these 3 sources.

Let us calculate the lead shielding to reduce the ^{24}Na dose rate from 177 to 1 mrem/hr. Because the ^{24}Na gamma energy is so much higher than from the two other sources, this shield thickness will, for practical purposes, absorb all the other gammas. The number of half value layers, n, needed to attenuate the ^{24}Na gammas is

$$\frac{I}{I_0} = \frac{1}{177} = \frac{1}{2^n}$$

$n = 7.5$ HVL

To be conservative, the calculated thickness of a HVL will be based on the 2.75 MeV gamma. From Table 5.2, we find, by interpolation μ (Pb, 2.75 MeV) = 0.486 cm^{-1}

$$\text{HVL} = \frac{0.693}{\mu} = \frac{0.693}{0.486 \text{ cm}^{-1}} = 1.43 \text{ cm}$$

To account for buildup, add 1.5 HVL, for a total trial shield thickness of

t = (1.5 + 7.5) HVL × 1.42 cm/HVL = 12.9 cm

Now calculate the attenuation of the 2.75 MeV gamma. The unshielded dose rate at 0.75 m is estimated with the specific gamma ray constant (equation 6.18):

$$\Gamma = 0.5\sum f_i E_i = 0.5 \times 2.75 = 1.37 \frac{\text{mrem} \cdot \text{m}^2}{\text{mCi} \cdot \text{hr}}$$

(equation 10.1)

$$\dot{H} = \frac{\Gamma \times A}{d^2} = \frac{1.37 \dfrac{\text{mrem} \cdot \text{m}^2}{\text{mCi} \cdot \text{hr}} \times 54 \text{ mCi}}{(0.75 \text{ m})^2} = 131.5 \frac{\text{mrems}}{\text{hr}}$$

The buildup factor, B, for a lead shield 6.3 relaxation lengths thick (μt = 0.486 × 12.9 = 6.3) is 3.5 (Fig. 10.9). The shielded dose rate is

$$\dot{H} = \dot{H}_0 B e^{-\mu t}$$

$$\dot{H} = 131.5 \frac{\text{mrems}}{\text{hr}} \times 3.5 e^{-6.3} = 0.85 \frac{\text{mrems}}{\text{hr}}$$

If we make a similar calculation for the 1.37 MeV gamma, we find the dose rate to be 0.05 mrem/hr. For the other two radionuclides, a 12.9 cm thick lead shield reduces the radiation for practical purposes to zero. The required shield thickness is 12.9 cm of lead (5").

10.21 Design a spherical shield for a 1×10^{11} Bq (2.7 Ci) ^{90}Sr "point" source so that the dose equivalent rate at the surface will not exceed 2 mSv (200 millirem) per hour. What is the dose equivalent rate at a distance of 1 meter from the shielded source? **10.21**

Assume that ^{90}Y is in equilibrium with the ^{90}Sr. ^{90}Y emits a 2.27 MeV beta. Using equation 5.2 to find the range of the beta:

$R = 412 \times (E\text{ MeV})^{1.265 - 0.0954\ \ln(E)}$

$R = 412 \times (2.27)^{1.265 - 0.0954 \times \ln(2.27)} = 1090\text{ mg/cm}^2 = 1.09\text{ g/cm}^2$ is the density thickness required.

Example 10.9 lists the density of polyethylene as: $\rho = 0.95 \frac{\text{g}}{\text{cm}^3}$

Calculating the thickness of polyethylene required to shield the ^{90}Y betas;

$$\frac{1.09\text{g}}{\text{cm}^2} \times \frac{\text{cm}^3}{0.95\text{ g}} = 1.1\text{cm}$$

A significant amount of bremsstrahlung is produced by the polyethylene shielding and a layer of lead is used to shield the bremsstrahlung. First, calculate the amount of bremsstrahlung produced. The effective "Z" of polyethylene, assuming for this case, the formula for polyethylene is CH_2, is calculated using equation 10.34;

$$N_H = 1\text{ cm}^3 \times \frac{0.95\text{ g}}{\text{cm}^3} \times \frac{1\text{ mol}}{14\text{ g}} \times \frac{6.02 \times 10^{23}\text{ molecules}}{\text{mol}} \times \frac{2\text{ atoms}}{\text{molecule}} = 8 \times 10^{22}\,\frac{\text{atoms}}{\text{cm}^3}$$

$$N_C = 1\text{ cm}^3 \times \frac{0.95\text{ g}}{\text{cm}^3} \times \frac{1\text{ mol}}{14\text{ g}} \times \frac{6.02 \times 10^{23}\text{ molecules}}{\text{mol}} \times \frac{1\text{ atoms}}{\text{molecule}} = 4 \times 10^{22}\,\frac{\text{atoms}}{\text{cm}^3}$$

C = 6
H = 1

$$Z_{effective} = \frac{N_1 Z_1^2 + N_2 Z_2^2}{N_1 Z_1 + N_2 Z_2} = \frac{\left[8 \times 10^{22}\,\frac{\text{atoms}}{\text{cm}^3} \times 1^2\right] + \left[4 \times 10^{22}\,\frac{\text{atoms}}{\text{cm}^3} \times 6^2\right]}{\left[8 \times 10^{22}\,\frac{\text{atoms}}{\text{cm}^3} \times 1\right] + \left[4 \times 10^{22}\,\frac{\text{atoms}}{\text{cm}^3} \times 6\right]} = 4.75$$

Bremsstrahlung production is now estimated using equation 5.11:
$E_{Y-90} = 2.27$ MeV

$$f_{Y-90} = 3.5 \times 10^{-4} ZE = 3.5 \times 10^{-4} \times (4.75) \times 2.27 = 3.8 \times 10^{-3}$$

The average energy of the betas from the ^{90}Sr - ^{90}Y source is 0.18 + 0.93 = 1.11 MeV/transformation.

$$E_\beta = 1 \times 10^{11}\,\text{Bq} \times \frac{1\frac{\text{trans}}{\text{sec}}}{\text{Bq}} \times 1.11\frac{\text{MeV}}{\text{d}} = 1.11 \times 10^{11}\,\frac{\text{MeV}}{\text{sec}}$$

The amount of this beta energy that is converted to x-rays is

$$E_X = f \times E_\beta = 3.8 \times 10^{-3} \times 1.11 \times 10^{11}\,\frac{\text{MeV}}{\text{s}} \times 1.6 \times 10^{-13}\,\frac{\text{J}}{\text{MeV}}$$

$$E_X = 6.75 \times 10^{-5}\,\frac{\text{J}}{\text{s}}$$

If the source is surrounded by 1.1 cm of plastic, then the x-ray energy flux at the plastic surface is

$$\phi_{XE} = \frac{6.75 \times 10^{-5}\,\frac{\text{J}}{\text{s}}}{4\pi(1.1\text{ cm})^2} = 4.44 \times 10^{-6}\,\frac{\text{J}}{\text{cm}^2 \cdot \text{s}}$$

The dose rate from this flux is calculated from

$$\dot{H} = \frac{\phi_{XE}\,\frac{\text{J}}{\text{cm}^2 \cdot \text{s}} \times \mu_{en}\,\frac{\text{cm}^2}{\text{g}} \times 3.6 \times 10^3\,\frac{\text{s}}{\text{h}}}{0.001\frac{\text{J/g}}{\text{Gy}} \times 1\frac{\text{Gy}}{\text{Sv}} \times \frac{1\text{ Sv}}{10^3\text{ mSv}}}$$

Using μ_{en} (muscle, 2.27 MeV) = 0.0249 cm^2/g (Table 5.3), we find that

$$\dot{H} = 398.1 \frac{\text{mSv}}{\text{h}}$$

We wish to reduce the dose rate with the lead shield by a factor of

$$\frac{\dot{H}}{\dot{H}_0} = \frac{2}{398.1} = 5.02 \times 10^{-3}$$

Combining both inverse square dispersion and attenuation by the shield, but excluding buildup, we can calculate a minimum shield thickness t

$$\frac{\dot{H}}{\dot{H}_0} = 5.02 \times 10^{-3} = \left(\frac{1.1}{t + 1.1}\right)^2 \text{e}^{-\mu t}$$

Using μ (Pb, 2.27 MeV) = 0.506 cm^{-1} (Table 5.2) we find that t = 4.2 cm. To account for buildup, increase t to 5 cm, and then using a buildup factor B (Pb, 2.27 MeV, μt = 2.53) = 1.82 (RHH, Fig. 10.9), calculate the resulting attenuation

$$\frac{\dot{H}}{\dot{H}_0} = 1.82 \left(\frac{1.1}{5 + 1.1}\right)^2 \text{e}^{-2.53} = 4.7 \times 10^{-3}$$

This is slightly better than the design criterion of 5.02 × 10^{-3}. Therefore, the shielding requirements are
1.1 cm polyethylene and 5 cm lead.

Solutions for Chapter 11

INTERNAL RADIATION PROTECTION

11.1 A health physicist finds that a radiochemist was inhaling $Ba^{35}SO_4$ particles that were leaking out of a faulty glove box. The radiochemist had been inhaling the dust, whose mean radioactivity concentration was 3.3 MBq/m^3 (9×10^{-5} mCi/cm^3), for a period of 2 hr. Using the ICRP 3 compartment lung model, calculate the absorbed dose to the lung during the 13 week period and during the 1 year period immediately following inhalation. **11.1**

T_R = 87 days

Since no particle size is given, the ICRP default value of 1 μm AMAD particles is used. Assuming conditions of light work, Appendix C gives a volume of 9.6 m^3 of air inhaled in an 8 hour day. Assume that the person inhales approximately 10 m^3 of air. Calculate the inhaled activity:

$$2 \text{ hrs} \times 3.3 \frac{\text{MBq}}{\text{m}^3} \times \frac{1 \times 10^6 \text{ Bq}}{\text{MBq}} \times \frac{10 \text{ m}^3}{8 \text{ hr}} = 8.25 \times 10^6 \text{ Bq} \text{ is the total inhaled activity}$$

The elimination constant for each of the compartments is calculated next. Table 8.5, Figure 8.4 or ICRP 26 give the following depositions of inhaled 1 μm AMAD particles:

	Deposition	Fraction in lung	Total activity	Activity in lung
N-P	30%	0	8.25×10^6 Bq	0
T-B	8%	0.08	8.25×10^6 Bq	6.6×10^5 Bq
P	25%	0.25	8.25×10^6 Bq	2.1×10^6 Bq
			Total deposited in lung	2.7×10^6 Bq

Clearance rates from the various lung compartments depend on the solubility class. $BaSO_4$ is in class w, moderate solubility (ICRP, Health Physics, 12:173, 1966, 10 CFR 20 Appendix B). Class w particles are assigned biological removal half times, T_B, as shown in the table below. For all the particles in the TB region, and for 40% of those in the P region, $T_B \leq 1$ day. Since these clearance half times <<< 87 days, the effective clearance half time, T_E is the same as T_B. The effective clearance rate constant for these particles is:

$$\lambda_E = \frac{0.693}{T_E}$$

For 60% of the particles deposited in the P region, whose T_B = 50 days, the effective T_E is calculated from equation 6.54:

$$T_E = \frac{T_R \times T_B}{T_R + T_B} = \frac{87 \text{ days} \times 50 \text{ days}}{87 \text{ days} + 50 \text{ days}} = 32 \text{ days}$$

$$\lambda_E = \frac{0.693}{T_{1/2}} = \frac{0.693}{32 \text{ day}} = 0.022 \text{ d}^{-1}$$

Region	% cleared	$A_S(0)$, Bq	T_B, d	T_E, d	λ_E, d^{-1}
TB	50	0.5 x 6.6 x 10^5	0.01	0.01	69.3
TB	50	0.5 x 6.6 x 10^5	0.2	0.2	3.47
P	40	0.4 x 2.61 x 10^6	1	1	0.693
P	60	0.6 x 2.1 x 10^6	50	32	0.022

The dose from the activity in the lung is given by the product of the accumulated activity, $\tilde{A}$ Bq·d and the dose conversion factor, DCF Gy/Bq·d.

$$D = \tilde{A} \text{ Bq·d} \times \text{DCF}, \frac{\text{Gy}}{\text{Bq} \cdot \text{d}}$$

The cumulated activity for a single compartment is (equation 6.91)

$$\tilde{A} = \frac{A_S(0)}{\lambda}\left(1 - e^{-\lambda t}\right)$$

and for n compartments

$$\tilde{A} = \sum^{n} \frac{A_{Si}(0)}{\lambda_i}\left(1 - e^{-\lambda_i t}\right)$$

During the first 13 weeks, all the compartments but the last will be emptied, that is $e^{-\lambda t} \cong 0$ for the first 3 compartments(Note that the equation is in 2 lines):

$$\tilde{A}(13 \text{ weeks}) = \frac{(0.5)\times 6.6\times 10^5\,\text{Bq}}{69.3\ \text{d}^{-1}} + \frac{(0.5)\times 6.6\times 10^5\,\text{Bq}}{3.47\ \text{d}^{-1}} +$$
$$+\frac{(0.4)\times 2.1\times 10^6\,\text{Bq}}{0.693\ \text{d}^{-1}} + \frac{(0.6)\times 2.1\times 10^6\,\text{Bq}}{0.022\ \text{d}^{-1}}\left(1 - e^{-0.022\times 91}\right)$$

$$\tilde{A}(13 \text{ weeks}) = 5.1\times 10^7\ \text{Bq}\cdot\text{d}$$

After 1 year, $e^{-0.022 \times 365} \cong 0$, and the last term becomes $0.6 \times 2.1 \times 10^6$ Bq/0.022 d^{-1}, which leads to a 1 year cumulated activity

$$\tilde{A}(1 \text{ yr}) = 5.9\times 10^7\ \text{Bq}\cdot\text{d}$$

Sulfur 35 emits a single beta whose mean energy is 0.049 MeV, and no gammas. Using a lung weight of 1 kg (Appendix C), the DCF is calculated

$$\frac{\text{mGy}}{\text{Bq}\cdot\text{d}} = \frac{1\dfrac{\text{t}}{\text{s}\cdot\text{Bq}}\times 8.64\times 10^4\,\dfrac{\text{s}}{\text{d}}\times 4.9\times 10^{-2}\,\dfrac{\text{MeV}}{\text{t}}\times 1.6\times 10^{-13}\,\dfrac{\text{J}}{\text{MeV}}}{1\ \text{kg}\times 1\dfrac{\text{J/kg}}{\text{Gy}}\times\dfrac{1\ \text{Gy}}{10^3\,\text{mGy}}}$$

$$\text{DCF} = 6.8\times 10^{-7}\ \frac{\text{mGy}}{\text{Bq}\cdot\text{d}}$$

Therefore

$$D(13\ \text{wk}) = 5.1\times 10^7\ \text{Bq}\cdot\text{d}\times\ 6.8\times 10^{-7}\ \frac{\text{mGy}}{\text{Bq}\cdot\text{d}} = 35\ \text{mGy}$$

$$D(1\ \text{yr}) = 5.9\times 10^7\ \text{Bq}\cdot\text{d}\times\ 6.8\times 10^{-7}\ \frac{\text{mGy}}{\text{Bq}\cdot\text{d}} = 40\ \text{mGy}$$

11.2

11.2 A tank, of volume 100 L, contained ^{85}Kr gas at a pressure of 10.0 kg/cm^2. (9.71 atmospheres). The specific activity of the krypton is 20 Ci/g. The tank is in an unventilated storage room, at a temperature of 27°C, whose dimensions are 3 × 3 × 2 m. As a result of a very small leak, the gas leaked out until the pressure in the tank was 9.9 kg/cm^2. A man unknowingly then spent 1 h in the storage room. Assume the half saturation time for krypton solution in the body fluids to be 3 min. Henry's law constant for Kr in water at body temperature is 2.13 × 10^7. Calculate (a) the immersion dose, (b) the internal dose due to the inhaled krypton. The partition of Kr in water to Kr in fat is 1:10.

First, calculate the activity of the escaped gas:

The original number of moles of labeled Kr in the tank is calculated with the ideal gas law.

$$PV = nRT$$

$$n = \frac{PV}{RT} = \frac{9.71 \text{ atm} \times 100 \text{ liters}}{0.082 \frac{\text{liter} \cdot \text{atm}}{\text{mole} \cdot \text{K}} \times 300 \text{ K}} = 39.4 \text{ moles}$$

The amount of Kr gas that escaped, Q, is

$$Q = \frac{(10.0 - 9.9)\frac{\text{kg}}{\text{cm}^2}}{10.0\frac{\text{kg}}{\text{cm}^2}} \times 39.4 \text{ mol} = 0.394 \text{ mole}$$

The specific activity of the tagged Kr is 20 Ci/g, while the specific activity of ^{85}Kr is calculated with equation 4.31.

$$SA = \frac{A_{Ra} T_{Ra}}{A_{Kr-85} T_{Kr-85}} = \frac{226 \times 1620 \text{ yr}}{85 \times 10.3 \text{ yr}} = 418.2 \frac{\text{Ci}}{\text{g}}$$

The fraction of Kr that is ^{85}Kr is

$$f = \frac{20 \, \text{Ci}/\text{g}}{418.2 \, \text{Ci}/\text{g}} = 0.0478$$

The molecular weight of the tagged Kr is

$(0.478 \times 85) + 0.9522 \times 83.8 = 83.86$ g/mole

and the molar concentration of ^{85}Kr activity is 83.86 g/mole × 20 Ci/g = 1677 Ci/ mole.

The atmospheric concentration of ^{85}Kr activity in the room is

$$C = \frac{\text{activity}}{\text{volume}} = \frac{0.394\text{mole} \times 3.7 \times 10^{10}\ \frac{\text{Bq}}{\text{Ci}}}{3\text{ m} \times 3\text{ m} \times 2\text{ m} \times} = 1.36 \times 10^{12}\ \frac{\text{Bq}}{\text{m}^3}\left(36.7\frac{\text{Ci}}{\text{m}^3}\right)$$

Krypton 85 emits one beta per transformation, $E_{max} = 0.672$ MeV, $\bar{E} = 0.246$ MeV, and a gamma photon in only 0.41% of the transformations. Thus, only the beta will deliver a significant dose to the skin, which is calculated with equation 6.38:

$$\dot{D}_b = 2.45 \times 10^{-7} \times C \times \bar{E} \times e^{-\mu\beta(0.007)}$$

The absorption coefficient, μ_b is given by equation 6.21:

$$\mu_b = 18.6(E_{max} - 0.036)^{-1.37} = 34.6\ \text{cm}^2/\text{g}$$

$$\dot{D}_b = 2.45 \times 10^{-7} \times 1.36 \times 10^{12}\ \frac{\text{Bq}}{\text{m}^3} \times 0.246\ \text{MeV} \times e^{-34.6\times(0.007)} = 64 \times 10^3\ \frac{\text{mGy}}{\text{hr}}$$

$$\dot{D}_b = 6.4 \times 10^3\ \frac{\text{rads}}{\text{hr}}$$ is the external dose rate to skin.

$$D_b = \dot{D}_b \times t = 6.4 \times 10^3\ \frac{\text{rads}}{\text{hr}} \times 1\ \text{hr} = 6.4 \times 10^3\ \text{rad}$$

SYSTEMIC INTERNAL DOSE

Calculate the dose to from ^{85}Kr in the body fluids (water in the body) and in the body fat. Start by computing the molar concentration of the ^{85}Kr in the air:

$$\frac{36.7\,\frac{\text{Ci}}{\text{m}^3}}{418.2\,\frac{\text{Ci}}{\text{g}}} \times \frac{1\text{ mole}\,^{85}\text{Kr}}{85\text{ g}} \times \frac{1\text{ m}^3}{1\times 10^6\text{ cm}^3} = 1.03\times 10^{-9}\,\frac{\text{mole}\,^{85}\text{Kr}}{\text{cm}^3}$$

Now compute the concentration of natural krypton in the air. The concentration of naturally occurring krypton in the atmosphere is approximately 1 ppm (CRC). Using the ideal gas law, we find the molar volume of air at 25°C to be:

$$\frac{V}{n} = \frac{RT}{P} = \frac{0.082\,\frac{\text{liter}\cdot\text{atm}}{\text{mole}\cdot\text{K}} \times 298\text{ K}}{1\text{ atm}} = 24.4\,\frac{\text{liters}}{\text{mole}},$$

and the molar concentration of naturally occurring Kr is

$$\frac{1\text{ mole Kr}}{10^6\text{ mole air}} \times \frac{\text{mole air}}{24.4\text{ liters air}} \times \frac{1\text{ liter air}}{1000\text{ cm}^3\text{air}} = 4.1\times 10^{-11}\,\frac{\text{mole Kr}}{\text{cm}^3\text{air}}.$$

The concentration in the room of the ^{85}Kr is much greater than naturally occurring Kr. Thus, naturally occurring Kr is ignored when calculating permeation of ^{85}Kr into body fat. Using values calculated earlier for ^{85}Kr:

$$\frac{0.394\text{ mole }^{85}\text{Kr escaped}}{18\text{ m}^3} \times \frac{24.4\text{ liters air}}{\text{mole air}} \times \frac{\text{m}^3\text{ air}}{1000\text{ liter air}} = 5.34\times 10^{-4}\text{moles }^{85}\text{Kr/mole air}$$

Calculate the amount of ^{85}Kr which permeates the water in the body. The saturation concentration of a gas in water is given by Henry's Law (equation 8.16)

$$p(gas) = K\,\frac{n_g}{n_g + n_s}$$

Since the total pressure of a gas mixture equals the sum of the partial pressures of its constituents, the partial pressure of the Kr in the air is

$$\frac{p(\text{Kr})}{760\text{ mm}} = \frac{5.3\times 10^{-4}\text{ mole Kr}}{1\text{ mole air}}$$

$p(\text{Kr}) = 0.41$ mm Hg

Henry's Law constant, $K = 2.13 \times 10^7$ mm Hg for Kr at 38ºC (Table 8.16). The molar concentration of water is

$$n_s = \frac{1000 \frac{\text{g H}_2\text{O}}{\text{liter}}}{18 \frac{\text{g H}_2\text{O}}{\text{mole}}} = 55.56 \frac{\text{moles H}_2\text{O}}{\text{liter H}_2\text{O}}$$

Substituting these values into Henry's Law, we have

$$0.41 \text{ mm} = 2.13 \times 10^7 \text{ mm} \times \frac{n_g}{n_g + 55.56 \frac{\text{moles}}{\text{liter}}}$$

$$n_g = 1.06 \times 10^{-6} \frac{\text{moles Kr}}{\text{liter bodyfluid}}$$

A 70 kg reference man's water content is 43 L, and the total ^{85}Kr content in the man's body fluids is

$$1.06 \times 10^{-6} \frac{\text{moles Kr}}{\text{liter bodyfluid}} \times \frac{43 \text{ liters bodyfluid}}{\text{body}} \times 1677 \frac{\text{Ci}}{\text{mole Kr}} = 7.6 \times 10^{-2} \text{ Ci}$$

To find the quantity in the fat, recall from the problem that the partition ratio is 1:10, yielding:

$$\frac{X \frac{\text{moles Kr gas}}{\text{kg fat}}}{1.06 \times 10^{-6} \frac{\text{moles Kr gas}}{\text{liter bodyfluid}} \times \frac{1 \text{ liter body fluid}}{1 \text{ kg}}} = \frac{10}{1}$$

$$X = 1.06 \times 10^{-5} \frac{\text{moles gas}}{\text{kg fat}}$$

From Appendix C, the quantity of fat in the body is 13.5 kg, so the total quantity of activity in the fat is:

$$1.06 \times 10^{-5} \frac{\text{moles Kr}}{\text{kg fat}} \times \frac{13.5 \text{ kg}}{\text{body}} \times 1677 \frac{\text{Ci}}{\text{moles Kr}} = 0.24 \text{ Ci activity in the fat.}$$

Adding the activity from the body fluids (water) and fat:

7.6×10^{-2} Ci + 0.24 Ci = 0.316 Ci

$0.316 \text{ Ci} \times \frac{3.7 \times 10^{10} \text{Bq}}{\text{Ci}} = 1.17 \times 10^{10}$ Bq is the total activity deposited in the body.

Assume that the activity is uniformly distributed throughout the body. Calculate the dose rate using equation 6.47:

$$\dot{D}_S(\beta) = \frac{(q)\text{Bq} \times \frac{1\frac{\text{t}}{\text{s}}}{\text{Bq}} \overline{E} \frac{\text{MeV}}{\text{trans}} 1.6 \times 10^{-13} \frac{\text{J}}{\text{MeV}} \times \frac{3600 \text{ sec}}{\text{hr}}}{(m)\text{kg} \times 1 \frac{\text{J}}{\text{kg}} \Big/ \text{Gy}}$$

Substituting
$q = 1.17 \times 10^{10}$ Bq
$\overline{E} = 0.246$ MeV
$m = 70$ kg (Appendix C)

into the equation and solving for the dose rate, we get

$$\dot{D}_S(\beta) = 3.9 \times 10^{-4} \frac{\text{Gy}}{\text{min}} = 3.9 \times 10^{-2} \frac{\text{rads}}{\text{min}}$$

Since the half saturation time is 3 minutes, the man's saturation dose rate, D_S, will not be reached until about 15 to 18 minutes after the start of inhalation. His dose during inhalation, D_I, therefore is given by equation 11.17

$$D_I = \dot{D}_S \left[t - \frac{1}{k}(1 - e^{-kt}) \right]$$

where k, the saturation rate constant equals 0.693/3 minutes = 0.231 min^{-1}.

$$D_I = 3.9 \times 10^{-2} \frac{\text{rads}}{\text{min}} \times \left[60 \text{ min} - \frac{1}{0.231 \text{ min}^{-1}} \times (1 - \text{e}^{-0.231 \times 60}) \right] = 2.17 \text{ rads}$$

The dose from exhalation is described by equation 6.58;

$$D_E = \frac{\dot{D}_S}{\lambda} = \frac{0.039 \ \frac{\text{rads}}{\text{min}}}{0.231 \ \text{min}^{-1}} = 0.17 \text{ rads}$$

So that the total systemic internal dose is:

2.17 rads + 0.17 rads = 2.34 rads

DOSE TO LUNGS

Calculate the dose to the lungs from the ^{85}Kr residing in the lungs. Appendix C gives the mass of each lung as 1 kg, and the mean volume of air in the lungs as 2.7 liters {since the functional residual capacity is 2.2 liters (Appendix C) and the person is performing light activity, 20 L/min and 20 breaths/min = 1 liter/breath but a breath is air in and air out, so the mean breath is 0.5 liter.}

$$q = 2.7 \text{ liters} \times \frac{1\times 10^{-3} \ \text{m}^3}{1 \text{ liter}} \times 1.36 \times 10^{12} \ \frac{\text{Bq}}{\text{m}^3} = 3.6 \times 10^9 \text{ Bq}$$

$\overline{E} = 0.246$ MeV
$m = 1$ kg (Appendix C)

Calculate the dose using equation 6.47:

$$\dot{D}(\beta) = \frac{(q)\text{Bq} \times \frac{1\frac{\text{t}}{\text{s}}}{\text{Bq}} \overline{E} \frac{\text{MeV}}{\text{t}} 1.6 \times 10^{-13} \frac{\text{J}}{\text{MeV}} \times \frac{3600 \text{ s}}{\text{hr}}}{(m)\text{kg} \times 1\frac{\text{J}}{\text{kg}} \Big/ \text{Gy}}$$

$$\dot{D}(\beta) = \frac{3.6 \times 10^9 \text{ Bq} \times \frac{1\frac{\text{t}}{\text{s}}}{\text{Bq}} \times 0.246 \frac{\text{MeV}}{\text{t}} \times 1.6 \times 10^{-13} \frac{\text{J}}{\text{MeV}} \times \frac{3600 \text{ s}}{\text{hr}}}{1 \text{ kg} \times 1\frac{\text{J}}{\text{kg}} \Big/ \text{Gy}}$$

$\dot{D}(\beta) = 0.52 \frac{\text{Gy}}{\text{hr}} = 52 \frac{\text{rads}}{\text{hr}}$ is the dose rate to the lungs from the ^{85}Kr breathed into the lungs. So that one hour in the ^{85}Kr atmosphere gives 52 rads to the lung.

After inhalation of ^{85}Kr has ceased, the lung will continue to be irradiated as the radiokrypton in the body, 1.17×10^{10} Bq, is released at a rate ot 0.231 per minute. The mean residence time in the lung of this activity is

$$t = \frac{1}{k} = \frac{1}{0.231\ \text{min}^{-1}} = 4.33\ \text{min}$$

The dose to the lung during the washout is

$$D(\text{washout}) = \dot{D} \times t$$

$$D(\text{washout}) = \frac{1.17 \times 10^{10}\ \text{Bq} \times \frac{60\ \text{tpm}}{\text{Bq}} \times 0.246 \frac{\text{MeV}}{\text{t}} \times 1.6 \times 10^{-13}\ \frac{\text{J}}{\text{MeV}}}{1\ \text{kg} \times 1 \frac{\text{J}}{\text{kg}} \Big/ \text{Gy}} \times 4.33\ \text{min}$$

$D(\text{washout}) = 0.12\ \text{Gy} = 12\ \text{rad}$

Total dose to the lung = 52 rads + 12 rad

$D(\text{lung}) = 64$ rads

It should be noted that the external dose is very much greater than the internal dose. This is true for all the rare gases except radon. Thus, the DAC for these gases is based on submersion rather than inhalation.

11.3

11.3 If the man in problem 2 turned on a small ventilation fan of capacity 100 ft^3/min as he entered the room, calculate his immersion and inhalation doses.

$$100 \frac{\text{ft}^3}{\text{min}} \times \frac{\text{m}^3}{35.3\ \text{ft}^3} = 2.83 \frac{\text{m}^3}{\text{min}}$$

The volume of the room is $3 \times 3 \times 2 = 18\ \text{m}^3$

Calculate the turnover rate;

$$k = \frac{2.83 \frac{\text{m}^3}{\text{min}}}{18\ \text{m}^3} = 0.16 \text{ room changes per minute}$$

Finding the concentration at the end of the 60 minute (1 hour) period with equation 11.18:

$C_0 = 36.6\frac{\text{Ci}}{\text{m}^3}$ (from problem 11.2)
$k = 0.16\ \text{min}^{-1}$
$t = 60$ min

$$C = C_0 e^{-kt} = 36.6\frac{\text{Ci}}{\text{m}^3}\text{e}^{-0.16 \times 60} = 2.5 \times 10^{-3}\frac{\text{Ci}}{\text{m}^3}$$

Now calculate the average concentration in the room (note that on a semilog graph, the decrease in concentration would describe a straight line. The average concentration.):

$$\overline{C} = \text{antilog}\left(\frac{\log(C_0) - \log(C)}{2}\right) = \sqrt{C_0 \times C} = \sqrt{36.6\frac{\text{Ci}}{\text{m}^3} \times 2.5 \times 10^{-3}\frac{\text{Ci}}{\text{m}^3}} = 0.3\frac{\text{Ci}}{\text{m}^3}$$

Now find the ratio of this to the original concentration:

$\dfrac{0.3\frac{\text{Ci}}{\text{m}^3}}{36.6\frac{\text{Ci}}{\text{m}^3}} = 8.2 \times 10^{-3}$ is the fraction of the unventilated dose that will be received with fan on.

The external dose to the skin would then be (from problem 11.2):

6.4×10^3 rads $\times\ 8.2 \times 10^{-3}$ =52.5 rads

The systemic body dose would be: 2.4 rads $\times\ 8.2 \times 10^{-3} = 2 \times 10^{-2}$ rads

The inhalation dose to the lungs would be: 52 rads $\times\ 8.2 \times 10^{-3} = 0.4$ rads

11.4 An accidental discharge of ^{89}Sr into a reservoir resulted in a contamination level of 37 Bq (10^{-3} μCi) per cm^3 of water. **11.4**

(a) Using the *basic* radiological health criterion of the ICRP, would this water be acceptable for drinking purposes for the general public if the turnover half time of the water in the reservoir is 30 days?

(b) If the water were ingested continuously, what maximum body burden would be reached?

(c) How long after ingestion started would this maximum occur?

(d) What would be the absorbed dose during the first 13 weeks of ingestion?

(e) What would be the absorbed dose during the first year?
(f) What would be the absorbed dose during 50 years following the start of ingestion?

$$\text{Reservoir} \xrightarrow{\lambda_{reservoir}} \text{Man} \xrightarrow{\lambda_{man}} \text{Excretion and Transformation}$$

(b) (c) Find an expression for the quantity of activity (q) in man at any given time from the activity in the reservoir.

C_0 = Reservoir concentration at time zero.
q = quantity in man
$q = 0$ at $t = 0$
λ_r = Removal rate from the reservoir
λ_m = Removal rate from man
$f_w = 0.21$ = Fraction of intake deposited in bone by ingestion. See ICRP 2 , p. 176. Note that FGR 11 (p.48) and ICRP 61 (p.11) only address the fraction absorbed into the blood from intake with this term and NOT the fraction absorbed in the bone.

$$\text{daily intake} = 2200\frac{\text{mL}}{\text{day}} \times C_0 \times f_w \times e^{-\lambda_r t}$$

$$\text{daily elimination} = \lambda_m \times q$$

$$\frac{dq}{dt} = \text{daily intake} - \text{daily elimination} = \left(2200\frac{\text{mL}}{\text{day}} \times C_0 \times e^{-\lambda_r t} \times f_w\right) - (\lambda_m \times q)$$

let K represent

$$K = 2200\frac{\text{mL}}{\text{day}} \times C_0 \times f_w$$

Substituting for the value K;

$$\frac{dq}{dt} = \left(K \times e^{-l_r t}\right) - (l_m \times q)$$

$$\frac{dq}{dt} + (\lambda_m q) = \left(K e^{-\lambda_r t}\right)$$

The above equation is the form

$$\frac{dy}{dx} + Py = Q$$

Where

$y = q$
$x = t$
$P = 1_m$
$Q = Ke^{-\lambda_r t}$

The solution of the differential equation, using the integrating factor method described in the textbook on pages 108 and 109 is

$$q = \frac{K}{\lambda_m - \lambda_r}\left(e^{(-\lambda_r)t} - e^{-(\lambda_m)t}\right)$$

The above expression will give the quantity of the activity in man (body burden) at any given time after starting to drink the water.

The time after start of continuous ingestion to the maximum body burden is given by equation 4.57:

$$t = t_{max} = \frac{\ln\left(\frac{\lambda_m}{\lambda_r}\right)}{(\lambda_m - \lambda_r)}$$

Since the biological half life of ^{89}Sr is is about 50 years (ICRP 2) and its radiological half life is 50.3 days (ICRP 2), its effective half life is also about 50.3 days, and the effective elimination constant is (equation 6.52):

$$\lambda_m = \frac{0.693}{T_E} = \frac{0.693}{50.3 \text{ days}} = 0.0138 \text{ d}^{-1}$$ is the elimination rate of ^{89}Sr from man.

The turnover half time of the reservoir (T_{res}) is 30 days, so its effective turnover half time, T_r (equation 6.54) is:

$$T_r = \frac{T_{res} \times T_B}{T_{res} + T_B} = \frac{30 \times 50.3}{30 + 50.3} = 18.8 \text{ days}$$

and its elimination rate constant

$$\lambda_r = \frac{0.693}{T_r} = \frac{0.693}{18.8 \text{ days}} = 0.0368 \text{ d}^{-1}$$

Find t_{max};

$$t_{max} = \frac{\ln\left(\frac{\lambda_m}{\lambda_r}\right)}{(\lambda_m - \lambda_r)} = \frac{\ln\left(\frac{0.0138 \text{ days}^{-1}}{0.0368 \text{ days}^{-1}}\right)}{(0.0138 \text{ days}^{-1} - 0.0368 \text{ days}^{-1})} = 42.6 \text{ days}$$

(c) The maximum body burden will occur after 42.6 days of continuous intake. Now find the maximum body burden, solving first for K;

$C_0 = 37 \frac{\text{Bq}}{\text{mL}}$

$f_w = 0.21$ (From ICRP 2, p.176) (Fraction reaching organ of reference by ingestion)

$$K = 2200 \frac{\text{mL}}{\text{day}} \times C_0 \times f_w = 2200 \frac{\text{mL}}{\text{day}} \times 37 \frac{\text{Bq}}{\text{mL}} \times 0.21 = 1.7 \times 10^4 \frac{\text{Bq}}{\text{day}} \text{ initial uptake}$$

(b) Calculate the activity in the human body of Sr-89 at the time of maximum body burden (42.6 days).

$K = 17094 \frac{\text{Bq}}{\text{day}}$ is the uptake

$\lambda_r = 0.0368 \text{ d}^{-1}$

$\lambda_m = 0.0138 \text{ d}^{-1}$

$t = 42.6$ days

$$q(t) = \frac{K}{\lambda_m - \lambda_r}\left(e^{(-\lambda_r)t} - e^{-(\lambda_m)t}\right)$$

$$q = \frac{17094 \dfrac{\text{Bq}}{\text{day}}}{0.0138\ \text{days}^{-1} - 0.0368\ \text{days}^{-1}} \times \left(e^{-\left(0.0368\ \text{days}^{-1}\right) \times 42.6\ \text{days}} - e^{-\left(0.0138\ \text{days}^{-1}\right) \times 42.6\ \text{days}} \right)$$

$$q = 2.6 \times 10^5\ \text{Bq}$$

The maximum body burden would be 2.6×10^5 Bq reached after 42.6 days.

Calculation of the absorbed dose

(d) The dose over a time period *t* to the skeleton from skeletal deposit of ^{89}Sr (99% of the body's Sr content is in the skeleton) is calculated from

$$H = \int_0^t \dot{H}\, dt$$

The instantaneous dose rate $\dot{H}$ due to a skeletal burden of *q* Bq is:

$$\dot{H} = \frac{q\ \text{Bq} \times 1 \dfrac{\text{tps}}{\text{Bq}} \times \overline{E}\, \dfrac{\text{MeV}}{\text{t}} \times 1.6 \times 10^{-13} \dfrac{\text{J}}{\text{MeV}} \times 8.64 \times 10^4 \dfrac{\text{sec}}{\text{day}}}{w\ \text{kg} \times 1 \dfrac{\text{J}}{\text{kg}} \Big/ \text{Gy} \times \dfrac{1\ \text{Gy}}{\text{Sv}}}$$

Substituting $\overline{E}$ (^{89}Sr) = 0.583 MeV (NRHH) and *w*(skeleton) = 7 kg, and combing constants we find that

$$\dot{H} = q\ \text{Bq} \times \text{A} \frac{\text{Sv}}{\text{d} \cdot \text{Bq}}$$

$$\dot{H} \frac{\text{Sv}}{\text{d}} = 1.151 \times 10^{-9} \frac{\text{Sv}}{\text{d} \cdot \text{Bq}} \times q\ \text{Bq}$$

Therefore

$$H = A \int_0^t q(t) \times dt$$

Substituting the expression for *q* (*t*) into the integral yields

$$H = A \int_0^t \frac{K}{\lambda_m - \lambda_r} \left(e^{(-\lambda_r)t} - e^{-(\lambda_m)t} \right) dt$$

Integrating, we obtain

$$H = \frac{AK}{\lambda_m - \lambda_r}\left\{\left[\frac{1}{\lambda_r}\left(1 - e^{(-\lambda_r)t}\right)\right] - \left[\frac{1}{\lambda_m}\left(1 - e^{-(\lambda_m)t}\right)\right]\right\}$$

Substituting

$$K = 1.7 \times 10^4 \frac{\text{Bq}}{\text{day}} \text{ (uptake)}$$

$$\lambda_r = 0.0368 \text{ d}^{-1}$$

$$\lambda_m = 0.0138 \text{ d}^{-1}$$

$$A = 1.15 \times 10^{-9} \frac{\text{Sv}}{\text{Bq} \cdot \text{day}}$$

we have

$$H = -8.5 \times 10^{-4} \, [\, 27.17(1 - e^{-0.0368t}) - 72.46(1 - e^{-0.0138t})]$$

Solving for t = 91 days (13 weeks), we find

H (91 days) = 2.19×10^{-2} Sv = 21.9 mSv (2,190 mrems)

For t = 365 days (1 year) and for t = 50 years, $e^{-0.0368t}$ and $e^{-0.0138t}$ <<< 1, therefore,

H (1 yr, 50 yr) = -8.56×10^{-4} [27.17 – 72.46]

(e)(f) H (1 yr, 50 yr) = 3.88×10^{-2} Sv = 38.8 mSv (3,880 mrems)

The fact that the 1 year and 50 year doses are the same means that all the dose was absorbed during the first year.

(a) The basic radiological health criterion limits the dose to members of the public to less than or equal to 1/50 of the occupational limit. For an individual organ or tissue such as the skeleton, this corresponds to 1/50 × 500 mSv = 10 mSv. In this case, the calculated dose is 39 mSv. Therefore, the water is not acceptable for public consumption at this level of contamination.

11.5

11.5 Nickel carbonyl $Ni(CO)_4$ has a maximum permissible atmospheric concentration of 1 part per billion (ppb) based on its chemical toxicity. A chemist is going to use this compound tagged with ^{63}Ni. The specific activity of the nickel is 2.5×10^8 Bq/g (6.75 mCi/g). The industrial hygienist is planning to limit the atmospheric concentration of $Ni(CO)_4$ in the lab to 0.5 ppb. Will this restriction meet the requirement for the radioactivity DAC of 3×10^{-7} μCi/mL?

Determine if enough Ni is ^{63}Ni to change the molecular weight used in converting to moles.

The specific activity of ^{63}Ni is given by equation 4.31, where;

$$SA = \frac{A_{Ra} \times T_{Ra}}{A_{Ni-63} \times T_{Ni-63}} = \frac{226 \times 1620 \text{ yr}}{63 \times 92 \text{ yr}} = 63.2\frac{\text{Ci}}{\text{g}}$$

$$f(^{63}\text{Ni}) = \frac{SA\ ^{*}\text{Ni}}{SA\ ^{63}\text{Ni}} \quad \frac{6.75 \times 10^{-3}\frac{\text{Ci}}{\text{g}}}{63.2\frac{\text{Ci}}{\text{g}}} = 1.07 \times 10^{-4}$$

Very few of all Ni atoms in the compound are ^{63}Ni. Therefore, the atomic weight of *Ni will be about the same as Ni, 58.71.

Calculate the number of mCi per mole of compound;

$$\frac{58.71 \text{ g Ni}}{\text{mole NiCO}_4} \times \frac{6.75 \text{ mCi}}{\text{g Ni}} = 396.3\frac{\text{mCi}}{\text{mole NiCO}_4}$$

0.5 parts per billion, is the same as 0.5 moles of $Ni(CO)_4$ per 1 billion moles air. Converting to air concentration:

2.45×10^4 mL per mole air at STP, 760 mm Hg and 25°C

$$\frac{0.5 \text{ mol NiCO}_4}{10^9 \text{ mol air}} \times 396.3\frac{\text{mCi}}{\text{mol NiCO}_4} \times \frac{\text{mol air}}{2.45 \times 10^4 \text{ mL}} \times \frac{10^3\ \mu\text{Ci}}{\text{mCi}} = 8.1 \times 10^{-9}\frac{\mu\text{Ci}}{\text{mL}} \text{ is}$$

the airborne concentration corresponding to 0.5 ppb. Yes, the restriction is met with these requirements.

11.6 Chlorine 36 tagged chloroform, $CHCl_3$, whose specific activity is 100 μCi/mole, is to be used under such conditions that 100 mg/hr may be lost by evaporation. The experiment is to be done in a laboratory of dimensions 15′×10′×8′. **11.6**

The lab is ventilated at a rate of 100 ft^3/min.

(a) Do any special measures have to be taken in order to control the atmospheric concentration of the ^{36}Cl to 10% of its DAC (DAC = 1 × 10^{-6} μCi/mL)?

Calculate the volume of the room:

15 × 10 × 8 = 1200 ft^3 is the volume of the room.

$\frac{100\ \text{ft}^3}{\text{min}}$ is the flow rate in the room. Converting to metric units;

$$k = \frac{100\ \text{ft}^3}{\text{min}} \times \frac{\text{m}^3}{35.314\ \text{ft}^3} = 2.83 \frac{\text{m}^3}{\text{min}}$$

First, find the specific activity of ^{36}Cl and compare it to the specific activity listed in the problem to find the fraction of chlorine atoms that are ^{36}Cl:

Equation 4.31 is used with the following data:

$$SA(^{36}\text{Cl}) = \frac{A_{Ra}T_{Ra}}{A_{Cl-36}T_{Cl-36}} = \frac{226 \times 1620\ \text{yr}}{36 \times 3.08 \times 10^5\ \text{yr}} = 3.3 \times 10^{-2}\ \frac{\text{Ci}}{\text{g}}$$

$$\frac{3.3 \times 10^{-2}\ \text{Ci}}{\text{g}} \times \frac{1 \times 10^6\ \mu\text{Ci}}{\text{Ci}} \times \frac{36\ \text{g}}{\text{mole}\ ^{36}\text{Cl}} \times \frac{3\ \text{mole}\ ^{36}\text{Cl}}{1\ \text{mole CHCl}_3} = 3.56 \times 10^6\ \frac{\mu\text{Ci}}{\text{mole}}$$ if all the Cl atoms were ^{36}Cl.

Computing the fraction of ^{36}Cl tagged:

$$\frac{100 \frac{\mu\text{Ci}}{\text{mole}}}{3.56 \times 10^6 \frac{\mu\text{Ci}}{\text{mole}}} = 2.81 \times 10^{-5}\ \frac{\text{moles}\ ^{36}\text{Cl}}{\text{mole Cl}}$$

The molecular weight is not significantly affected by the ^{36}Cl.

The molecular weight of $CHCl_3$ is (Appendix B);
C = 12
H = 1
Cl = (3) × 35.45 = 106.35
Total for $CHCl_3$ = 12 + 1 + 106.35 = 119.35

Finding the steady state concentration in the room, with a loss rate of 100 mg/hr: The rate of generation of the radioactive $CHCl_3$ vapor, G, is

$$G = \frac{100 \text{ mg}}{\text{hr}} \times \frac{\text{g}}{1000 \text{ mg}} \times \frac{\text{mole}}{119.35 \text{ g}} \times \frac{100 \ \mu\text{Ci}}{\text{mole}} \times \frac{1 \text{ hr}}{60 \text{ min}} = 0.0014 \frac{\mu\text{Ci}}{\text{min}}$$

The steady state concentration, where the rate of generation is equal to the rate of removal is (equation 11.26):

$$C = \frac{G}{Q} = \frac{1.4 \times 10^{-3} \frac{\mu\text{Ci}}{\text{min}}}{100 \frac{\text{ft}^3}{\text{min}} \times \left(\frac{1 \text{ m}}{3.28 \text{ ft}}\right)^3 \times 10^6 \frac{\text{mL}}{\text{m}^3}} = 4.94 \times 10^{-10} \frac{\mu\text{Ci}}{\text{mL}}$$ is the steady state

concentration in the room. This is much less than 0.1 × DAC ($1 \times 10^{-6} \frac{\mu\text{Ci}}{\text{mL}}$).

Therefore no special controls are needed.

(b) To what concentration of chloroform, in parts per million, does the radiological DAC correspond for this compound? Compare this concentration to the chemical PEL for chloroform.

Since 100 μCi/mole produces $4.94 \times 10^{-10} \frac{\mu\text{Ci}}{\text{cm}^3}$, calculate the number of moles per mL are in the room;

$$\frac{4.94 \times 10^{-10} \frac{\mu\text{Ci}}{\text{cm}^3}}{100 \frac{\mu\text{Ci}}{\text{mole}}} \times \frac{1\text{cm}^3}{\text{mL}} = 4.94 \times 10^{-12} \frac{\text{moles CHCl}_3}{\text{mL}}$$ is the concentration in the room.

Standard air at 760 mm and 25°C has 24.5×10^3 mL/mole air. Combining this information;

$$4.94 \times 10^{-12}\,\frac{\text{moles CHCl}_3}{\text{mL}} \times 24.5 \times 10^3\,\frac{\text{mL}}{\text{mole air}} = 1.2 \times 10^{-7}\,\frac{\text{moles CHCl}_3}{\text{mole air}}$$

Just like when converting to percent, where you multiply the fraction by 100, here where the result must be expressed in parts per million, the answer is multiplied by 1 million:

$1.2 \times 10^{-7}\,\frac{\text{moles CHCl}_3}{\text{mole air}} \times 1 \times 10^6 = 0.12$ ppm, compare with the OSHA P.E.L of 50 ppm (29 CFR 1910.1000)

11.7

11.7 For the purpose of estimating hazards from toxic vapors or gases of high molecular weight, it is sometimes *incorrectly* assumed that settling of the vapor is determined by the specific gravity of the pure vapor, which is defined as

$$\frac{\text{Molecular weight of the pure vapor}}{\text{"Molecular weight" of air}}$$

instead of the correct specific gravity given by

$$\frac{\text{Molecular weight of air and vapor mixture}}{\text{"Molecular weight" of air}}.$$

(a) If the vapor pressure of benzene (benzol), C_6H_6, is 160 mm Hg at 20°C, calculate the correct specific gravity of a saturated air mixture of benzene vapors and compare it to the specific gravity of the pure vapor.

MW of $C_6H_6 = 78$
Air is approximately 20% oxygen and 80% Nitrogen
"MW" of air = (0.2 × 32) + (0.8 × 28) = 28.8

$$\text{Specific Gravity of the pure vapor} = \frac{MW_{C_6H_6}}{MW_{air}} = \frac{78}{28.8} = 2.71$$

Specific Gravity of mixture =

$$\frac{\dfrac{VP_{C_6H_6}}{\text{atmospheric pressure}} MW_{C_6H_6} + \dfrac{P_{atm} - VP_{C_6H_6}}{\text{atmospheric pressure}} MW_{air}}{MW_{air}}$$

$$\text{Specific Gravity of mixture} = \frac{\frac{160}{760} \times 78 + \frac{760-160}{760} \times 28.8}{28.8} = 1.36$$

(b) If the chemical PEL for benzene is 10 ppm by volume, calculate the specific gravity of an air–benzene mixture of this concentration.

Specific Gravity of mixture

$$= \frac{\left(\text{ppm}_{C_6H_6} \times 10^6\right)\text{MW}_{C_6H_6} + \left[1 - \left(\text{ppm}_{C_6H_6} \times 10^6\right)\right]\text{MW}_{\text{air}}}{\text{MW}_{\text{air}}}$$

$$\text{Specific Gravity of mixture} = \frac{\left(10 \times 10^6\right) \times 78 + \left[1 - \left(10 \times 10^6\right)\right] \times 28.8}{28.8}$$

$= 1.00002$

(c) What is the maximum specific activity of ^{14}C–tagged benzene in order that one half the radiological DAC for ^{14}C (DAC = 1×10^{-6} $\mu Ci/cm^3$) not be exceeded by a benzene concentration of 10 ppm?

Note that standard air contains $24.5 \times 10^3 \dfrac{cm^3}{\text{mole air}}$ at 25°C and 760 mm Hg.

Half of the DAC is calculated as;

$$1 \times 10^{-6}\ \frac{\mu Ci}{cm^3} \times 0.5 \times 24.5 \times 10^3 \frac{cm^3}{\text{mole air}} = 0.01225 \frac{\mu Ci}{\text{mole air}}$$

Convert concentration in ppm to moles;

$$10\text{ ppm} = 10 \times 10^{-6} \frac{\text{mole } C_6H_6}{\text{mole air}}$$

Combining the two;

$$\frac{0.01225 \frac{\mu Ci}{\text{mole air}}}{10 \times 10^{-6} \frac{\text{mole } C_6H_6}{\text{mole air}}} = 1.225 \times 10^3 \frac{\mu Ci}{\text{mole } C_6H_6}$$

$$1.225 \times 10^3 \frac{\mu Ci}{\text{mole } C_6H_6} \times \frac{1 \text{ mole}}{1000 \text{ millimole}} = 1.2 \frac{\mu Ci}{\text{millimole } C_6H_6}$$

11.8

11.8 Iodine 131 is to be continuously released to the environment through a chimney whose effective height is 100 m, and whose discharge rate is 100 m^3/min. The average wind speed is 2 m.p.s. and the lapse rate is stable.
(a) At what maximum rate may the radioiodine be discharged if the maximum downwind ground level concentration is not to exceed 10% of the ICRP's DAC of 700 Bq/m^3 (2 × 10^{-8} mCi/cm^3).
(b) How far from the chimney will this maximum occur?

Calculating part (b) first is required to answer part (a). Looking at table 11.10, stable lapse rate and a 2 m/sec wind implies category D. The maximum ground concentration occurs on plume centerline, using equation 11.7:

$H = 100$ m

$$\sigma_z = \frac{H}{\sqrt{2}} = \frac{100 \text{ m}}{\sqrt{2}} = 70.7 \text{ m}$$

(b) Careful examination of figure 11.8 shows that $\sigma_z = 70.7$ m at a downwind distance of 3.1 × 10^3 m.

(a) Calculating the maximum rate of discharge, Q, is done using equation 11.5 (assuming the I–131 is a gas, and total reflection by the ground does occur);

$$\chi = 0.1 \times \left(700 \frac{\text{Bq}}{\text{m}^3}\right) = 70 \frac{\text{Bq}}{\text{m}^3}$$ is the maximum desired ground concentration.

$$\chi(x, y) = \frac{Q}{\pi \sigma_y \sigma_z \mu} e^{-\frac{1}{2}\left(\frac{y^2}{\sigma_y^2} + \frac{H^2}{\sigma_z^2}\right)}$$

$y = 0$ since the maximum is on the centerline;
$\sigma_y = 2.1 \times 10^2$ m (from fig. 11.7, at 3.1 × 10^3 m, "D" stability category)
$\sigma_z = 70.7$ m (calculated above)
$H = 100$ m is the effective stack height
$\mu = 2$ m/sec

$$70 \frac{\text{Bq}}{\text{m}^3} = \frac{Q \frac{\text{Bq}}{\text{sec}}}{\pi \times (2.1 \times 10^2 \text{ m}) \times (70.7 \text{ m}) \times 2 \frac{\text{m}}{\text{sec}}} e^{-\frac{1}{2} \times \left(\frac{0}{(2 \times 10^2)^2} + \frac{100^2}{70.7^2}\right)}$$

$Q = 1.8 \times 10^7 \dfrac{\text{Bq}}{\text{sec}}$ is the maximum discharge rate of ^{131}I to meet 10% of the DAC.

11.9 Inhalation exposure is often described as the product of atmospheric concentration and time, as in units of Bq×s/m^3. Using the ICRP assumptions that 23% of inhaled iodine is deposited in the thyroid, and that the thyroid weighs 20 g, calculate the dose corresponding to an acute exposure of 1 Bq×s/m^3 of (a) ^{131}I, (b)^{133}I. (c) Assuming that the other 77% of the inhaled iodine is absorbed into the blood and is bound to the protein, calculate the total body doses due to the protein–bound iodine. **11.9**

Reference person (appendix C) breaths 20 liters per minute during light activity.

$$1\frac{\text{Bq}\cdot\text{s}}{\text{m}^3} \times 20\frac{\text{liters}}{\text{min}} \times \frac{1\,\text{min}}{60\,\text{sec}} \times \frac{1\ \text{m}^3}{10^3\,\text{liters}} = 3.33 \times 10^{-4}\ \text{Bq}$$

The numerical values for the parameters needed to solve this problem, effective half life, T_E and effective absorbed energy per transformation, E_E, may be found in various sources, including several ICRP publications. Although the exact numbers differ somewhat among the sources, all are estimates based on mathematical models, and are approximately the same. ICRP 2 concisely lists these values for easy reference, and are tabulated below for use in the solution of the problem. The effective elimination rate constant, λ_E, is not listed in ICRP 2, but is calculated with equation 6.52; $\lambda_E = 0.693/T_E$.

	^{131}I			^{133}I		
	T_E,D	λ_E,d^{-1}	E_E, MeV/t	T_E, d	λ_E,d^{-1}	E_E, MeV/t
Thyroid	7.6	0.09	0.23	0.87	0.8	0.54
Body	7.6	0.09	0.44	0.87	0.8	0.84

The dose is calculated from equation 6.58

$$D = \frac{\dot{D}_0}{\lambda_E}, \text{ and}$$

$\dot{D}_0$, the initial dose rate, is calculated with equation 6.47:

$$\dot{D}_0 = \frac{q\ \text{Bq} \times 1\frac{\text{tps}}{\text{Bq}} \times E_E\ \frac{\text{MeV}}{\text{t}} \times 1.6\times10^{-13}\ \frac{\text{J}}{\text{MeV}} \times 8.64\times10^{4}\ \frac{\text{sec}}{\text{day}}}{m\ \text{kg} \times 1\frac{\text{J}}{\text{kg}}\Big/\text{Gy}}$$

For the case of ^{131}I in the thyroid:

$$\dot{D}_0 = \frac{(3.33\times10^{-4}\times0.23)\text{Bq} \times 1\frac{\text{tps}}{\text{Bq}} \times 0.23\frac{\text{MeV}}{\text{t}} \times 1.6\times10^{-13}\ \frac{\text{J}}{\text{MeV}} \times 8.64\times10^{4}\ \frac{\text{s}}{\text{d}}}{0.02\ \text{kg} \times 1\frac{\text{J}}{\text{kg}}\Big/\text{Gy}}$$

$$\dot{D}_0 = 1.22\times10^{-11}\ \frac{\text{Gy}}{\text{day}}$$

The dose to the thyroid is

$$D\ (\text{thyroid},\ ^{131}\text{I}) = \frac{\dot{D}_0}{\lambda_E} = \frac{1.22\times10^{-11}\ \frac{\text{Gy}}{\text{day}}}{0.09\ \text{day}^{-1}} = 1.35\times10^{-10}\ \text{Gy}$$

The dose to the body from ^{131}I is (Note the equation is split into two lines)

$$D = \frac{1}{0.09\ \text{d}^{-1}} \times$$

$$\times \frac{(3.33\times10^{-4}\times0.77)\text{Bq} \times 1\frac{\text{tps}}{\text{Bq}} \times 0.44\frac{\text{MeV}}{\text{t}} \times 1.6\times10^{-13}\ \frac{\text{J}}{\text{MeV}} \times 8.64\times10^{4}\ \frac{\text{s}}{\text{d}}}{70\ \text{kg} \times 1\frac{\text{J}}{\text{kg}}\Big/\text{Gy}}$$

$$D\ (\text{body},\ ^{131}\text{I}) = 2.48\times10^{-13}\ \text{Gy}$$

For the case of ^{133}I (Note that the equation is split into two lines)

$$D(\text{thyroid, } {}^{133}\text{I} = \frac{1}{0.8\ \text{d}^{-1}} \times$$

$$\times \frac{(3.33 \times 10^{-4} \times 0.23)\text{Bq} \times 1\dfrac{\text{tps}}{\text{Bq}} \times 0.54\dfrac{\text{MeV}}{\text{t}} \times 1.6 \times 10^{-13}\dfrac{\text{J}}{\text{MeV}} \times 8.64 \times 10^{4}\dfrac{\text{s}}{\text{d}}}{0.02\ \text{kg} \times 1\dfrac{\text{J}}{\text{kg}}\Big/\text{Gy}}$$

D (thyroid, ^{133}I) = 3.57×10^{-11}Gy

$$D(\text{body, } {}^{133}\text{I} = \frac{1}{0.8\ \text{d}^{-1}} \times$$

$$\times \frac{(3.33 \times 10^{-4} \times 0.77)\text{Bq} \times 1\dfrac{\text{tps}}{\text{Bq}} \times 0.84\dfrac{\text{MeV}}{\text{t}} \times 1.6 \times 10^{-13}\dfrac{\text{J}}{\text{MeV}} \times 8.64 \times 10^{4}\dfrac{\text{s}}{\text{d}}}{70\ \text{kg} \times 1\dfrac{\text{J}}{\text{kg}}\Big/\text{Gy}}$$

D (body, ^{133}I) $= 5.32 \times 10^{-14}$ Gy

In summary, the doses are

	^{131}I	^{133}I
Thyroid	1.4×10^{-10} Gy	3.6×10^{-11} Gy
Body	2.5×10^{-13} Gy	5.32×10^{-14} Gy

11.10 Disposal of animal carcasses in a biomedical research institution is by incineration. If the incinerator requires 34 kg air per minute, how much ^{131}I activity may be incinerated per 40 hour week, assuming all the iodine in the animal carcasses is volatilized, if the 10 CFR 20 limit of 2×10^{-10} µCi/mL in the effluent air is not to be exceeded? **11.10**

The 10CFR20 atmospheric limits for inhalation are based on the volume of air that a person inhales during a year, at a nominal temperature of 25ºC. The density of air at STP = 1.293 kg/m^3. At 25ºC, this corresponds to

$$\rho(\text{air, } 25^\circ\text{C}) = 1.293\frac{\text{kg}}{\text{m}^3} \times \frac{273}{273 + 25} = 1.185\frac{\text{kg}}{\text{m}^3}$$

$$\frac{34\text{ kg}}{\text{min}} \times \frac{1\text{ m}^3}{1.185\text{ kg}} \times \frac{1 \times 10^6\text{ mL}}{\text{m}^3} = 2.87 \times 10^7\ \frac{\text{mL air}}{\text{min}}$$

$$\frac{2 \times 10^{-10}\ \mu\text{Ci}}{\text{mL}} \times \frac{2.87 \times 10^7\text{ mL air}}{\text{min}} \times \frac{60\text{ min}}{\text{hr}} \times \frac{40\text{ hr}}{\text{week}} = 13.8\frac{\mu\text{Ci}}{\text{week}}$$

BUT, 10 CFR 20 effluent limits are based on continuous (168 hr/wk) exposure. Therefore, for a week the maximum activity that may be sent up the chimney is

$$13.8\ \frac{\mu\text{Ci}}{40\text{ hr}} \times 168\ \frac{\text{hr}}{\text{week}} = 58\ \frac{\mu\text{Ci}}{\text{week}}$$

11.11

11.11 A graphite moderated reactor is cooled by passing 680,000 kg air per hour through the core. The mean temperature in the core is 300°C, and the thermal neutron flux is 5×10^{13} neutrons/cm^2/sec. If the air spends an average of 10 sec in the reactor core, what is the rate of production of ^{41}Ar? If the chimney through which the air is discharged is 100 meters high and has an orifice diameter of 2 meters; and the temperature of the effluent air is 170°C, while the ambient temperature is 30°C on a sunny day and if the mean wind velocity is 2 m/sec, at what distance from the chimney will the ground level concentration of ^{41}Ar be a maximum? What will be the value of this maximum concentration (in Bq/m^3)? How does this figure compare to the DAC for ^{41}Ar?

The production rate of ^{41}Ar activity is given by equation 5.59:

$$A = \lambda N = \phi\frac{\text{neutrons}}{\text{cm}^2 \cdot \text{sec}} \times \sigma\frac{\text{cm}^2}{\text{atom}} \times n\frac{\text{atoms}}{\text{sec}}\left(1 - e^{-\lambda t}\right)$$

The number, n, of ^{40}Ar atoms that pass through the core is calculated: Argon comprises 0.934 volume percent of air, and 99.6% of all Ar is ^{40}Ar. Therefore consider all the Ar to be ^{40}Ar. We will use the mean molecular weight of all the gases in air, 28.8, as the "molecular weight" of air.

$$n = \frac{6.8 \times 10^5\ \frac{\text{kg}}{\text{h}} \times 10^3\ \frac{\text{g}}{\text{kg}}}{28.8\frac{\text{g}}{\text{mol air}}} \times 9.34 \times 10^{-3}\ \frac{\text{mol Ar}}{\text{mol air}} \times 6.02 \times 10^{23}\ \frac{\text{atoms Ar}}{\text{mole Ar}} \times \frac{1\text{ h}}{3600\text{ s}}$$

$n = 3.7 \times 10^{25}$ atoms/sec

The radioactive decay constant, λ, for ^{41}Ar is

$$\lambda = \frac{0.693}{T} = \frac{0.693}{110\ \text{min} \times 60\dfrac{\text{s}}{\text{min}}} = 1.05 \times 10^{-4}\ \text{sec}^{-1}$$

The cross section for thermal neutron capture at 20ºC (293K), σ_0, is 0.64 barns (CRC). σ at the core temperature of 300ºC (573K) is calculated with equation 5.53, modified to account for the fact that the mean σ of a thermal neutron energy distribution is $1.128\sigma_0$.

$$\sigma_{573\ \text{K}} = \frac{\sigma_{293\ \text{K}}}{1.128}\sqrt{\frac{273\ \text{K}}{T}} = \frac{0.64 \times 10^{-24}\,\text{cm}^2}{1.128}\sqrt{\frac{293\ \text{K}}{573\ \text{K}}} = 4.1 \times 10^{-25}\ \text{cm}^2$$

Substituting these values into the activation equation, we have

$$A = 5 \times 10^{13}\ \frac{\text{n}}{\text{cm}^2 \cdot \text{s}} \times 4.1 \times 10^{-25}\ \frac{\text{cm}^2}{\text{atom}} \times 3.7 \times 10^{25}\ \frac{\text{atoms}}{\text{s}}\left(1 - e^{-1.05\times10^{-4}\,\text{s}^{-1}\times 10\ \text{s}}\right)$$

$A = 8 \times 10^{11}$ Bq/s

Maximum ground level concentration, χ_{max}, occurs at the downwind distance where (equation 11.7):

$$\sigma_z = \frac{H}{\sqrt{2}}$$

H, the effective chimney height, equation 11.6, is

$$H = h + d\left(\frac{v}{\mu}\right)^{1.4} \times \left(1 + \frac{\Delta T}{T}\right)$$

v, the effluent velocity is given by

$$v = \frac{Q\dfrac{\text{m}^3}{\text{s}}}{A\ \text{m}^2} = \frac{1}{\dfrac{\pi}{4}(2\ \text{m})^2} \times \frac{6.8 \times 10^5\ \dfrac{\text{kg}}{\text{h}}}{\left(1.293 \times \dfrac{273}{273 + 170}\right)\dfrac{\text{kg}}{\text{m}^3} \times 3600\dfrac{\text{s}}{\text{h}}}$$

$v = 75.5$ m/s

Substituting into the equation for *H* gives

$$H = 100\text{ m} + 2\text{ m} \times \left(\frac{75.5\dfrac{\text{m}}{\text{sec}}}{2\dfrac{\text{m}}{\text{sec}}}\right)^{1.4} \times \left(1 + \frac{140\text{ K}}{443\text{ K}}\right) = 523\text{ m}$$

$$\sigma_z = \frac{H}{\sqrt{2}} = \frac{523\text{ m}}{\sqrt{2}} = 370\text{ m}$$

The given atmospheric conditions give stability category A. Figure 11.8, Curve A, shows that σ_z = 370 m at a downwind distance of 800 m. The ground level concentration is given by equation 11.5.

$$\chi = \frac{Q}{\pi\sigma_y\sigma_z\mu} e^{-\frac{1}{2}\left(\frac{H^2}{\sigma_z^2}\right)}$$

σ_z = 370 m
σ_y = 170 m (Fig. 11.8)

$$\chi(800{,}0) = \frac{8\times 10^{11}\dfrac{\text{Bq}}{\text{sec}}}{\pi\times(170\text{ m})\times(370\text{ m})\times 2\dfrac{\text{m}}{\text{sec}}} \times e^{-\frac{1}{2}\times\left(\frac{523^2}{370^2}\right)}$$

$$\chi(800{,}0) = 7.4\times 10^5\,\frac{\text{Bq}}{\text{m}^3}$$

This does not consider decay during travel time. Considering only the 800 m distance downwind, at a wind speed of 2 m/s, the travel time is 400 seconds, or 6.7 minutes. The maximum ground level concentration, therefore is (equation 4.18);

$$\chi_{\max} = 7.4\times 10^5\,\frac{\text{Bq}}{\text{m}^3}\times e^{-\frac{0.693}{110\text{ min}}\times 6.7\text{ min}} = 7.1\times 10^5\,\frac{\text{Bq}}{\text{m}^3}$$

$$7.1\times 10^5\,\frac{\text{Bq}}{\text{m}^3}\times\frac{1\times 10^6\,\mu\text{Ci}}{3.7\times 10^{10}\,\text{Bq}}\times\frac{1\text{ m}^3}{1\times 10^6\,\text{mL}} = 2\times 10^{-5}\,\frac{\mu\text{Ci}}{\text{mL}}$$

Compare this with the value in 10 CFR 20, Appendix B, table 2, column 1, for effluent concentrations, 1×10^{-8} μCi/mL, or the occupational DAC in 10 CFR 20, Appendix B, Table 1, column 3, of 3×10^{-6} μCi/mL. The effluent concentration exceeds the applicable NRC standards for these atmospheric conditions.

11.12 About 10^{13} Bq (270 Ci) of ^{14}C waste is generated per year from biomedical sources in the United States. If this waste will continue to be generated at the same annual rate, **11.12**

(a) What will be the resultant steady state quantity of ^{14}C waste?

Under steady state conditions:

Amount generated per year = Amount decayed per year

$$G = \lambda \times A_{SS}$$

$$\lambda = \frac{0.693}{T_{1/2}} = \frac{0.693}{5720} = 1.21 \times 10^{-4} \text{ yr}$$

$$A_{SS} = \frac{G}{\lambda} = \frac{10^{13}\ \frac{\text{Bq}}{\text{y}}}{1.21 \times 10^{-9}\ \text{y}^{-1}} = 8.26 \times 10^{16}\ \text{Bq}$$

(b) How long will it take until 99% of the steady state inventory is reached?

The buildup towards secular equilibrium (steady state) is given by a variant of equation 4.38

$$A = A_{ss}(1 - e^{-\lambda t})$$

where A_{SS} is the steady state activity, A is the activity at time t after the start of buildup.

$$\frac{A}{A_{SS}} = 0.99 = 1 - e^{-\lambda t}$$

$$e^{-\lambda t} = 1 - 0.99 = 0.01$$

Solving for t, we have:

$$t = \frac{\ln(0.01)}{-1.21 \times 10^{-4}\,\text{yr}^{-1}} = 3.8 \times 10^4\ \text{yr}$$

11.13

11.13 Analysis of albacore in the Pacific Ocean for ^{137}Cs from nuclear bomb fallout showed the mean concentration to be 2.74 Bq/kg (7.4 pCi/kg) wet weight during the period 1965 to 1971. Calculate the committed dose equivalent due to the consumption of 1 kg albacore per week for 1 year.

$$\text{Daily intake} = \frac{2.74\ \text{Bq}}{\text{kg}} \times \frac{1\ \text{kg}}{\text{wk}} \times \frac{1\ \text{wk}}{7\ \text{days}} = 0.391 \frac{\text{Bq}}{\text{day}}$$

Cs-137 elimination follows a two compartment model (ICRP 30), one with a 2 day half life, the other having a 110 day half life. Ten percent of the ingested activity is deposited in the 2 day half life compartment and 90% is deposited in the long lived compartment.

The committed dose equivalent is

$$H = \tilde{A}\ \text{Bq} \cdot \text{d} \times S \frac{\text{Sv}}{\text{Bq} \cdot \text{d}}$$

First, we will calculate $\tilde{A}$.
The ^{137}Cs body burden, $q(t)$ at any time after the start of continuous intake is given by a variant of equation 8.40

$$q(t) = q_{01}\left(1 - e^{-\lambda_1 t}\right) + q_{02}\left(1 - e^{-\lambda_2 t}\right)$$

where q_{01} and q_{02} are the steady state activities in the respective compartments, and

$$q_{02} = 9q_{01}$$

$$\lambda_1 = \frac{0.693}{2\ \text{days}} = 0.347\ \text{day}^{-1}$$

$$\lambda_2 = \frac{0.693}{110\ \text{days}} = 6.3 \times 10^{-3}\ \text{day}^{-1}$$

At steady state:

Amount deposited per day = amount eliminated per day

All the ingested Cs is absorbed and deposited in the body. Therefore, the daily deposited activity is

$$q_{\text{in}} = 2.74\frac{\text{Bq}}{\text{kg}} \times 1\frac{\text{kg}}{\text{wk}} \times \frac{1\text{ wk}}{7\text{ d}} = 0.391\frac{\text{Bq}}{\text{d}}$$

$$q_{out} = \lambda_1 q_{01} + \lambda_2 q_{02} = \lambda_1 q_{01} + \lambda_2 \times 9q_{01} = q_{01}(\lambda_1 + 9\lambda_2)$$

$$0.391\frac{\text{Bq}}{\text{day}} = q_{01}(\lambda_1 + 9\lambda_2) = q_1\left[0.347\text{ day}^{-1} + 9 \times 6.3 \times 10^{-3}\text{day}^{-1}\right]$$

$$q_{01} = 0.97\text{ Bq}$$
$$q_{02} = 9 \times q_{01} = 8.73\text{ Bq}$$

The total cumulated activity is

$$\tilde{A} = \tilde{A}(\text{ingestion}) + \tilde{A}(\text{elimination})$$

$\tilde{A}(\text{ingestion})$ is given by a variant of equation 11.17:

$$\tilde{A}(\text{ingestion}) = q_0\left[t_i - \frac{1}{\lambda_1}\left(1 - e^{-\lambda t}\right)\right]$$

and $\tilde{A}(\text{elinmination})$ is given by a variant of equation 6.58

$$\tilde{A}(\text{elinmination}) = \frac{q}{\lambda}$$

For compartment 1, the short lived compartment, q at the end of the 365 day ingestion period will equal q_0. Substituting the values for compartment 1, we have

$$\tilde{A}_1 = 0.97\text{ Bq} \times \left[365\text{ day} - \frac{1}{0.347\text{day}^{-1}} \times \left(1 - e^{-0.347\text{day}^{-1} \times 365\text{ day}}\right)\right] + \left[\frac{0.97\text{ Bq}}{0.347\text{day}^{-1}}\right]$$

$\tilde{A}_1 = 354 \text{ Bq} \cdot \text{day}$

For compartment 2, $q(365)$, the activity after 365 days ingestion is

$$q(365) = 8.73 \text{ Bq} \times \left(1 - e^{-0.0063 \times (365)}\right) = 7.85 \text{ Bq}$$

Substituting the values for compartment 2, we have

$$\tilde{A}_2 = 8.73 \text{ Bq}\left[365 \text{ day} - \frac{1}{6.3 \times 10^{-3}\text{day}^{-1}}\left(1 - e^{-6.3\times10^{-3}\text{day}^{-1} \times 365 \text{ day}}\right)\right] + \frac{7.85 \text{ Bq}}{6.3 \times 10^{-3}\text{day}^{-1}}$$

$\tilde{A}_2 = 3186 \text{ Bq·day}$

The total cumulated activity is

$$\tilde{A} = \tilde{A}_1 + \tilde{A}_2$$

$$\tilde{A} = 354 + 3186 = 3540 \text{ Bq·d}$$

The S(body←body) factor for ^{137}Cs is 9.1×10^{-11} Sv/Bq·d (MIRD Pamphlet No. 11 or page 222 of the text). The dose equivalent due to eating the ^{137}Cs contaminated seafood is calculated using equation 6.97;

$$H = \tilde{A} \times S = 3.54 \times 10^3 \text{ Bq}\times\text{day} \times 9.1 \times 10^{-11}\frac{\text{Sv}}{\text{Bq} \cdot \text{day}}$$

$$H = 3.2 \times 10^{-7} \text{ Sv}$$

11.14

11.14 Krypton gas, tagged with ^{85}Kr to a specific activity of 1.3×10^{11} Bq/mole, (3.5 Ci/mole), will be transferred from a tank into another vessel at a rate of 0.1 cm^3/min (at 25°C and 760 torr) through plastic tubing. There is a remote possibility that the tubing connection will break, and the gas will escape into the laboratory. If the laboratory dimensions are 3 m × 4 m × 3 m, what must be the minimum ventilation rate if the steady state concentration is not to exceed 1/10 of the 10 CFR 20 limit of 3.7×10^5 Bq/m^3 (1×10^{-5} μCi/mL)?

The steady state concentration in a ventilated room is given by equation 11.26

$$C = \frac{\text{Generation rate}}{\text{Ventilation rate}} = \frac{G}{Q}$$

Molar volume of gas at 273 K = $2.24 \times 10^4 \frac{\text{mL}}{\text{mole}}$

Calculate G, the rate of generation;

$$G = 0.1 \frac{\text{mL}}{\text{min}} \times \frac{1}{2.24 \times 10^4 \frac{\text{mL}}{\text{mole}}} \times 1.3 \times 10^{11} \frac{\text{Bq}}{\text{mole}} \times \frac{273\ \text{K}}{(273 + 25)\ \text{K}} = 5.32 \times 10^5 \frac{\text{Bq}}{\text{min}}$$

Calculate the maximum concentration allowed (10% of 10 CFR 20 limit);

$$C = 0.1 \times 3.7 \times 10^5 \frac{\text{Bq}}{\text{m}^3} = 3.7 \times 10^4 \frac{\text{Bq}}{\text{m}^3}$$

$$Q = \frac{G}{C} = \frac{5.32 \times 10^5 \frac{\text{Bq}}{\text{min}}}{3.7 \times 10^4 \frac{\text{Bq}}{\text{m}^3}} = 14.4 \frac{\text{m}^3}{\text{min}}$$

Solutions for Chapter 12

CRITICALITY

12.1 Cooling water circulates through a water boiler reactor core at a rate of 4 L/min through a coiled stainless steel tube of 6.4 mm inside diameter and 213 cm in length. The concentration of Na and Cl in the water is 5 atoms each per million molecules H_2O. What is the concentration of induced Na and Cl radioactivity in the cooling water after a single passage through the reactor core if the mean thermal flux is 10^{11} neutrons per cm^2/s and the mean temperature in the core is 80°C? **12.1**

The number of radioactive atoms/L produced by thermal neutron irradiation of N target atoms/L during an irradiation time t seconds is:

$$n = N\frac{\text{targets}}{\text{L}} \times \sigma\frac{\text{cm}^2}{\text{target}} \times \phi\frac{\text{neutrons}}{\text{cm}^2\cdot\text{s}} \times t \text{ sec}$$

Since the irradiation time of one passage through the core is much less than the half life of the activated isotopes, the resulting activity is :

$$A = \lambda \text{ sec}^{-1} \times n$$

To correct for the cross section at a different temperature, the following equation is applied to the cross sections (Ethrington):

$$\sigma = \sigma_0\frac{1}{1.128}\sqrt{\frac{293\text{K}}{(273+80)\text{K}}} = \sigma_0 \times 0.808$$

The following reactions and their associated parameters are used for this problem. Also listed is the number of target atoms per liter for each element, which were calculated as shown below.

Reaction	Cross Sections		N	Activated Isotopes	
	σ_0,b	σ, b	targets/L	$T_{1/2}$	λ, S^{-1}
$^{23}Na\ (n,\gamma)^{36}Cl$	0.53	0.43	1.625×10^{20}	15 h	1.28×10^{-5}
$^{35}Cl(n,\gamma)^{36}Cl$	43.6	35.2	1.23×10^{20}	3.08×10^{5} y	7.13×10^{-14}
$^{35}Cl(n,p)^{35}S$	0.489	0.40	1.23×10^{20}	87 d	9.22×10^{-8}
$^{37}Cl(n,\gamma)^{38}Cl$	0.423	0.34	4.0×10^{19}	37.5 m	3.08×10^{-4}

Calculate the number of atoms of each nuclide present per cm^3.

H_2O, with density of 0.97 g/cm^3 (CRC) at 80°C, and a MW of 18 g/mole;

$$\frac{6.03 \times 10^{23} \text{ molecules}}{\text{mole}} \times \frac{1 \text{ mole}}{18 \text{ g}} \times \frac{970 \text{ g}}{\text{L}} = 3.25 \times 10^{25} \frac{\text{molecules } H_2O}{\text{L}}$$

Since there are 5 atoms ^{23}Na and Cl for every million molecules of water;

$$3.25 \times 10^{25} \frac{\text{molecules } H_2O}{\text{L}} \times \frac{5 \text{ atoms } ^{23}\text{Na}}{10^6 \text{ molecules } H_2O}$$

$$= 1.625 \times 10^{20} \frac{\text{atoms } ^{23}\text{Na and Cl}}{\text{L}}$$

There are two isotopes of Cl; 75.4% ^{35}Cl and 24.6% ^{37}Cl, whose concentrations are

$$0.754 \times 1.625 \times 10^{20} \frac{\text{atoms Cl}}{\text{L}} = 1.23 \times 10^{20} \frac{\text{atoms } ^{35}\text{Cl}}{\text{L}}$$

and

$$0.246 \times 1.625 \times 10^{20} \frac{\text{atoms Cl}}{\text{L}} = 4.0 \times 10^{19} \frac{\text{atoms } ^{37}\text{Cl}}{\text{L}}$$

Calculate the irradiation time that is, the time that the water spends in the reactor;

distance = velocity × time

and $\text{velocity} = \dfrac{\text{volumetric flow rate}}{\text{area}}$

therefore: $\text{distance} = \dfrac{\text{volumetric flow rate}}{\text{area}} \times t$

$$213\ \text{cm} = \frac{4000 \dfrac{\text{cm}^3}{\text{min}}}{\pi/4\left(0.64\ \text{cm}\right)^2 \times 60 \dfrac{\text{sec}}{\text{min}}} \times t$$

$t = 1.03$ seconds

For the case of ^{24}Na, the induced atomic concentration after a single passage through the reactor core:

$$n = N \frac{\text{targets}}{\text{L}} \times \sigma \frac{\text{cm}^2}{\text{target}} \times \phi \frac{\text{neutrons}}{\text{cm}^2 \cdot \text{sec}} \times t\ \text{sec}$$

$$n = 1.625 \times 10^{20} \frac{\text{targets}\ ^{23}\text{Na}}{\text{L}} \times 0.43 \times 10^{-24} \frac{\text{cm}^2}{\text{atom}^{23}\text{Na}} \times 10^{11} \frac{\text{neutrons}}{\text{cm}^2 \cdot \text{sec}} \times 1.03\ \text{sec}$$

$n = 7.2 \times 10^6$ atoms ^{24}Na/L

and the activity is

$\text{Activity} = \lambda \times n$

Activity (^{24}Na) $= 1.28 \times 10^{-5}\ \text{sec}^{-1} \times 7.2 \times 10^6 = 92$ Bq/L

By similar calculations, we find that for the other activations:

^{36}Cl: $\text{l}n = 7.13 \times 10^{-14}\ \text{sec}^{-1} \times 1.23 \times 10^{20} \times 35.2 \times 10^{-24} \times 10^{11} \times 1.03$

$= 3.2 \times 10^{-5} \dfrac{\text{Bq}}{\text{L}}$

^{35}S: $\ln = 9.22 \times 10^{-8} \times 1.23 \times 10^{20} \times 0.40 \times 10^{-24} \times 10^{11} \times 1.03$

$= 0.47 \frac{\text{Bq}}{\text{L}}$

^{38}Cl: $\ln = 3.08 \times 10^{-4} \times 4 \times 10^{19} \times 0.34 \times 10^{-24} \times 10^{11} \times 1.03$

$= 431 \frac{\text{Bq}}{\text{L}}$

12.2

12.2 If the cooling water in problem 1 circulates through a heat exchange reservoir containing 400 L (including the water in pipes between the core and the reservoir), what will be the concentration of induced activity in the reservoir after 7 days operation of the reactor?

The rate of change of activity in the reservoir is:

$$\frac{dQ}{dt} = \text{Activity rate in } - \text{activity rate out}$$

For the ith isotope, let:

$K_i \frac{\text{Bq}}{\text{min}}$ = the activation rate of the ith isotope.

Q_i Bq = quantity of the ith isotope in the system at any time t

$\lambda_i \text{ min}^{-1}$ = radionuclide decay constant for the ith isotope

$\frac{Q_i \text{ Bq}}{400 \text{ L}}$ = concentration at any time t

$$\text{rate into reservoir } = K\frac{\text{Bq}}{\text{min}} + \left(\frac{Q\text{ Bq}}{400\text{ L}} \times \frac{4\text{ L}}{\text{min}}\right)$$

$$\text{rate out of reservoir} = \left(\frac{Q\text{ Bq}}{400\text{ L}} \times \frac{4\text{ L}}{\text{min}}\right) + \lambda \text{ min}^{-1} \times Q\text{ Bq}$$

Replacing words with the above equations:

$$\frac{dQ}{dt} = \left\{ K\frac{\text{Bq}}{\text{min}} + \left(\frac{Q\ \text{Bq}}{400\ \text{L}} \times \frac{4\ \text{L}}{\text{min}} \right) \right\} - \left\{ \left(\frac{Q\ \text{Bq}}{400\ \text{L}} \times \frac{4\ \text{L}}{\text{min}} \right) + \lambda\ \text{min}^{-1} \times Q\ \text{Bq} \right\}$$

Combining terms;

$$\frac{dQ}{dt} = K\frac{\text{Bq}}{\text{min}} - \lambda\ \text{min}^{-1} \times Q\ \text{Bq}$$

$$\frac{dQ}{dt} = K - \lambda \times Q$$

$$\frac{dQ}{K - \lambda \cdot Q} = dt$$

$$\int_0^Q \frac{dQ}{K - \lambda \cdot Q} = \int_0^t dt$$

$Q = \frac{K}{\lambda}\left(1 - e^{-\lambda t}\right)$, the activity for each individual isotope after irradiation time t.

Calculate the activity of ^{24}Na. A value for K is calculated using the information in problem 12.1;

$$K = 92\frac{\text{Bq}}{\text{L}} \times \frac{4\ \text{L}}{\text{min}} = 368\frac{\text{Bq}}{\text{min}}$$

$$\lambda = \frac{0.693}{15\ \text{hr} \times \frac{60\ \text{min}}{1\ \text{hr}}} = 7.7 \times 10^{-4}\ \text{min}^{-1} = 1.11\ \text{d}^{-1}$$

Putting values into the equation and solving for $t = 1 \times 10^4$ min (7 days):

$$Q = \frac{K}{\lambda}\left(1 - e^{-\lambda \times t}\right) = \frac{368\frac{\text{Bq}}{\text{min}}}{7.7 \times 10^{-4}\ \text{min}^{-1}}\left(1 - e^{-7.7\times10^{-4}\times1\times10^{4}}\right) = 4.78 \times 10^{5}\ \text{Bq}\ ^{24}\text{Na}$$

Since Q was defined as the activity in the total system, the concentration is:

$$C = \frac{4.78 \times 10^5\,\text{Bq}}{400\text{ L}} \times \frac{1\text{ liter}}{1000\text{ mL}} = 1.2 \times 10^3\,\frac{\text{Bq}}{\text{L}} = 32\,\frac{\text{pCi}}{\text{mL}}$$

the activity concentrations for the other activated radioisotopes are calculated in a similar manner, and the results are tabulated below. The values for C_i and λ are taken from problem 12.1.

Isotope	$C_i, \frac{\text{Bq}}{\text{L}}$	$K, \frac{\text{Bq}}{\text{min}} = 4C_i$	λ, min^{-1}	Q, Bq	C $\frac{\text{Bq}}{\text{L}}$	C $\frac{\text{pCi}}{\text{mL}}$
^{24}Na	92	368	7.7×10^{-4}	4.78×10^5	1.2×10^3	32
^{36}Cl	3.2×10^{-5}	1.28×10^{-4}	4.3×10^{-12}	1.3	3.2×10^{-3}	8.6×10^{-5}
^{35}S	0.47	1.88	5.5×10^{-6}	1.83×10^4	46	1.2
^{38}Cl	431	1724	0.0185	9.32×10^4	233	6.3

12.3

12.3 If the tank of problem 12.2 is spherical, what will be the surface dose rate due to the induced radioactivity one week after the start of operation?

$\Gamma(^{24}\text{Na})$ is listed in Table 6.3 as $1.84\frac{\text{R}\cdot\text{m}^2}{\text{Ci}\cdot\text{h}}$, which becomes, using 0.95 rad/R

$$\Gamma(^{24}\text{Na}) = 1.84\frac{\text{R}\cdot\text{m}^2}{\text{Ci}\cdot\text{h}} \times 10^3\,\frac{\text{mR}}{\text{R}} \times 10^4\,\frac{\text{cm}^2}{\text{m}^2} \times 10^{-12}\,\frac{\text{Ci}}{\text{pCi}} \times 0.95\frac{\text{mrad}}{\text{mR}}$$

$$\Gamma(^{24}\text{Na}) = 175 \times 10^{-5}\,\frac{\text{mrad}\cdot\text{cm}^2}{\text{pCi}\cdot\text{h}}$$

$\Gamma(^{38}\text{Cl})$ is not listed. It may be estimated by a variant of equation 6.18.

$$\Gamma = 4.75 \times 10^{-6} \sum f_i E_i\,\frac{\text{mrad}\cdot\text{cm}^2}{\text{pCi}\cdot\text{hr}}$$

$$\Gamma = 4.75 \times 10^{-6}\,(0.38 \times 1.6 + 0.47 \times 2.17) = 7.73 \times 10^{-6}\,\frac{\text{mrad}\cdot\text{cm}^2}{\text{pCi}\cdot\text{hr}}$$

Only ^{24}Na and ^{38}Cl are gamma emitters, and thus contribute to the surface dose. Use equation 10.37 to find the dose rate at the surface of the sphere;

$$\dot{D} = \frac{1}{2} \times C \times \Gamma \times \frac{4\pi}{\mu} \times \left(1 - e^{-\mu \cdot r}\right)$$

$$C = \frac{\text{activity}}{\text{volume}}$$

Calculate the radius of a 400 liter spherical tank:

$$V = \frac{4}{3}\pi r^3$$

$$r = \left(\frac{3}{4\pi}V\right)^{\frac{1}{3}} = \left(\frac{3}{4\times\pi}\times 400\ \text{L}\times\frac{1000\ \text{cm}^3}{\text{L}}\right)^{\frac{1}{3}} = 45.7\ \text{cm}$$

The values in the table below for concentration, C, are from problem 12.2, and the mean linear absorption coefficients in water, $\bar{\mu}$, are from the data in Table 5.3.

Isotope	$C\ \frac{\text{pCi}}{\text{cm}^3}$	γ MeV	f	$\Gamma\ \frac{\text{mrad}\cdot\text{cm}^2}{\text{pCi}\cdot\text{hr}}$	$\bar{\mu}$, cm^{-1}	$\dot{D}\ \frac{\text{mrad}}{\text{h}}$	$\dot{D}\ \frac{\mu\text{Gy}}{\text{h}}$
^{24}Na	32	1.37	1	1.75×10^{-5}	0.026	9.409×10^{-2}	0.94
		2.75	1				
^{38}Cl	6.3	1.6	0.38	7.73×10^{-6}	0.027	8.033×10^{-3}	0.08
		2.17	0.47				

Substituting the values from the table into the surface dose rate equation gives, for ^{24}Na

$$\dot{D} = \frac{1}{2}\times 32\frac{\text{pCi}}{\text{cm}^3}\times 1.75\times 10^{-5}\ \frac{\text{mrad}\cdot\text{cm}^2}{\text{pCi}\cdot\text{h}}\times\frac{4\pi}{0.026\ \text{cm}^{-1}}\times\left(1-e^{-0.026\times 45.7}\right)$$

$$\dot{D}(^{24}\text{Na}) = 9.409\times 10^{-2}\ \frac{\text{mrad}}{\text{h}}$$

and for ^{38}Cl, we find

$$\dot{D}(^{38}\text{Cl}) = 8.033\times 10^{-3}\ \frac{\text{mrad}}{\text{h}}$$

$$\dot{D} = \dot{D}(^{24}\text{Na}) + \dot{D}(^{38}\text{Cl}) = (9.409 + 0.8033)\times 10^{-2} = 0.1\ \frac{\text{mrad}}{\text{h}} = 1\ \frac{\mu\text{Gy}}{\text{h}}$$

The resulting dose at the surface at the tank is 0.1 mrads/hr = 1 μGy/hr. Note that this is also the maximum (equilibrium) dose rate at a NaCl concentration of 5 NaCl atoms per 10^6 H_2O molecules.

12.4

12.4 A research reactor, after going critical for the first time, operates at a power level of 100W for 4 h. How much fission product activity does the reactor contain at the following times after shutdown of the reactor?
Using equation 12.23b;

$$A = 1.46 \times P \times \left[(\tau - t)^{-0.2} - \tau^{-0.2}\right]$$

t = total time
t = operation time in days = 4 hr = 4/24 day = 0.167 day
$\tau - t$ = cooling time
P = 100 W

(a) 1 h
τ = 1 hr + 4 hr = 5/24 day = 0.208 day

$A = 1.46 \times 100\ \text{W} \times \left[(0.208\ \text{d} - 0.167\ \text{d})^{-0.2} - (0.208\ \text{d})^{-0.2}\right] = 75.4$ Ci present after 1 hr

(b) 8 h
τ = 8 hr + 4 hr = 0.5 day

$A = 1.46 \times 100\ \text{W} \times \left[(0.5\ \text{d} - 0.167\ \text{d})^{-0.2} - (0.5\ \text{d})^{-0.2}\right] = 14.2$ Ci after 8 hr

(c) 7 days
τ = 7 days + 4 hr = 7 day + 4/24 day = 7.167 days

$A = 1.46 \times 100\ \text{W} \times \left[(7.167\ \text{d} - 0.167\ \text{d})^{-0.2} - (7.167\ \text{d})^{-0.2}\right] = 0.46$ Ci after 7 days

(d) 30 days
τ = 30 days + 4 hr = 30 day + 0.167 day = 30.167 day

$A = 1.46 \times 100\ \text{W} \times \left[(30.167\ \text{d} - 0.167\ \text{d})^{-0.2} - (30.167\ \text{d})^{-0.2}\right] = 0.08$ Ci after 30 days

12.5 A research reactor, after going critical for the first time, operates at a power level of 100 W for 4 hr. How many curies of fission product activity does that core contain? **12.5**

Equation 12.23

$$A = 1.46 \times P \times \left[(\tau - t)^{-0.2} - \tau^{-0.2}\right] \text{ Ci},$$

is valid only for times greater than or equal to 10 seconds after shutdown. Therefore, the activity in the reactor can be approximated by graphing the activity from times 10 - 60 seconds after shutdown, and then extrapolating the curve back to $t = 0$. Substituting
$t = 4$ hours = 1/6 day
$\tau - t = 10 \text{ seconds} = 1.16 \times 10^{-4}$ day
into the equation, we have

$$A = 1.46 \times 100 \times \left[\left(1.16 \times 10^{-4}\right)^{-0.2} - (1/6)^{-0.2}\right] = 686 \text{ Ci}$$

The calculated activity for the other times, until 60 seconds after shutdown, are tabulated and plotted below. The extrapolated curve intersects the $t = 0$ axis at 1000 Ci.

Sec	Ci
10	686
15	616
20	570
25	536
30	509
35	488
40	469
45	453
50	440
55	427
60	416

From the following graph an activity of 1000 Ci is extrapolated.

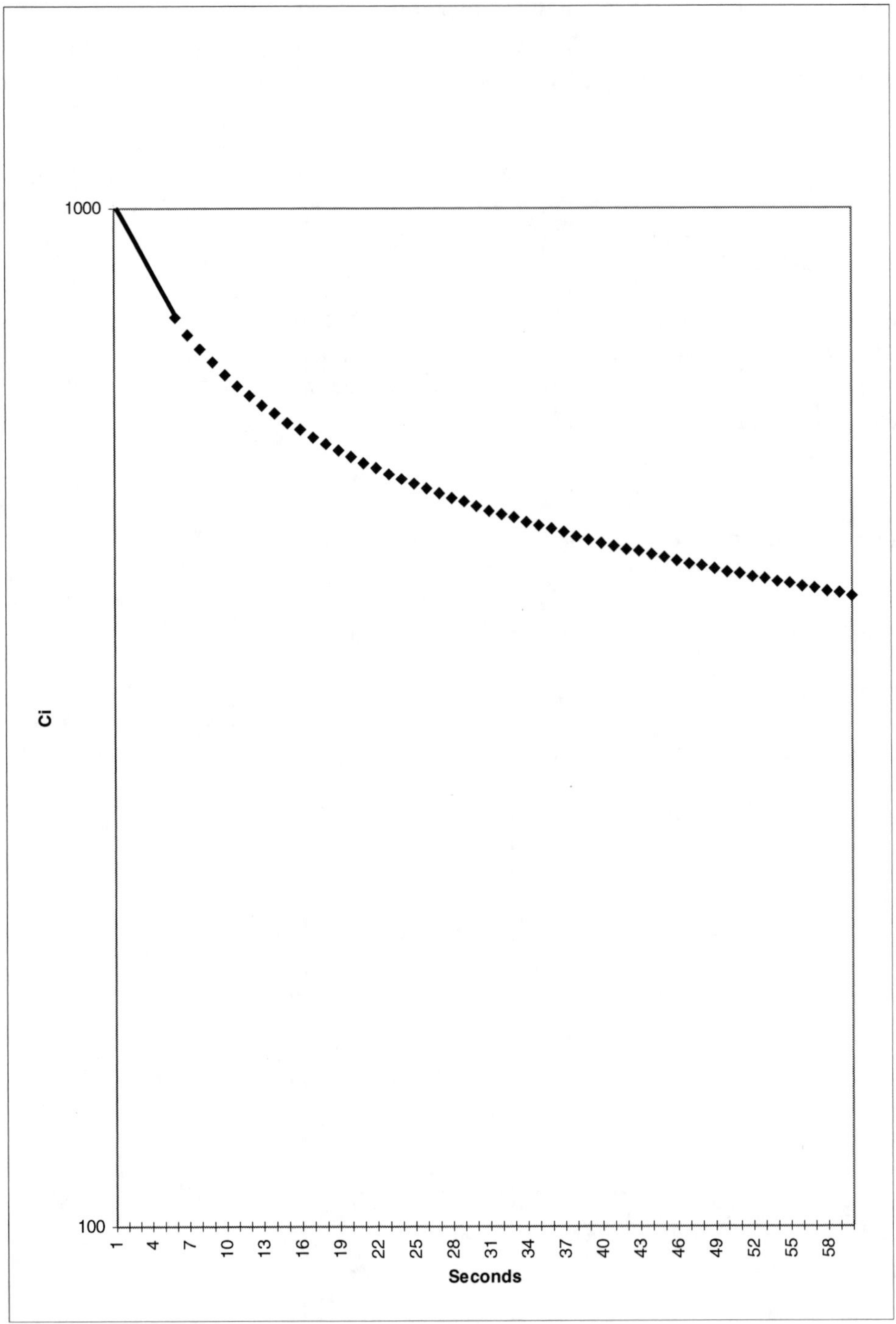
1000
100
Ci
1
4
7
10
13
16
19
22
25
28
31
34
37
40
43
46
49
52
55
58
Seconds

12.6 An accidental criticality occurred in an aqueous solution in a half filled mixing tank 25 cm diameter by 100 cm high. The energy released during the burst was estimated as 1800 J. Assuming that, on the average, each disintegration of a fission product is accompanied by a 1 MeV γ-ray, estimate the γ–ray dose rate at the surface of the tank (which maintained its integrity during the criticality) and at a distance of 25 feet from the tank at 1 min, 1 hr, 1 day, and 1 week after the criticality. **12.6**

According to Chapter 12, approximately 190 MeV per fission is released.

$$\frac{190 \text{ MeV}}{\text{fission}} \times 1.6 \times 10^{-13} \frac{\text{J}}{\text{MeV}} \times X \text{ fissions} = 1800 \text{ J}$$

$X = 5.92 \times 10^{13}$ fissions required to produce 1800 J energy.

Equation 12.3b can be used to estimate the activity at a given time after a criticality. Combine this information with the number of fissions required to produce 1800 J energy.

$$A = 1.03 \times 10^{-16}\, T^{-1.2} = 1.03 \times 10^{-16}\, T^{-1.2} \frac{\text{Ci}}{\text{fission}} \times 5.92 \times 10^{13} \text{ fissions}$$

$$A = 6.1 \times 10^{-3}\, T^{-1.2} \text{ Ci}$$

Calculate the activity at each time: ΔT, after criticality

$$\Delta T = 1 \text{ min} = 1 \text{ min} \times \frac{1 \text{ day}}{1440 \text{ min}} = 6.94 \times 10^{-4} \text{ day}$$

$A = 6.1 \times 10^{-3}\, \Delta T^{-1.2} \text{ Ci} = 6.1 \times 10^{-3}\, (6.94 \times 10^{-4} \text{ day})^{-1.2} \text{ Ci} = 37.6$ Ci is the activity present 1 minute after criticality.

The average dose rate within the tank is calculated with equation 6.68

$$\dot{D}(t) = C(t) \times \Gamma \times \overline{g}$$

Since the surface dose rate is one half the average within the tank, the surface dose rate is

$$\dot{D}_s(t) = \frac{1}{2} C(t) \times \Gamma \times \overline{g}$$

$C(t)$, the concentration at time t, is

$$C(t) = \frac{A(t)}{\text{vol.}} = \frac{A(t)}{\frac{\pi}{4}(25\text{ cm})^2 \times 50\text{ cm}} = \frac{A(t)}{2.45 \times 10^4\text{ cm}^3}$$

$$\Gamma = 0.5\sum f_i E_i \frac{\text{R} \cdot \text{m}^2}{\text{Ci} \cdot \text{hr}} = 0.5 \times 1 \times 1 \frac{\text{R} \cdot \text{m}^2}{\text{Ci} \cdot \text{hr}} \times 10^4 \frac{\text{cm}^2}{\text{m}^2} \times 0.95 \frac{\text{rad}}{\text{R}}$$

$$\Gamma = 4.75 \times 10^3 \frac{\text{rad} \cdot \text{cm}^2}{\text{Ci} \cdot \text{hr}}$$

$\bar{g}$, the mean geometry factor = 132.5 cm for a 25 cm diameter by 50 cm tall cylinder of water (Table 6.4).

The unshielded surface dose rate at time t after criticality is:

$$\dot{D}_s(t) = \frac{1}{2} \times \frac{A(t)}{2.45 \times 10^4\text{ cm}^3} \times 4.75 \times 10^3 \frac{\text{rad} \cdot \text{cm}^2}{\text{Ci} \cdot \text{hr}} \times 132.5\text{ cm}$$

$$\dot{D}_s(t) = 12.4 \frac{\text{rad}}{\text{Ci} \cdot \text{hr}} \times A(t)\text{ Ci}$$

At $\Delta T = 1$ minute,

$$\dot{D}_s(1\text{ min}) = 12.4 \frac{\text{rad}}{\text{Ci} \cdot \text{hr}} \times 37.6\text{ Ci} = 466 \frac{\text{rads}}{\text{hr}}$$

At a distance of 25 feet (762 cm), the 25 cm diameter by 50 cm tall tank can be considered a "point" source. The dose rate may therefore be calculated with equation 10.1

$$\dot{D}(t) = \frac{\Gamma}{d^2} \times A(t) = \frac{4.75 \times 10^3 \frac{\text{rad} \cdot \text{cm}}{\text{Ci} \cdot \text{hr}}}{(762\text{ cm})^2} \times A(t)$$

$$\dot{D}(t) = 8.18 \times 10^{-3} \frac{\text{rad}}{\text{Ci} \cdot \text{hr}} \times A\text{ Ci}$$

For 1 minute after criticality, the dose rate at 25 feet is

$$\dot{D}_{25}(1\text{ min}) = 8.18 \times 10^{-3}\,\frac{\text{rad}}{\text{Ci}\cdot\text{hr}} \times 37.6\text{ Ci} = 0.31\frac{\text{rad}}{\text{hr}} = 3.1 \times 10^{-3}\,\frac{\text{Gy}}{\text{hr}}$$

If we repeat these calculations for the dose rates at the later times post criticality, we obtain

		D (surface)		*D* (25 ft)	
ΔT	$A(t)$, Ci	rad/hr	Gy/hr	rad/hr	Gy/hr
1 m (1/1440 d)	37.6	466	4.66	0.31	3.1×10^{-3}
1 h (1/24 d)	0.276	3.4	0.034	2.3×10^{-3}	2.3×10^{-5}
1 d	6.1×10^{-3}	7.6×10^{-2}	7.6×10^{-4}	5×10^{-5}	5×10^{-7}
1 wk (7 d)	5.9×10^{-4}	7.3×10^{-3}	7.3×10^{-5}	4.8×10^{-6}	4.8×10^{-8}

12.7 A slab of pure natural uranium metal weighing 1 kg is irradiated in a thermal neutron flux of 10^{12} neutrons per cm^2/sec for 24 days at a temperature of 150°F. If the fission yield for ^{131}I is 2.8%, how many millicuries of ^{131}I will be extracted 5 days after the end of the irradiation? **12.7**

The activity of a fission product whose yield is *f* per fission is given by a variant of equation 5.59. If the fission product decays for a time t_d after the end of neutron activation, then the activity is

$$A = \frac{f\phi\sigma n}{3.7 \times 10^7}\left(1 - e^{-\lambda t_i}\right)\left(e^{-\lambda t_d}\right)\text{ mCi}$$

σ, the fission cross section at 65.6°C (150°F) is calculated from σ_0 (^{235}U, 20°C) = 586 b using a variant of equation 5.53. A "not one over v" factor, 0.974, must be used in calculating σ (65.6°C), as well as the 1/1.128 factor to account for the fact that the mean σ in a Maxwellian distribution is greater than the most probable σ.

$$\sigma(T) = \frac{\sigma_0}{1.128} \times \text{not }{}^{1}\!/_{\text{v}} \times \sqrt{\frac{T_0}{T}}$$

$$\sigma\,(65.6°\mathrm{C}) = \frac{586\ \mathrm{b}}{1.128} \times 0.974 \times \sqrt{\frac{273° + 20°}{273° + 65.6°}} = 471\ \mathrm{b}$$

n, the number of ^{235}U target atoms is

$$n = 1000\ \mathrm{g\ U} \times \frac{0.72\ \mathrm{g}\ ^{235}\mathrm{U}}{100\ \mathrm{g\ U}} \times \frac{6.02 \times 10^{23}\ \mathrm{atoms}\ ^{235}\mathrm{U/mole}}{235\ \mathrm{g}\ ^{235}\mathrm{U/mole}}$$

$$n = 1.84 \times 10^{22}\ \mathrm{atoms}\ ^{235}\mathrm{U}$$

$$\lambda\,(^{131}\mathrm{I}) = \frac{0.693}{T\,(^{131}I)} = \frac{0.693}{8\ \mathrm{d}} = 0.087\ \mathrm{d}^{-1}$$

Substituting these values into the activity equation for 24 days irradiation and 5 days decay, we have

$A=$

$$\frac{2.8 \times 10^{-2} \times 10^{12}\ \frac{\mathrm{n}}{\mathrm{cm}^2 \cdot \mathrm{s}} \times 4.71 \times 10^{-22}\ \mathrm{cm}^2 \times 1.84 \times 10^{22}\ \mathrm{atoms}}{3.7 \times 10^{7}\ \mathrm{dps/mCi}} \left(1 - e^{-0.08 \times 24}\right)\left(e^{-0.087 \times 5}\right)$$

$A = 3.72 \times 10^{3}\ \mathrm{mCi}$

12.8 **12.8** What is the uranium concentration of uranyl sulfate UO_2SO_4 aqueous solution that can go critical if the uranium is enriched to
(a) 10%
For criticality, $k = \eta \varepsilon p f = 1$

Eta (η), the mean number of fission neutrons per neutron absorbed in uranium, is calculated from equation 12.7 and from the data in Example 12.2 in the text. These data can also be found in various nuclear references.

$$\eta = \frac{\sigma_{f5}}{\sigma_{a5} + \left(\frac{N_8}{N_5}\right) \times \sigma_{a8}} v$$

where

σ_{f5} = 549 b fission cross section ^{235}U
σ_{a5} = 650 b absorption cross section ^{235}U
σ_{a8} = 2.8 b absorption cross section ^{238}U

$\frac{N_8}{N_5} = \frac{90}{10} = 9$ = molar ratio of U-8 to U-5 atoms in 10% enriched U

$v = 2.5$ for ^{235}U = average number of neutrons per fission

$$\eta = \frac{549}{650 + (0.9) \times 2.8} \times 2.5 = 2.03$$

The fast fission factor, ε, can be assumed to be 1, since this is a homogeneous assembly. Additionally, p, the resonance escape probability, is also assumed to be 1, since the molar ratio of moderator to feul is very high (Example 12.2 in the text book discusses each of these factors in more detail).

The value of f, the thermal utilization factor that will lead to criticality, $k_\infty = 1$ is

$k_\infty = \eta \varepsilon p f$
$1 = 2.03 \times 1 \times 1 \times f$
$f = 0.4926$

The dependency of f on the composition of the aqueous UO_2SO_4 solution is given by equation 12.14

$$f = \frac{\sigma_{a5} M_5 + \sigma_{a8} M_8}{\sigma_{a5} M_5 + \sigma_{a8} M_8 + \sigma_{aH_2O} M_{H_2O} + \sigma_{aO_2SO_4} M_{O_2SO_4}}$$

where
M_5 = moles U-5 per mole water
M_8 = moles U-8 per mole water
M_{O2SO4} = moles O_2SO_4 per mole water
σ_{H2O} = absorption cross section of H_2O = 0.664 b (Text, p. 526)
σ_{O2SO4} = absorption cross section of O_2SO_4 = 0.491 b (Text, p. 526)
M_{H2Or} = mole water per mole water = 1

If M = the number of moles of UO_2SO_4 per mole H_2O to attain criticality, then for 10% enrichment,

$\text{U-5}/\text{U} = 0.1$, $\text{U-8}/\text{U} = 0.9$, the number of moles per mole of H_2O for each of the components of the UO_2SO_4 solution is given in the table below.

Component	σ_a b	moles	σ_a × moles
H_2O	0.664	1	0.664
O_2SO_4	0.491	M	0.491M
U-5	650	0.1M	65M
U-8	2.8	0.9M	2.52M

Substituting these values into equation 12.14 gives

$$f = \frac{65\,M + 2.52\,M}{65\,M + 2.52\,M + 0.664 + 0.491\,M} = 0.4296$$

$M = 0.00745$ mole 10% enriched UO_2SO_4 per mole of water for criticality.

The molecular weight of the enriched uranium is

(235 × 0.1) + (238 × 0.9) = 237.7 g/mole of enriched uranium.

and the molecular weight of the UO_2SO_4 solution is

237.7 + (2 × 16) + 32 + (4 × 16) = 365.7 g/mole UO_2SO_4

The concentration of 10% enriched UO_2SO_4 required to attain criticality:

$$365.7\,\frac{\text{g}}{1\text{ mol UO}_2\text{SO}_4} \times 7.45 \times 10^{-3}\,\frac{\text{mol UO}_2\text{SO}_4}{\text{mol H}_2\text{O}} \times \frac{1\text{ mol H}_2\text{O}}{18\text{ g}} \times 10^3\,\frac{\text{g}}{1\text{ L}}$$

$$= 151.4\,\frac{\text{g UO}_2\text{SO}_4}{\text{L H}_2\text{O}}$$

(b) The calculations for 90% enriched UO_2SO_4 are made in a similar manner, using the values for η and for f appropriate to 90% enrichment

$$\eta = \frac{\sigma_{f5}}{\sigma_{a5} + \left(\frac{N_8}{N_5}\right) \times \sigma_{a8}} v = \frac{549}{650 + \left(\frac{10}{90}\right) \times 2.8} 2.5 = 2.11$$

The value of f needed for criticality ($k_\infty = 1$) is

$1 = \eta\varepsilon pf$
$1 = 2.11 \times 1 \times 1 \times f$

If we substitute equation 12.14 for *f* into the criticality equation, we have

$$1 = 2.11 \times \frac{\sigma_{a5} M_5 + \sigma_{a8} M_8}{\sigma_{a5} M_5 + \sigma_{a8} M_8 + \sigma_{aH_2O} M_{H_2O} + \sigma_{aO_2SO_4} M_{O_2SO_4}}$$

By letting M = the number of moles of 90% enriched UO_2SO_4, we obtain the following values to substitute into the equation above:

Component	σ_a b	moles	$\sigma_a \times$ moles
H_2O	0.664	1	0.664
O_2SO_4	0.491	M	0.491 M
U5	650	0.9 M	585
U8	2.8	0.1 M	0.28 M

Substituting these values into the equation, we have

$$1 = 2.11 \times \frac{585M + 0.28M}{585M + 0.28M + 0.664 + 0.491M}$$

$M = 1.023 \times 10^{-3}$ mole UO_2SO_4

The molecular weight of 90% enriched uranium is

$(235 \times 0.9) + (238 \times 0.1) = 235.3$

and the molecular weight of 90% enriched UO_2SO_4 is

$235.3 + (2 \times 16) + 32 + (4 \times 16) = 363.3$

The concentration of 90% enriched UO_2SO_4 required in the aqueous solution to attain criticality is

$$C = 363.3 \frac{\text{g}}{\text{mol UO}_2\text{SO}_4} \times 1.023 \times 10^{-3} \frac{\text{mol UO}_2\text{SO}_4}{1 \text{ mol H}_2\text{O}} \times \frac{1 \text{ mol H}_2\text{O}}{18 \text{ g}} \times \frac{1000 \text{ g}}{1 \text{ L}}$$

$$C = 20.64 \frac{\text{g UO}_2\text{SO}_4}{\text{L H}_2\text{O}}$$

12.9

12.9 Calculate η for ^{239}Pu, given that the fission cross section is 664 barns and the non–fission absorption cross section is 361 barns.

Eta (η), the number of fission neutrons per neutron, is given by equation 12.7:

$$\eta = \frac{\text{fission cross section}}{\text{total cross section}} \times \text{number of neutrons per fission} = \frac{\sigma_f}{\sigma_{total}} \times \nu$$

For Pu, ν = 3.0 neutrons per fission (p. 522 in text)

$$\eta\left(^{239}\text{Pu}\right) = \frac{664}{664+361} \times 3.0 = 1.94 \frac{\text{fission neutrons}}{\text{fission}}$$

12.10

12.10 The blood plasma from a worker who was overexposed during a criticality accident had a ^{24}Na activity of 37 Bq (0.001 μCi) per mL 15 hr after the accident. The accidental excursion lasted 10 msec. What was the absorbed dose due to (a) the ^{14}N(n,p)^{14}C reaction and (b) the autointegral gamma ray dose due to the n,γ reaction of the hydrogen. All the Na in nature is ^{23}Na. The thermal neutron activation cross section at 20°C is 0.53 barns, and $T_{1/2}(^{24}\text{Na})$ = 15hr.

The neutron flux during the criticality is calculated from the initial induced activity. The number, n, of the ^{24}Na atoms per mL that were made radioactive by the ^{23}Na(n, γ)^{24}Na reaction during the 10 millisecond exposure is given by

$$n = N \frac{^{23}\text{Na atoms}}{\text{mL}} \times \phi \frac{\text{neutrons}}{\text{cm}^2 \cdot \text{s}} \times \sigma \frac{\text{cm}^2}{\text{atom}} \times t \text{ sec}$$

The initial activity of these ^{24}Na atoms is given by

$$A = \lambda n$$

Since we had 37 Bq/mL at exactly 1 half life (T = 15 h) after the criticality, the initial activity was 74 Bq.

$$74\ \mathrm{s}^{-1} = \frac{0.693}{15\ \mathrm{h} \times 3600 \frac{\mathrm{s}}{\mathrm{h}}} \times n$$

$n = 5.77 \times 10^6$ atoms ^{24}Na

N, the number of ^{23}Na target atoms, is determined by the NaCl concentration in the blood, 9 mg/mL (ICRP 23):

$$N = \frac{6.02 \times 10^{23} \frac{\text{atoms Na}}{\text{mol}}}{58.5\ \mathrm{g} \frac{\text{NaCl}}{\text{mol}}} \times 9 \times 10^{-3} \frac{\text{g NaCl}}{\text{mL blood}} = 9.3 \times 10^{19} \frac{\text{atoms }^{23}\text{Na}}{\text{mL blood}}$$

The activation cross section for 2200 m/sec neutrons, σ_0 (20°C) is corrected to 37°C by a variant of equation 5.53

$$\sigma(37^\circ\mathrm{C}) = \frac{\sigma_0}{1.128}\sqrt{\frac{T_0}{T}} = \frac{0.53\ \mathrm{b}}{1.128} \times \sqrt{\frac{273+20}{273+37}} = 0.46\ \mathrm{b}$$

Substituting these values into the activation equation, we have (note equation is in split into two lines)

$$5.77 \times 10^6 \frac{\text{atoms }^{24}\text{Na}}{\text{mL}} =$$

$$9.3 \times 10^{19} \frac{\text{atoms }^{23}\text{Na}}{\text{mL}} \times \phi \frac{\mathrm{n}}{\mathrm{cm}^2 \cdot \mathrm{s}} \times 0.46 \times 10^{-24} \frac{\mathrm{cm}^2}{\text{atom }^{23}\text{Na}} \times 10 \times 10^{-3}\ \mathrm{s}$$

$$\phi = 1.35 \times 10^{13} \frac{\mathrm{n}}{\mathrm{cm}^2 \cdot \mathrm{sec}}$$

a) The absorbed dose due to the ^{14}N (n,p) ^{14}C reaction is the product of the dose rate, equation 6.105, and the 10×10^{-3} second exposure time

$$D = \dot{D} \times t = \frac{\phi N\sigma \times Q \times 1.6 \times 10^{-13} \frac{\text{J}}{\text{MeV}}}{1 \frac{\text{J}/\text{kg}}{\text{Gy}}} \times t$$

where

$$\phi = 1.35 \times 10^{13} \frac{\text{n}}{\text{cm}^2 \cdot \text{sec}}$$

$N = 1.49 \times 10^{24}$ nitrogen atoms/kg tissue (Table 6.12)
$\sigma = 1.75 \times 10^{-24}$ cm^2 (page 225 in text)
$Q = 0.63$ MeV = energy released per (n,p) reaction (page 616 in text)
$t = 10 \times 10^{-3}$ sec

$$D(\text{n, p}) =$$

$$\frac{1.35 \times 10^{13} \frac{\text{n}}{\text{cm}^2 \cdot \text{s}} \times 1.49 \times 10^{24} \frac{\text{atoms}}{\text{kg}} \times 1.75 \times 10^{-24} \frac{\text{cm}^2}{\text{atom}} \times 0.63 \text{ MeV} \times 1.6 \times 10^{-13} \frac{}{\text{M}}}{1 \frac{\text{J}/\text{kg}}{\text{Gy}}}$$

$$D(\text{n, p}) = 35.5 \times 10^{-3} \text{ Gy}$$

(b) The absorbed dose rate from the ^{1}H(n, γ)^{2}H reaction is calculated by combining the (n, γ) reaction rate, equation 6.106

$$A = \phi \times N_H \times \sigma_H$$

where
ϕ = neutron flux
$N_H = 5.98 \times 10^{25}$ hydrogen atoms per kg (Table 6.12)
$\sigma_H = 0.33 \times 10^{-24}$ cm^2 (text, p. 252)

with the equation for a uniformly distributed gamma emitter, equation 6.82

$$\dot{D} = \frac{A}{m} \times \Phi \times \Delta$$

where

A/m = Bq/kg
Φ = 0.278 (Table 6.8) = absorbed fraction for 2.23 MeV gamma uniformly distributed throughout the body
Δ = dose rate in an infinite mass whose specific activity is 1 Bq/kg

$$\Delta = 2.23\frac{\text{MeV}}{\text{d}} \times 1.6 \times 10^{-13}\,\frac{\text{J}}{\text{MeV}} \times 1\frac{\text{dps}}{\text{Bq}} \times 1\frac{\text{Gy}}{1\ \text{J/kg}}$$

$$\Delta = 3.57 \times 10^{-13}\,\frac{\text{Gy/s}}{\text{Bq/kg}}$$

The absorbed dose is the product of the absorbed dose rate and the exposure time

$$D(\text{n},\gamma) = \dot{D}(\text{n},\gamma) \times t$$

$$D(\text{n},\gamma) = (\phi N_H \sigma_H)\frac{\text{"Bq"}}{\text{kg}} \times \Phi \times \Delta\frac{\text{Gy/s}}{\text{Bq/kg}} \times t \text{ sec}$$

Note that the equation is split into two lines:

$$D(\text{n},\gamma) = 1.35 \times 10^{13}\,\frac{\text{n}}{\text{cm}^2 \cdot \text{s}} \times 5.98 \times 10^{25}\,\frac{\text{atoms}}{\text{kg}} \times 0.33 \times 10^{-24}\,\frac{\text{cm}^2}{\text{atom}} \times$$

$$\times 0.278 \times 3.57 \times 10^{-13}\,\frac{\text{Gy/s}}{\text{Bq/kg}} \times 0.01 \text{ sec}$$

$$D(\text{n},\gamma) = 0.264 \text{ Gy}$$

Note that this problem only considers the dose from the thermal portion of the neutron spectrum.

12.11 (a) For the case where $k = 1.0025$, and an initial number of 1000 neutrons, how many neutrons will be present after 10 generations? **12.11**

Equation 12.5 gives the multiplication factor

$$k_{eff} = \frac{N_{f+1}}{N} = 1.0025 \frac{\text{neutrons}}{\text{neutron}} \Big/ \text{generation}$$

To find the number of neutrons after 10 generations (n = 10);

$$N_{fn} = (k_{eff})^{n\text{-}1} N_0 = (1.0025)^9 \times (1000) = 1023 \text{ neutrons}$$

(b) After how many generations will the neutron flux be doubled?

$$N_n = (k_{eff})^{n\text{-}1} N_0$$

$$2000 = (1.0025)^{n\text{-}1} \times (1000)$$

Solve for n;

$$2 = (1.0025)^{n\text{-}1}$$

$$n = \frac{\log 2}{\log 1.0025} + 1 = 279 \text{ generations}$$

12.12

12.12 At 20 minutes after a criticality accident the dose rate in a laboratory from the fission products was 15 Gy/hr (1500 rad/hr). If the laboratory ventilation system was shut down at the time of the criticality, how long would it take before a person could enter the laboratory if his dose equivalent during a 15 minute exposure time is not to exceed 50 mGy (5 rad)?

$$T_1 = 20 \text{ min} \times \frac{1 \text{ hr}}{60 \text{ min}} = 0.33 \text{ hr}$$

$$\dot{D}_1 = 15 \frac{\text{Gy}}{\text{hr}}$$

$$\dot{D}_2 = \frac{50 \text{ mGy}}{15 \text{ min}} = \frac{50 \text{ mGy}}{15 \text{ min}} \times \frac{60 \text{ min}}{\text{hr}} \times \frac{1 \text{ Gy}}{1000 \text{ mGy}} = 0.2 \frac{\text{Gy}}{\text{hr}}$$

Equation 12.4 is used to determine the time:

$$\frac{\dot{D}_2}{\dot{D}_1} = \frac{T_2^{-1.2}}{T_1^{-1.2}}$$

$$\dot{D}_2 = \dot{D}_1 \left(\frac{T_1}{T_2} \right)^{1.2}$$

Inserting values and solving for T_2:

$$0.2 \frac{\text{Gy}}{\text{hr}} = 15 \frac{\text{Gy}}{\text{hr}} \times \left(\frac{0.33 \text{ hr}}{T_2} \right)^{1.2}$$

T_2 = 12.17 hrs. = 730 minutes after the accident, OR 710 minutes after the first measurement (730 – 20 = 710)

12.13 A transient burst of 1×10^{15} fissions in an unshielded accumulation of fissile materials causes a total dose equivalent of 0.25 Sv (25 rem) at a distance of 2 meters. If the neutron to gamma dose equivalent ratio is 9, what were the absorbed doses from the gammas and from the neutrons? **12.13**

The dose equivalent is found using 10CFR20 quality factors. The quality factor for gamma rays is 1. The quality factor for fast neutrons (all neutrons are born fast, Chapter 5) is 10. The equation representing the dose equivalent is:

$$H = Q \times D$$

$$\frac{H(n)}{H(\gamma)} = 9$$

$$H(\gamma) + H(n) = 0.25 \text{ Sv}$$

Replacing $H(n)$,

$$9H(\gamma) + H(\gamma) = 0.25 \text{ Sv}$$

$$H(g) = 0.025 \text{ Sv}$$

$$H(\text{n}) = 0.250 \text{ Sv} - 0.025 \text{ Sv} = 0.225 \text{ Sv}$$

$$D(g) = 0.025 \text{ Sv} \times 1 \frac{\text{Gy}}{\text{Sv}} = 25 \text{ mGy}$$

$$D(n) = 0.225 \text{ Sv} \times \frac{1 \text{ Gy}}{10 \text{ Sv}} = 0.0225 \text{ Gy} = 22.5 \text{ mGy}$$

12.14

12.14 The composition, by weight percent, of a concrete mix used in reactor shielding consists of oxygen, 52.17%, Si: 34.0%, Ca: 4.4%, Al: 3.5%, Na: 1.6%, Fe: 1.5%, K: 1.3%, H: 1.0%. The density of the concrete is 2.35 g/cm^3.
(a) Find and tabulate the thermal (2200 m/s) absorption cross section for each element.
(b) Calculate the linear attenuation coefficient (macroscopic cross section) of the concrete.

The microscopic cross section (σ_a in barns), for each element is tabulated in the table below (CRC).

To calculate the total macroscopic cross section for the concrete, the macroscopic cross section for each isotope of each element in the concrete is calculated, then the total summed. The values were calculated in the table below in the following manner;

From equation 5.23, the macroscopic cross section, Σ, is

$$\Sigma = \sum \sigma_i N_i$$

For each element, N, the number of atoms present per cm^3, must be calculated, and then multiplied by the microscopic cross section. Using O as an example

$$N_i, \text{ atoms/cm}^3 = \frac{6.02 \times 10^{23} \dfrac{\text{atoms}}{\text{mole}}}{A_i \dfrac{\text{g}}{\text{mole}}} \times f_i \times 2.35 \frac{\text{g}}{\text{cm}^3} = 1.42 \times 10^{24} \times \frac{f_i}{A_i}$$

$$N(0) = 1.42 \times 10^{24} \times \frac{0.522}{16} = 4.63 \times 10^{22} \frac{\text{atoms}}{\text{cm}^3}$$

$$\sigma(0) \times N(0) = 2.8 \times 10^{-28} \times 4.63 \times 10^{22} = 1.29 \times 10^{-5} \text{ cm}^{-1}$$

Element	f, wt. Fraction, abundance in concrete	σ_i cm^2 × 10^{-24} Cross section, b	A_I, $\frac{g}{mole}$	N_i, at/cc	$\sigma_I \times N_i$, cm^{-1} Cross Section
Oxygen	5.22E-01	2.80E-04	16	4.63E22	1.29E-05
Silicon	3.40E-01	1.70E-01	28	1.72E22	2.91E-03
Calcium	4.40E-02	4.30E-01	40.1	1.56E22	6.67E-04
Aluminum	3.50E-02	2.30E-01	27	1.84E21	4.22E-04
Sodium	1.60E-02	5.25E-01	23	9.88E20	5.17E-04
Iron	1.50E-02	2.56E+00	55.9	3.81E20	9.72E-04
Potassium	1.30E-02	2.10E+00	39.1	4.72E20	9.88E-04
Hydrogen	1.00E-02	3.32E-01	1	1.42E22	4.70E-03
				Sum	1.12E-02

The macroscopic cross section for this concrete is 1.1×10^{-2} cm^{-1}

12.15 The ^{131}I fission yield is 2.77%. What is the ^{131}I activity in the core of a power reactor that has been operating at a power level of 3000 MW (t) for **12.15**
(a) 8 days
(b) 30 days
(c) 60 days
(d) 180 days?

The fission product activity at time t after start of neutron irradiation is given by a variant of equation 4.38.

$$A(t) = K \times (1 - e^{-\lambda t})$$

where K is the production rate of the fission product.

$$K = 3.3 \times 10^{10} \frac{\frac{\text{fissions}}{\text{sec}}}{\text{W}} \times 3 \times 10^{9}\,\text{W} \times 2.77 \times 10^{-2} \frac{^{131}\text{I}}{\text{fission}} = 2.74 \times 10^{18} \frac{^{131}\text{I}}{\text{sec}}$$

$$\lambda(^{131}\text{I}) = \frac{0.693}{T} = \frac{0.693}{8\ \text{d}} = 0.087\ \text{d}^{-1}$$

Substituting these values into the inventory equation, we have

$$A(t) = 2.74 \times 10^{18} \frac{^{131}\text{I}}{\text{sec}} \times \left(1 - e^{-0.087 \times t}\right) \text{ dps (or Bq)}$$

and in mCi, the activity is

$$A(t) = \frac{2.74 \times 10^{18} \text{ s}^{-1}}{3.7 \times 10^{10} s^{-1} \cdot \text{Ci}^{-1}} \times \left(1 - e^{-0.087 \times t}\right)$$

$$A(t) = 7.4 \times 10^{7} \frac{^{131}\text{I}}{\text{sec}} \times \left(1 - e^{-0.087 \times t}\right) \text{Ci}$$

For $t = 8$ days

$$A(8) = 7.4 \times 10^{7} \frac{^{131}\text{I}}{\text{sec}} \times \left(1 - e^{-0.087 \times 8}\right) = 3.7 \times 10^{7} \text{ Ci} = 37 \text{ MCi}$$

By similar calculations for the other operating times, we have

t, days	Bq	MCi
8	1.37E+18	37.01
30	2.54E+18	68.54
60	2.72E+18	73.64
180	2.74E+18	74.05

12.16

12.16 Tritium is produced in a nuclear reactor in ternary fission, in which one ^{3}H nucleus is produced in every 10^4 fissions. What is the tritium activity in a reactor that had been operating at a mean power level of 3000 MW(t) for 2 years?

The activity of a fission product in the core of a reactor that had been operating at a power level of *P* watts for a time *t* is given by

$A(t) = K(1 - e^{-\lambda t})$ dps (or Bq)

where K = production rate of the fission product, atoms/second.

$$K = P \text{ watts} \times 3.3 \times 10^{10} \frac{\text{fiss}}{\text{s} \cdot \text{W}} \times f \frac{\text{atoms}}{\text{fiss}}$$

$$K = 3 \times 10^{9} \text{ W} \times 3.3 \times 10^{10} \frac{\text{fiss}}{\text{s} \cdot \text{W}} \times 1 \times 10^{-4} \frac{\text{atoms}}{\text{fiss}} = 9.9 \times 10^{15} \frac{\text{atoms}}{\text{s}}$$

$$\lambda(^{3}\text{H}) = \frac{0.693}{T} = \frac{0.693}{12.3 \text{ yr}} = 0.056 \text{ y}^{-1}$$

$$A(2 \text{ y}) = 9.9 \times 10^{15} \text{ s}^{-1} \times \left(1 - \text{e}^{-0.056 \times 2 \text{ yr}}\right) = 1.1 \times 10^{15} \text{ Bq}$$

In terms of curies,

$$A(2 \text{ y}) = \frac{1.1 \times 10^{15} \text{ Bq}}{3.7 \times 10^{10} \frac{\text{Bq}}{\text{Ci}}} = 2.9 \times 10^{4} \text{ Ci}$$

Solutions for Chapter 13

EVALUATION OF PROTECTIVE MEASURES

13.1 A series of measurements with threshold detectors showed the following spectral distribution of neutrons: **13.1**

Energy	Percent neutrons
Thermal	40
1000 eV	20
10,000 eV	10
0.1 MeV	10
1 MeV	10
10 MeV	10

When 500 mg ^{32}S was irradiated for 2 h in this field and then counted in a 2π counter 24 h after the end of irradiation, the result was 500 counts/min. What is the dose rate in the neutron field?

The neutron dose rate depends on the neutron flux, ϕ, which is determined by measuring the induced activity. Fast neutron irradiation of ^{32}S produces ^{32}P, whose $T_{1/2}$ = 14.3 days:

$^{32}S(n, p)^{32}P$

The induced activity's relation to the flux after an irradiation time t_i is given by equation 5.59:

$$\lambda N = \phi \sigma n \left(1 - e^{-\lambda t}\right)$$

The induced activity, A, determined with a 50% counting efficiency (2π geometry) is

$$A = \frac{500 \text{ counts}}{\text{min}} \times \frac{2 \text{ dis}}{1 \text{ count}} \times \frac{1 \text{ min}}{60 \text{ sec}} = 16.67 \frac{\text{dis}}{\text{sec}}$$

Correcting for 24 hours decay, we have

$$16.67 \text{ dps} = A_0 e^{-0.002 \text{ h}^{-1} \times 24 \text{ h}}$$

$$A_0 = 17.5 \text{ dps}$$

σ (^{32}S, 10 MeV) = 0.4 barn (Garber, D.I. and Kinsey, R.R.:Neutron Cross Sections, BNL 325, 1976). Only the 10 MeV neutrons contribute to the activation reaction because the reaction has a neutron energy threshold of 1.5 MeV.

n, the number of ^{32}S target atoms is

$$n = 0.5 \text{ g} \times \frac{6.02 \times 10^{23} \text{ atoms/mole}}{32 \text{ g/mole}} = 9.4 \times 10^{21} \text{ atoms}$$

$$\lambda(^{32}\text{P}) = \frac{0.693}{T_{1/2}(^{32}\text{P})} = \frac{0.693}{14.3 \text{ d} \times 24 \text{ h/d}} = 2 \times 10^{-3} \text{ h}^{-1}$$

Substituting these values into the activation equation, we have

$$17.5 \text{ s}^{-1} = \phi \frac{\text{neut}}{\text{cm}^2 \cdot \text{s}} \times 0.4 \times 10^{-24} \frac{\text{cm}^2}{\text{atom}} \times 9.4 \times 10^{21} \text{ atoms}\left(1 - \text{e}^{-0.002 \text{ h}^{-1} \times 2 \text{ h}}\right)$$

$$\phi = 1.17 \times 10^6 \frac{\text{neut}}{\text{cm}^2 \cdot \text{s}}$$

Since 10 MeV neutrons constitute only 10% of the total neutron flux, the fluxes for the other neutrons are:

Energy	$\phi_i \times 10^6\ \dfrac{\text{neut}}{\text{cm}^2 \cdot \text{s}}$	$\phi\left(\dfrac{1\ \text{mSv}}{40\ \text{h}}\right)$	$\dot{H}_i,\ \dfrac{\text{mSv}}{\text{h}}$
Thermal	4.68	270	433
1,000 eV	2.34	280	209
10,000 eV	1.17	290	101
0.1 MeV	1.17	58	504
1 MeV	1.17	10	2925
10 MeV	1.17	8.5	3441

$$\dot{H} = \sum \dot{H}_i = 7613 \frac{\text{mSv}}{\text{h}} = 7.6 \frac{\text{Sv}}{\text{h}}$$

Column 3 in the table above, $\phi\left(\dfrac{1\ \text{mSv}}{40\ \text{h}}\right)$, which is taken directly from Table 9.5, gives the neutron fluence rates, or fluxes, for a 1 mSv dose from a 40 hour exposure. These fluxes thus lead to a dose rate of 1/40 of 1 mSv/h. The dose rate, $\dot{H}_i$, from each of these neutron fluxes is calculated by:

$$\frac{\phi_i}{\phi\left(\dfrac{1\ \text{mSv}}{40\ \text{h}}\right)} = \frac{\dot{H}_i \dfrac{\text{mSv}}{\text{h}}}{\dfrac{1}{40} \dfrac{\text{mSv}}{\text{h}}}$$

$$\dot{H}_i = \frac{1}{40} \times \frac{\phi_i}{\phi\left(\dfrac{1\ \text{mSv}}{\text{h}}\right)}$$

For the thermal neutrons, we have

$$\dot{H}(\text{thermal}) = \frac{1}{40} \times \frac{4.68 \times 10^6}{270} = 433 \frac{\text{mSv}}{\text{h}}$$

The dose rates from each of the other groups of neutrons were calculated similarly, and are listed in the table above. The dose rate in the neutron beam is

$$\dot{H} = \sum_{i=1} H_i = 7613 \frac{\text{mSv}}{\text{h}} = 7.6 \frac{\text{Sv}}{\text{h}}$$

13.2

13.2 A sealed ^{90}Sr source is leak tested. The wipe, counted in a 2π gas–flow counter, gave 155 counts in 5 min. The background was 130 counts in 5 min. At the 95% confidence level, is the source contaminated?

$n_g = 155$ counts
$t_g = 5$ min

$$r_g = \frac{155 \text{ counts}}{5 \text{ min}} = 31 \text{ cpm} = M_g$$

$n_b = 130$ counts
$t_b = 5$ min

$$r_b = \frac{130 \text{ counts}}{5 \text{ min}} = 26 \text{ cpm} = M_b$$

Using equation 9.49 to find the "t" value:

$$t = \frac{|M_g - M_b|}{\sqrt{\frac{r_g}{t_g} + \frac{r_b}{t_b}}} = \frac{|31-26|}{\sqrt{\frac{31}{5} + \frac{26}{5}}} = 1.48$$

Since this is a one tail test, a "t" value of 1.645 is required to determine whether $M_g > M_b$ at the 95% confidence level (as listed in chapter 9). There is no difference between the two counts at the 95% confidence level, and therefore the source is not contaminated.

13.3

13.3 An air sample on a filter paper was counted in a 2π gas flow counter, and gave 800 counts in 5 min. A background count gave 260 counts in 10 min. What was the standard deviation of the net counting rate?

$n_g = 800$ counts
$t_g = 5$ min

$$r_g = \frac{800 \text{ counts}}{5 \text{ min}} = 160 \text{ cpm}$$

$n_b = 260$ counts
$t_b = 10$ min

$$r_b = \frac{260 \text{ counts}}{10 \text{ min}} = 26 \text{ cpm}$$

Using equation 9.33 to find the standard deviation:

$$\sigma_n = \sqrt{\frac{r_g}{t_g} + \frac{r_b}{t_b}} = \sqrt{\frac{160}{5} + \frac{26}{10}} = 5.9 \text{ cpm}$$

$R_{net} = 160 \text{ cpm} - 26 \text{ cpm} = 134 \text{ cpm}$

134 ± 5.9 cpm

13.4 A radioisotope worker weighing 70 kg inadvertently drinks water containing 3.7 MBq (100 μCi) ^{22}Na. Following this accidental exposure, his body burden was measured by whole body counts made over a period of 2 months. The following retention function was fitted to the whole body counting data: **13.4**

$Q(t) = 1.8\exp(-0.082t) + 1.9\exp(0.052t)$ MBq

Calculate:
(a) The cumulative activity, in Bq days.

Equation 6.91

$$\tilde{A} = \frac{A_S(0)}{\lambda_E}$$

$\lambda_{E_1} = 0.082 \text{ d}^{-1}$

$\lambda_{E_2} = 0.052 \text{ d}^{-1}$

$A_{S_1}(0) = 1.8$ MBq

$A_{S_2}(0) = 1.9$ MBq

$$\tilde{A} = \frac{1.8 \text{ MBq}}{0.082 \text{ d}^{-1}} + \frac{1.9 \text{ MBq}}{0.052 \text{ d}^{-1}} = 58.5 \text{ MBq·d}$$

(b) The initial dose rate, assuming the ^{22}Na to be uniformly distributed throughout the body

According to Fig. 4.8, ^{22}Na emits a 0.544 MeV positron in 89.8% of the decays, and a 1.277 MeV gamma in every decay. The dose rate from an internally deposited radioisotope is given by equation 6.47:

$$\dot{D} = \frac{q\ \text{Bq} \times \dfrac{1\ \text{tps}}{\text{Bq}} \times \overline{E}\ \dfrac{\text{MeV}}{\text{t}} \times 1.6 \times 10^{-13}\ \dfrac{\text{J}}{\text{MeV}} \times 3600\ \dfrac{\text{sec}}{\text{hr}}}{m\ \text{kg} \times 1 \dfrac{\text{J}}{\text{kg}} \Big/ \text{Gy}}$$

In the case of ^{22}Na, 3 different radiations contribute to the dose: the 0.544 MeV positron ($\overline{E}$ = 0.216 MeV, NRHH), the 0.51 MeV annihilation photons (2 photons per positron), and the 1.277 MeV gamma. The effective energy per transformation, E_e, is the sum of these 3 contributions. In the calculation below for E_e,

f_i = the number of particles per transformation
$\phi(E)$ = The fraction of the gamma ray energy absorbed in the body (Table 6.8, Total body to Total body)

$$\overline{E}(\beta^+) = f \times \overline{E} = 0.898 \frac{\beta^+}{\text{t}} \times 0.216 \frac{\text{MeV}}{\beta^+} = 0.194\ \text{MeV/t}$$

$$E(\text{annih}) = f \times 0.511 \times \phi = 0.898 \frac{\beta^+}{\text{t}} \times 2 \frac{\gamma}{\beta^+} \times 0.511 \frac{\text{MeV}}{\gamma} \times 0.34 = 0.312\ \text{MeV/t}$$

$$E(\gamma) = f \times E_\gamma \times \phi = 1 \frac{\gamma}{\text{t}} \times 1.277 \frac{\text{MeV}}{\gamma} \times 0.31 = 0.396\ \text{MeV/t}$$

E_e = 0.194 MeV/t + 0.312 MeV/t + 0.396 MeV/t

$$E_e = 0.902 \frac{\text{MeV}}{\text{t}}$$

When we substitute 0.902 MeV/t for E_e and 70 kg for m in the equation for $\dot{D}$, we have

$$\dot{D} = \frac{3.7 \times 10^6\ \text{Bq} \times \dfrac{1\ \text{tps}}{\text{Bq}} \times 0.902 \dfrac{\text{MeV}}{\text{t}} \times 1.6 \times 10^{-13} \dfrac{\text{J}}{\text{MeV}} \times 3600 \dfrac{\text{sec}}{\text{hr}}}{70\ \text{kg} \times 1 \dfrac{\text{J}}{\text{kg}} \Big/ \text{Gy}}$$

$$\dot{D} = 2.74 \times 10^{-6} \frac{\text{Gy}}{\text{hr}} = 27.4 \frac{\mu\text{Gy}}{\text{hr}}$$

13.5 The maximum permissible skeletal burden of ^{90}Sr is 74 kBq (2 μCi). Calculate the number of transformations per minute per 24 hr urine sample that may be expected from one fourth of this skeletal burden if 0.05% per day is eliminated in the urine. 13.5

$$74\text{ kBq} \times \frac{1000\text{ Bq}}{1\text{ kBq}} \times \frac{1\frac{\text{trans}}{\text{sec}}}{1\text{ Bq}} \times \frac{60\text{ sec}}{\text{min}} = 4.44 \times 10^6 \frac{\text{trans}}{\text{min}}$$

One quarter of the burden would then be:

$$4.44 \times 10^6 \frac{\text{trans}}{\text{min}} \times 0.25 = 1.11 \times 10^6 \text{ tpm}$$

Only 0.05% is eliminated in the urine per day:

$$1.11 \times 10^6 \text{ tpm} \times \frac{0.05}{100} = 555 \text{ tpm}$$

13.6 Using the ICRP three compartment lung model and the data for the reference man, calculate the ratio of concentration of soluble 1 μm AMAD uranium particles in the air to uranium in the urine, Bq/m^3 air per Bq/L urine, for the case where a steady state has been attained through continuous inhalation of the uranium. 13.6

Figure 8.3 and Table 8.5 gives the details of deposition of material in the respiratory tract;

Region	Percent Deposition	Deposited fraction absorbed into body	Fraction inhaled absorbed into body
N—P	30%	0.5	0.15
T—B	8%	0.95	0.076
P	25%	1	0.25
		Total absorbed	0.476

The total fraction of the inhaled uranium absorbed into the body is 0.476.

Assume 1 Bq/m^3 exposure, and from Appendix C, a reference person breaths 20 m^3/day.

$$1\frac{\text{Bq}}{\text{m}^3} \times 20\frac{\text{m}^3}{\text{day}} = 20\frac{\text{Bq}}{\text{day}}$$

So a person would take in 20 Bq/day. Since only 0.476 is the fraction absorbed in the body;

$9.6\frac{\text{Bq}}{\text{day}} \times 0.476 = 4.6\frac{\text{Bq}}{\text{day}}$ is absorbed. Reference man excretes 1.4 liters per day (appendix C).

Under steady state conditions, intake = output

$$4.6\frac{\text{Bq}}{\text{d}} \times \frac{\text{d}}{1.4\ \text{L urine}} = 3.3\ \frac{\text{Bq}}{\text{L urine}}$$

For an exposure of 1 μm AMAD at 1 Bq/m^3, 3.3 Bq/liter of urine would be expected if we neglect the small fraction of uranium deposited for long term storage in the bones.

It is interesting to compare this with the older ICRP 2 two compartment model:

According to ICRP 2, only 25% of the material is absorbed into the body fluids. The total fraction of the uranium absorbed into the body is 0.25. As calculated earlier, a person would take in 20 Bq/day. Since only 0.25 if the fraction absorbed in the body;

$20\frac{\text{Bq}}{\text{d}} \times 0.25 = 5\frac{\text{Bq}}{\text{d}}$ is absorbed. Reference man excretes 1.4 liters per day (appendix C).

$$5\frac{\text{Bq}}{\text{d}} \times \frac{\text{d}}{1.4\ \text{L urine}} = 3.6\ \frac{\text{Bq}}{\text{L urine}}$$

For an exposure of 1 μm AMAD at 1 Bq/m^3, 3.6 Bq/L of urine would be expected using the ICRP 2 two compartment model. Compare this with the three compartment model result of 6.8 Bq/L and note the difference is about a factor of 2.

13.7 The body burden of ^{137}Cs at time t days following a single intake Q(0) is given by **13.7**

$$Q(t) = Q(0)\,(0.1e^{-0.693t} + 0.9e^{-0.011t}).$$

If the ratio of urinary to fecal excretion is 9:1, calculate the activity per 24 hr urine sample 1 day and 10 days after ingestion of 50,000 Bq (1.35 μCi) ^{137}Cs.

Solve for day 1

$Q(0) = 50{,}000$ Bq
$t = 1$ day

$$Q(t) = Q(0) \times (0.1 \times e^{-0.693t} + 0.9 \times e^{-0.011t})$$

$$Q(1) = 50{,}000 \times (0.1 \times e^{-0.693 \times 1} + 0.9 \times e^{-0.011 \times 1}) = 47008$$

The quantity still retained in the body is 47008 Bq, so the total quantity excreted (in both the urine and feces) is:
$50000 - 47008 = 3.0 \times 10^3$ Bq is the total activity excreted on day one after exposure.

Since the urinary to fecal activity ratio is 9:1 (the total excretion would be 10, the sum of both excretion pathways), the quantity in the urine would be 90% of the total.

$3.0 \times 10^3 \text{ Bq} \times \dfrac{9}{10} = 2.7 \times 10^3$ Bq is the expected activity in the urine on day 1.

The activity excreted during day 10, A (10), is the difference between the body burdens on day 9 and day 10:

$$A(10) = Q\,(9) - Q\,(10)$$

$$Q(9) = 50000 \times (0.1 \times e^{-0.693 \times 9} + 0.9 \times e^{-0.011 \times 9}) = 4.08 \times 10^4 \text{ Bq}$$

$$Q(10) = 50000 \times (0.1 \times e^{-0.693 \times 10} + 0.9 \times e^{-0.011 \times 10}) = 4.03 \times 10^4 \text{ Bq}$$

Subtract the activity in the body on day 9 from day 10 to determine the excretion.

$$4.08 \times 10^4 \text{ Bq} - 4.03 \times 10^4 \text{ Bq} = 500 \text{ Bq}$$

Since 90% of the total is excreted in the urine, the activity in the urine would be:

$$500 \text{ Bq} \times \frac{9}{10} = 450 \text{ Bq}$$ is the activity expected in the urine on day ten

13.8 **13.8** A chemist accidentally inhaled a ^{14}C tagged organic solvent that is readily absorbed from the lungs. The solvent is known to concentrate in the liver. That part of the solvent which is eliminated before deposition in the liver leaves in the urine; the detoxification products are eliminated from the liver into the G.I. tract and into the urinary tract; 25% is eliminated in the urine and 75% in the feces. Following the inhalation, 24 hr urine samples were collected over a 2 week period and the following data were obtained:

Days after inhalation	1	2	3	4	5	6	8	10	12	14
kBq/sample	98	57	39	265	20	18	12	10	7.4	5.9

(a) How much activity was absorbed into the body?

The activity absorbed into the body is equal to the amount excreted; and the amount excreted is represented by the area under the excretion curve.

Graphing the data:

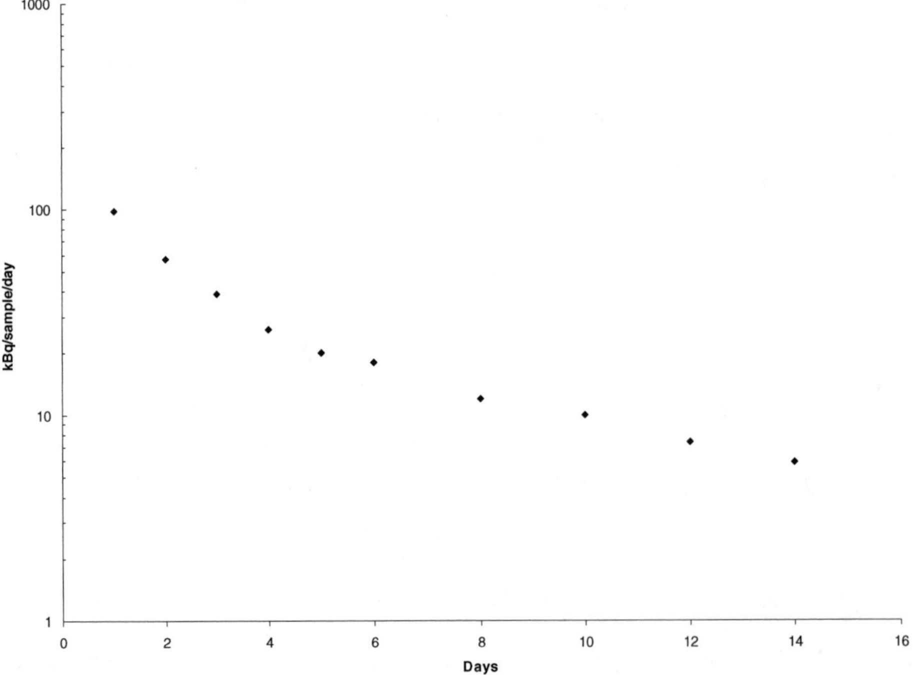

Since we know that clearance from the body follows first order kinetics, we plot the data on semi–log paper. Since the data fall on a curved line on semi–log paper, we know that several different compartments are being cleared at different rates. We note that the curve, after some time, eventually becomes a straight line. This means that all the shorter lived compartments have been cleared, and only the slowest clearing compartment is left. The intercept on the time = 0 axis of the extrapolated line represents the activity initially deposited in the longest lived compartment.

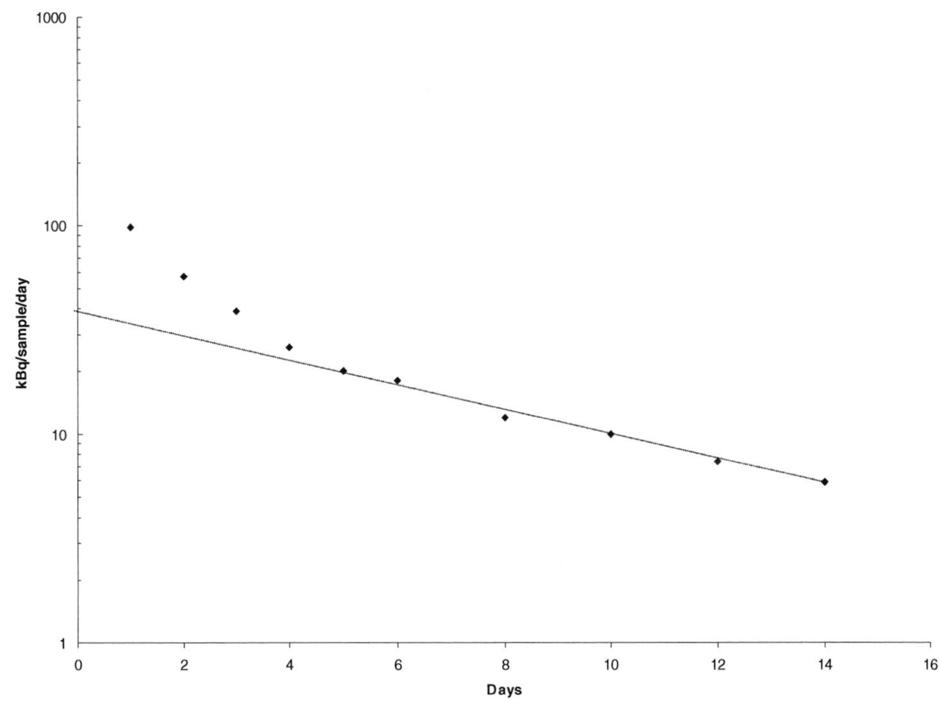

The extrapolated line intersects the t = 0 axis at 32 kBq. The slope of this line can be determined from its half clearance time, that is, the time until the urine activity reaches 16 kBq per sample. From the curve, we find the half clearance time to be 5.7 days. The slope of this line is computed:

$$\lambda = \frac{0.693}{5.7\ \text{d}} = 0.12\ \text{d}^{-1}$$

The equation representing the long term compartment of the clearance curve therefore is:

$$A(t)_{\text{urine}} = 32 \times e^{-0.12 \times t} \text{ kBq/day}$$

Since the clearance curve represents the sum of several compartments, the activity in the remaining compartments is determined by subtracting the contribution of the long term compartments from the total, and plotting these differences on semi–log paper; as shown in the table and graph below. In this case, the differences fall on a straight line, thus showing that there is only one rapidly cleared compartment. By extrapolating this rapid clearance component to zero, we find the intercept to be 128 kBq; the half clearance time for this compartment is 1.04 days, which yields a slope of 0.67 per day. The equation for the urinary clearance curve, which is the sum of 2 compartments is:

$$A(t)_{\text{urine}} = 128 \times e^{-0.67 \times t} + 32 \times e^{-0.12 \times t} \text{ Bq/day}$$

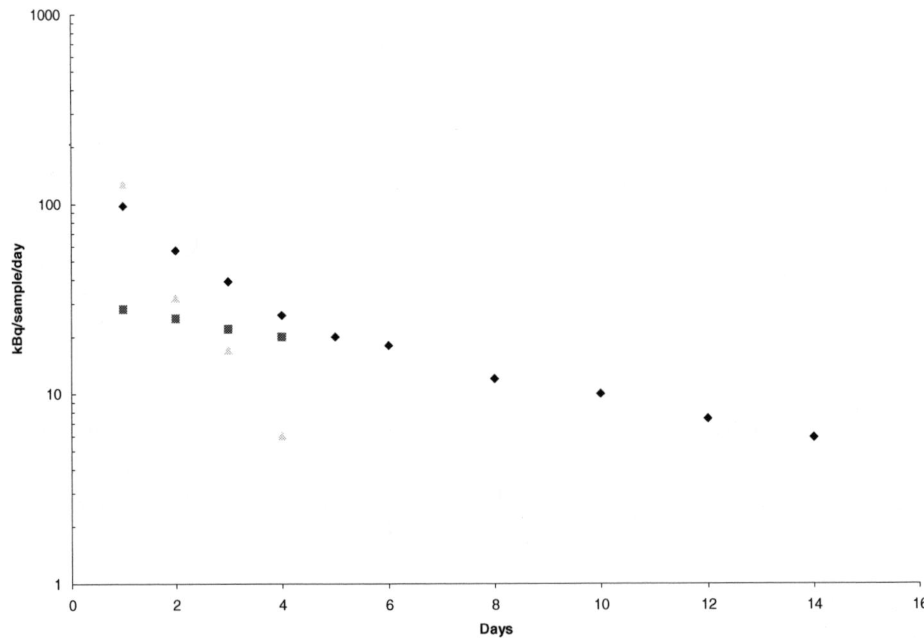

Day	Total activity in urine, Kbq/sample	Long term kBq/sample	Difference kBq/sample
1	98	28	128
2	57	25	32
3	39	22	17
4	26	20	6

The urinary activity of the slowly clearing compartment represents only 1/4 of the activity cleared from the liver. The total activity cleared from the liver is therefore four times that found in the urine. Thus, the intercept for the total "cleared" from the liver is 4 × 32, or 128 Bq. Therefore the curve representing the total clearance from the body is

$$A_T = 128 \times e^{-0.67 \times t} + 128 \times e^{-0.12 \times t}$$

The total activity absorbed into the body and eliminated by both the urine and feces is given by the area under the curve described by the above equation. Integrate to find the area:

$$A_T = \int_0^\infty 128 \times e^{-0.67 \times t} dt + \int_0^\infty 128 \times e^{-0.12 \times t} dt$$

$A_T = \dfrac{128 \text{ kBq}}{0.67} + \dfrac{128 \text{ kBq}}{0.12} = 191 \text{ kBq} + 1067 \text{ kBq} = 1258 \text{ kBq} = 1.3 \text{ MBq}$ is the total activity absorbed into the body.

(b) What was the dose to the body during the 13 weeks after inhalation?

The absorbed dose during a time interval t following a single acute intake is given by equation 6.57

$$D = \frac{\dot{D}_0}{\lambda}\left(1 - e^{-\lambda t}\right)$$

Where

λ = effective clearance rate

$\dot{D}_0$ = initial dose rate

$$\dot{D}_0 = \frac{q\ \text{kBq} \times 10^3\ \frac{\text{tps}}{\text{kBq}} \times \overline{E}\ \frac{\text{MeV}}{\text{t}} \times 1.6 \times 10^{-13}\ \frac{\text{J}}{\text{MeV}} \times 8.64 \times 10^4\ \frac{\text{sec}}{\text{day}}}{m\ \text{kg} \times \frac{1\text{J}}{\text{kg}} \Big/ \text{Gy}}$$

For the first compartment, in which $\overline{E}$ (^{14}C) = 0.049 MeV/t and whose $\lambda = 0.67\ \text{d}^{-1}$, liver weight = 1.8 kg, we have

$$\dot{D}_{01} = \frac{191\ \text{kBq} \times 10^3\ \frac{\text{tps}}{\text{kBq}} \times 0.049\ \frac{\text{MeV}}{\text{t}} \times 1.6 \times 10^{-13}\ \frac{\text{J}}{\text{MeV}} \times 8.64 \times 10^4\ \frac{\text{sec}}{\text{day}}}{(70 - 1.8)\ \text{kg} \times \frac{1\text{J}}{\text{kg}} \Big/ \text{Gy}}$$

$$\dot{D}_{01} = 1.92 \times 10^{-6}\ \frac{\text{Gy}}{\text{d}}$$

For compartment 2 (the liver weight = 1.8 kg)

$$\dot{D}_{02} = \frac{1067\ \text{kBq} \times 10^3\ \frac{\text{tps}}{\text{Bq}} \times 0.049\ \frac{\text{MeV}}{\text{t}} \times 1.6 \times 10^{-13}\ \frac{\text{J}}{\text{MeV}} \times 8.64 \times 10^4\ \frac{\text{sec}}{\text{d}}}{1.8\ \text{kg} \times \frac{1\text{J}}{\text{kg}} \Big/ \text{Gy}}$$

$$\dot{D}_{02} = 4.02 \times 10^{-4}\ \frac{\text{Gy}}{\text{d}}$$

The effective half life times of the ^{14}C in both compartments, 1 day and 5.8 days, are <<< 13 weeks (91 days). Therefore the body dose is

(b)

$$D(\text{body}) = \frac{\dot{D}_{01}}{\lambda_1} = \frac{1.92 \times 10^{-6}\ \frac{\text{Gy}}{\text{d}}}{0.67\ \text{d}^{-1}} = 2.87 \times 10^{-6}\ \text{Gy}$$

(c) The dose to the liver (compartment 2) is

$$D(\text{liver}) = \frac{\dot{D}_{02}}{\lambda_2} = \frac{4.0 \times 10^{-4}\ \frac{\text{Gy}}{\text{d}}}{0.12\ \text{d}^{-1}} = 3.35 \times 10^{-3}\ \text{Gy}$$

(d) The committed effective dose equivalent is calculated with equation 8.2, using w_T of 0.05 for the liver and 0.95 for the rest of the body, and 1 Gy = 1 Sv for beta radiation.

$$H_E = \sum w_T H_T$$
$$H_E = 0.95 \times 2.87 \times 10^{-6} + 0.05 \times 3.35 \times 10^{-3}$$
$$H_E = 1.7 \times 10^{-4}\ \text{Sv}$$

13.9 A health physicist samples waste water to ascertain that the water may be safely discharged into the environment. The water analysis is made by chemically separating the ^{90}Sr, allowing the ^{90}Y daughter to accumulate, then extracting and counting the ^{90}Y activity. The volume of the sample was 1 liter, the ^{90}Y ingrowth time was 7 days, and the ^{90}Y activity was determined 15 hr after extraction in an internal gas flow counter having an overall efficiency of 50%. The background counting rate, determined by a 60 minute count was 35 counts/min. The sample (including background) gave 2766 counts in 60 min. What was the ^{90}Sr concentration, at the 90% confidence level? **13.9**

Only counting error is considered.

Calculating the 90% confidence interval:

n_g = 2766 counts
t_g = 60 min

$$r_g = \frac{2766 \text{ counts}}{60 \text{ min}} = 46.1 \text{ cpm}$$

t_b = 60 min
r_b = 35 cpm
r_n = 46.1 – 35 = 11.1 cpm

Using equation 9.43 to find the standard deviation of the net count rate

$$\sigma_n = \sqrt{\frac{r_g}{t_{g1}} + \frac{r_b}{t_b}} = \sqrt{\frac{46.1}{60} + \frac{35}{60}} = 1.16 \text{ cpm}$$

The 90% confidence interval corresponds to 1.645 standard deviations, so the 90% confidence interval is:

1.16 × (1.645) = ±1.91 cpm is the interval associated with the average so the percent error, or coefficient of variation, is: Equation 9.39a

$$\% \text{ error} = CV = \frac{1.91 \text{ cpm}}{11.1 \text{ cpm}} = 0.17 = 17\%$$

The counter is only 50% efficient, so only half of the activity is counted, thus, multiplying the net number of counts by 2 will produce the number of decays;

$$2\frac{\text{dis}}{\text{count}} \times \frac{11.1 \text{ counts}}{\text{min}} \times \frac{1 \text{ min}}{60 \text{ sec}} \times \frac{1 \text{ Bq}}{\text{dps}} = 0.37 \text{ Bq}$$

Placing this value into equation 4.18 to account for the 15 hour delay before counting the ^{90}Y:

$$A = A_0 e^{-\lambda t}$$

$$0.37 \text{ Bq} = A_0 \times e^{-\left(\frac{0.693}{64 \text{ h}} \times 15\right)}$$

$A_0 = 0.435$ is the activity of the ^{90}Y at the start of the 15 hour extraction process. Now find the activity of the ^{90}Sr at the start of the 7 day (168 h) growth period using equation 4.40;

Q_A = activity of ^{90}Sr at the start of ingrowth period
Q_B = activity of ^{90}Y at end of 7 day ingrowth period (start of 15 hr period) = 0.435 Bq

$$\lambda_{Y-90} = \frac{0.693}{64 \text{ hr}} = 0.01083 \text{ hr}^{-1}$$

t = 7 days = 168 hr

$$Q_B = Q_A\left(1 - e^{-\lambda_B t}\right)$$

$$0.435 \text{ Bq} = Q_A\left(1 - e^{-0.01083 \text{ hr}^{-1} \times 168 \text{ hr}}\right)$$

$Q_A = 0.52$ Bq/L is the initial activity of ^{90}Sr isolated. Multiply this by the error calculated earlier (0.17) to obtain; $0.52 \times 0.17 = 0.09$.
0.52 ± 0.09 Bq/L is the 90% confidence interval of the ^{90}Sr concentration.

13.10 An air sample that was counted 4 hr after collection gave 1450 counts in 10 min. The background was counted for 30 min, and gave a rate of 45 counts/min. The sample was counted again 20 hr later, and gave 990 counts in 10 min; a 60 min background gave 2940 counts. If the volume of the air sample was 1.0 m^3, and if the counting geometry was 50%, calculate the atmospheric concentration of the long lived contaminant, Bq/m^3 and μCi/cm^3, and the 95% confidence limits. **13.10**

Calculating the 95% confidence limits:

At the 4 hour point;

n_{g1} = 1450 counts
t_{g1} = 10 min
r_{g1} = 145 cpm
t_{b1} = 30 min
r_{b1} = 45 cpm
$r_{n1} = r_{g1} - r_{b1}$ = 145 cpm – 45 cpm = 100 cpm at 4 hours

Twenty hours later;

n_{g2} = 990 counts
t_{g2} = 10 min
r_{g2} = 99 cpm
t_{b2} = 60 min
n_{b2} = 2940 counts

$$r_{b2} = \frac{2940 \text{ counts}}{60 \text{ min}} = 49 \text{ cpm}$$

$r_{n2} = r_{g2} - r_{b2}$ = 99 cpm – 49 cpm = 50 cpm at 20 hours later

Using equation 9.43 to find the standard deviations and equation 9.39a to find the coefficient of variation, CV:

$$\sigma(C_1) = \sqrt{\frac{r_{g1}}{t_{g1}} + \frac{r_{b1}}{t_{b1}}} = \sqrt{\frac{145}{10} + \frac{45}{30}} = 4$$

$$\mathrm{CV}(C_1)\frac{4 \text{ cpm}}{100 \text{ cpm}} = 0.04$$

$$\sigma(C_2) = \sqrt{\frac{r_{g2}}{t_{g2}} + \frac{r_{b2}}{t_{b2}}} = \sqrt{\frac{99}{10} + \frac{49}{60}} = 3.27 \text{ cpm}$$

After Δt = 20 hours, 10.6 hour ThB would have decreased, but the long lived contaminant would still be there. The count rate of the long lived contaminant, C_{LL} is given by equation 13.34:

$$C_{LL} = \frac{C_2 - C_1 e^{-\lambda \Delta t}}{1 - e^{-\lambda \Delta t}},$$

where
C_1 = the first net count rate = 100 cpm
C_2 = the second count rate = 50 cpm

$$\lambda = \frac{0.693}{T(\text{ThB})} = \frac{0.693}{10.6 \text{ hr}} = 0.0654 \text{ hr}^{-1}$$

Δt = time between C_1 and C_2 = 20 h

Substituting these values gives

$$C_{LL} = \frac{50 - 100 \times e^{-0.0654 \times (20)}}{1 - e^{-0.0654 \times (20)}} = 31.5 \text{ cpm}$$

$$\sigma_{C_{LL}} = \sqrt{\sigma^2(C_2) + \sigma^2(C_1 e^{-\lambda \Delta t})}$$

$$\sigma^2(C_2) = \frac{r_{g2}}{t_{g2}} + \frac{r_{b2}}{t_{b2}} = \frac{99}{10} + \frac{49}{60} = 10.76$$

$$\sigma^2(C_1 e^{-\lambda \Delta t}) = \left(CV(C_1) \times C_1 e^{-\lambda \Delta t}\right)^2 = \left(0.04 \times 100 e^{-0.0654 \times 20}\right)^2 = 1.17$$

Note that $\text{CV} = \dfrac{\sigma}{\text{mean}}$ (Equation 9.39a)

$$\sigma(C_{LL}) = \sqrt{10.76 + 1.17} = 3.45 \text{ cpm}$$

Therefore

C_{LL} = 31.5 ± 3.5 cpm

$$CV = \frac{\sigma}{\text{mean}} = \frac{3.5}{31.5} = 0.11$$

Since we have 50% geometry, the mean atmosphere concentration is

$$\overline{C}_{LL} = \frac{31.5\ \text{cpm} \times 2\dfrac{\text{tpm}}{\text{cpm}} \times \dfrac{1\ \text{Bq}}{60\ \text{tpm}}}{1\ \text{m}^3} = 1.05\frac{\text{Bq}}{\text{m}^3}$$

Since the CV = 0.11, $\sigma(\text{conc}) = 0.11 \times 1.05 = 0.12$, and the 95% confidence interval = $\pm 1.96\sigma = 0.23$

Therefore, $C_{LL} = 1.05 \pm 0.23\ \text{Bq/m}^3$

In traditional units, we have

$$C_{LL} = \frac{1.05\ \text{Bq}}{\text{m}^3} \times \frac{1\ \text{m}^3}{1 \times 10^6\ \text{mL}} \times \frac{\mu\text{Ci}}{3.7 \times 10^4\ \text{Bq}} = 2.84 \times 10^{-11}\ \frac{\mu\text{Ci}}{\text{mL}}$$

$$\sigma\left(\overline{C}_a\right) = CV \times \overline{C}_{LL} = 0.11 \times 2.84 \times 10^{-11} = 3.12 \times 10^{-12}\ \frac{\mu\text{Ci}}{\text{mL}}$$

The 95% confidence interval = $1.96\sigma = 1.96 \times 3.12 \times 10^{-12}\ \dfrac{\mu\text{Ci}}{\text{mL}}$

$$= 6.1 \times 10^{-12}\ \frac{\mu\text{Ci}}{\text{mL}}$$

$$C_{LL} = (28.4\ \pm 6.1) \times 10^{-12}\ \frac{\mu\text{Ci}}{\text{mL}}$$

13.11 A film badge worn by a worker in a fast neutron field showed the following distribution of proton recoil tracks among 100 random microscopic fields of $2 \times 10^{-4}\ \text{cm}^2$ each: **13.11**

Observed Tracks per Field	Frequency
0	40
1	40
2	18
3	2

(a) If 2600 tracks per square centimeter correspond to 1 mSv (100 mrems), what was the fast neutron dose?

Observed Tracks per Field, n	Frequency, f	$f \times n$
0	40	0
1	40	40
2	18	36
3	2	6
	Sum, $\sum f_i n_i$	82

$$\frac{82 \text{ tracks}}{100 \text{ fields} \times 2 \times 10^{-4} \text{cm}^2} = 4100 \frac{\text{tracks}}{\text{cm}^2}$$

Since 2600 tracks per square centimeter corresponds to 100 mrems,

$$\overline{H} = 4100 \frac{\text{tracks}}{\text{cm}^2} \times \frac{100 \text{ mrems}}{2600 \frac{\text{tracks}}{\text{cm}^2}} = 158 \text{ mrems}$$

$$\overline{H} = 158 \text{ mrems} \times \frac{1 \text{ mSv}}{100 \text{ mrems}} = 1.58 \text{ mSv}$$

(b) What is the 95% confidence limit of this measurement?

Equation 9.36 is used to find the standard deviation of the measurement;

$$\sigma = \sqrt{n} = \sqrt{82} = 9.06$$

The 95% confidence limit requires 1.96 standard deviations;

$$1.96 \times 9.06 = 17.75$$

The 95% coefficient of variation would be found using equation 9.39a:

$$95\% = \text{CV} = \frac{1.96\sigma}{\text{mean}} = \frac{17.75}{82} = 0.21$$

Giving a 95% confidence interval of: ± 0.21 × 158 mrems = ± 34.2 mrems

$H = 158 \pm 34$ mrems

$$95\%\text{s} = 34 \text{ mrems} \times \frac{1 \text{ mSv}}{100 \text{ mrems}} = 0.34 \text{ mSv}$$

$H = 1.58 \pm 0.34$ mSv

13.12 Using the three compartment ICRP lung model and the physiologic data for the reference person, compute the dose to the lungs and to the bone following a single acute exposure of 1 Bq·s (2.7×10^{-5} μCi·s) per cubic meter of respirable aerosol, MMAD = 2 μm, of (a) strontium titinate, (b) strontium chloride. **13.12**

(a) strontium titinate
Converting to Bq using a breathing rate of 10 liters per minute (rounded from Table 2 in Appendix C);

$1 \frac{\text{Bq} \cdot \text{sec}}{\text{m}^3} \times \frac{1 \text{ min}}{60 \text{ sec}} \times 10 \frac{\text{L}}{\text{min}} \times \frac{1 \text{ m}^3}{1000 \text{ L}} = 1.67 \times 10^{-4}$ Bq is the inhaled quantity of activity.

The ICRP three compartment model distributes activity with MMAD = 2 μm into the following compartments (Fig. 8.4):

Region of Deposition	Inhaled Activity, Bq	Fraction activity deposited in region	deposited actvity, Bq $A_S(0)$
N—P	1.67×10^{-4}	0.50	8.35×10^{-5}
T—B	1.67×10^{-4}	0.08	1.34×10^{-5}
P	1.67×10^{-4}	0.18	3.01×10^{-5}

N–P region deposition is cleared, and does not contribute significantly to the lung dose. The activity transferred to the blood and GI tract from the N–P region deposition are calculated later.

The dose to the lung is calculated from equation 6.97

$$H(\text{lung}) = \tilde{A}(\text{lung})\text{Bq}\cdot\text{d} \times S(\text{lung} \leftarrow \text{lung})\frac{\text{Sv}}{\text{Bq}\cdot\text{d}}$$

Clearance rates of particulates in the lung are given in Fig. 8.3. For $^{90}SrTiO_2$, which is class w (moderately soluble), the biological clearance rate = the effective clearance rate because $T_{1/2}$ (^{90}Sr) = 28 years. The activity deposited in each region, and for each clearance pathway, the fraction of the deposit, its retention half time *T* and clearance rate λ (0.693/*T*), are listed in the table below:

Region	Bq × 10^{-5}	*f*	T, d	λ, d^{-1}	To
N-P	8.35	0.1	0.01	69.3	Blood
		0.9	0.4	1.73	GI
T-B	1.34	0.5	0.01	69.3	Blood
		0.5	0.2	3.47	GI
P	3.01	0.4	1	0.693	GI
		0.4	50	0.0139	GI
		0.2	50	0.0139	Blood

The cumulated activity, $\tilde{A}$, for several compartments is given by a variant of equation 6.91

$$\tilde{A} = \sum_i \frac{A_i(0)}{\lambda_i}$$

If we substituted the values from the table above, we have

$$\tilde{A} = \frac{0.5 \times 1.34 \times 10^{-5}\,\text{Bq}}{69.3\ \text{d}^{-1}} + \frac{0.5 \times 1.34 \times 10^{-5}\,\text{Bq}}{3.47\ \text{d}^{-1}} + \frac{0.4 \times 3.01 \times 10^{-5}\,\text{Bq}}{0.693\ \text{d}^{-1}} + \frac{0.6 \times 3.01 \times 10^{-5}\,\text{Bq}}{0.0139\ \text{d}^{-1}}$$

$$\tilde{A} = 1.3 \times 10^{-3}\ \text{Bq}\times\text{day}$$

$$S(\text{lung} \leftarrow \text{lung}) = 4.2 \times 10^{-4}\frac{\text{rad}}{\mu\text{Ci}\cdot\text{hr}}\ \text{(MIRD Pamphlet 11)}$$

$$S = 4.2 \times 10^{-4} \frac{\text{rad}}{\mu\text{Ci} \cdot \text{hr}} \times \frac{1 \text{ Gy}}{100 \text{ rads}} \times \frac{1 \ \mu\text{Ci}}{3.7 \times 10^4 \text{ Bq}} \times \frac{1 \text{ Sv}}{1 \text{ Gy}} = 272 \times 10^{-9} \frac{\text{Sv}}{\text{Bq} \cdot \text{d}}$$

$$H = \tilde{A} \times S(\text{lung} \leftarrow \text{lung})$$

$$H = 1.33 \times 10^{-3} \text{ Bq} \cdot \text{d} \times 272 \times 10^{-9} \frac{\text{Sv}}{\text{Bq} \cdot \text{d}} = 3.6 \times 10^{-12} \text{ Sv}$$

According to the ICRP lung model, some of the inhaled ^{90}Sr is transferred from the lung to the blood, and some is transferred to the GI tract. Then,

30% from the blood goes to the bone
9% from the GI tract goes to the bone

From the N-P region, where 10% goes to the blood and 90% to the GI tract, the activity deposited in the bone is:

via blood: 8.35×10^{-5} Bq $\times$ 0.1 $\times$ 0.3 = 2.51×10^{-6} Bq
via GI: 8.35×10^{-5} Bq $\times$ 0.9 $\times$ 0.09 = 6.77×10^{-6} Bq

In a similar manner, we can calculate the contributions of the T-B and P regions to the bone, with the results that are tabulated below: The total activity deposited in the bone is 1.59×10^{-5} Bq

From	Via	Activity transferred, Bq	Deposition in bone, Bq,$\times 10^{-6}$
N-P	Blood	$8.35 \times 10^{-5} \times 0.1 \times 0.3$	2.51
	GI	$8.35 \times 10^{-5} \times 0.9 \times 0.09$	6.77
T-B	Blood	1.34×10^{-5}Bq $\times 0.5 \times 0.3$	2.01
	GI	1.34×10^{-5}Bq $\times 0.5 \times 0.09$	0.60
P	Blood	3.01×10^{-5}Bq $\times 0.2 \times 0.3$	1.81
	GI	3.01×10^{-5}Bq $\times 0.8 \times 0.09$	2.17
		Total transferred to bone	15.9×10^{-6} Bq

The dose equivalent to the bone is

$$H(\text{skeleton}) = \tilde{A}(\text{bone})\text{Bq} \cdot \text{d} \times S(\text{skeleton} \leftarrow \text{bone}) \frac{\text{Sv}}{\text{Bq} \cdot \text{d}}$$

The cumulated activity, $\tilde{A}$, is calculated using the ICRP value of 6400 days for the effective half life of ^{90}Sr in the bone.

$$\tilde{A}(\text{bone}) = \frac{A_S(0)}{\lambda_E} = \frac{A_S(0)}{0.693/T_E} = \frac{15.9\times10^{-6}\ \text{Bq}\times 6400\ \text{d}}{0.693} = 0.147\ \text{Bq}\cdot\text{d}$$

$$S(\text{skeleton}\leftarrow\text{bone}) = 8.45\times10^{-5}\ \frac{\text{rad}}{\mu\text{Ci}\cdot\text{h}}\times\frac{0.01\ \text{Gy}}{\text{rad}}\times\frac{1\ \mu\text{Ci}}{3.7\times10^{4}\ \text{Bq}}\times 24\frac{\text{h}}{\text{d}}\times\frac{1\ \text{Sv}}{\text{Gy}}$$

$$S(\text{skeleton}\leftarrow\text{bone}) = 5.48\times10^{-10}\ \frac{\text{Sv}}{\text{Bq}\cdot\text{d}}\quad\text{(MIRD 11)}$$

The dose to the skeleton is

$$H(\text{skeleton}) = 0.147\ \text{Bq}\cdot\text{d}\times 5.48\times10^{-10}\ \frac{\text{Sv}}{\text{Bq}\cdot\text{d}} = 8\times10^{-11}\ \text{Sv}$$

(b) strontium chloride
Since the MMAD is the same for each compound, the activity deposition is the same as for strontium titinate.

From Figure 8.4:

Region of Deposition	Total Activity in Bq	Fraction activity deposited in region	Activity deposited in the region in Bq $A_S(0)$
N-P	1.67×10^{-4}	0.50	8.35×10^{-5}
T-B	1.67×10^{-4}	0.08	1.34×10^{-5}
P	1.67×10^{-4}	0.18	3.01×10^{-5}

The dose to the lung from the inhaled $^{90}SrCl_2$ is calculated with equation 6.97

$$H(\text{lung}) = \tilde{A}(\text{lung})\text{Bq}\cdot\text{d}\times S(\text{lung}\leftarrow\text{lung})\frac{\text{Sv}}{\text{Bq}\cdot\text{d}}$$

The calculations for strontium chloride are very similar to part (a), except that it is a class D compound, and therefore has different retention half times in the lung. Since the radiological half life is long compared to the biological half life, only the

N–P region deposition is cleared, and does not contribute significantly to the lung dose in the N–P region, so the deposition dose is not calculated. The activity transferred to the blood and GI tract from the N–P region deposition are calculated later.

T–B region has 2 compartments, 95% clears at 0.01 days (l = 69.3 d^{-1}, Figure 8.3), and 5% clears with a half time of 0.2 d (l = 3.47 d^{-1}).

The dose to the lung from the inhaled $^{90}SrCl_2$ is calculated with equation 6.97

$$H(\text{lung}) = \tilde{A}(\text{lung}) \times S(\text{lung} \leftarrow \text{lung}) \frac{\text{Sv}}{\text{Bq} \cdot \text{d}}$$

The cumulated activity is calculated as in part (a), using the table below:

Region	Bq × 10^{-5}	f	T, d	λ, d^{-1}	To
N-P	8.35	0.5 0.5	0.01 0.01	69.3 1.73	Blood GI
T-B	1.34	0.95 0.05	0.01 0.2	69.3 3.47	Blood GI
P	3.01	1.0	0.5	1.39	Blood

$$\tilde{A}(\text{lung}) = \frac{A_i(0)}{\lambda_i} = \frac{0.95 \times 1.34 \times 10^{-5}\,\text{Bq}}{69.3\ \text{d}^{-1}} + \frac{0.05 \times 1.34 \times 10^{-5}\,\text{Bq}}{3.47\ \text{d}^{-1}} + \frac{3.01 \times 10^{-5}\,\text{Bq}}{1.39\ \text{d}^{-1}}$$

$$\tilde{A}\ (\text{lung}) = 2.19 \times 10^{-5}\ \text{Bq·d}$$

$$S(\text{lung} \leftarrow \text{lung}) = 2.72 \times 10^{-9} \frac{\text{Sv}}{\text{Bq} \cdot \text{d}}\ \text{(Adopted from MIRD 11)}$$

$$H(\text{lung}) = \tilde{A}(\text{lung}) \times S(\text{lung} \leftarrow \text{lung}) = 2.19 \times 10^{-5}\ \text{Bq·d} \times 2.72 \times 10^{-9} \frac{\text{Sv}}{\text{Bq} \cdot \text{d}}$$

$$H(\text{lung}) = 6 \times 10^{-14}\ \text{Sv}$$

The activity transferred from the lung to the bone too is calculated as in part (a), as shown in the table below:

From	Via	Activity transferred, Bq	Deposition in bone, Bq, × 10-6
N-P	Blood GI	$8.35 \times 10^{-5} \times 0.5 \times 0.3$ $8.35 \times 10^{-5} \times 0.5 \times 0.09$	12.53 3.76
T-B	Blood GI	1.34×10^{-5} Bq $\times 0.95 \times 0.3$ 1.34×10^{-5} Bq $\times 0.05 \times 0.09$	3.82 0.06
P	Blood	3.01 × 10-5 Bq × 0.05 × 0.3	9.03
		Total transferred to bone	29.2 × 10-6 Bq

$$H(\text{skeleton}) = \tilde{A}(\text{bone})\text{Bq}\cdot\text{d} \times S(\text{skeleton} \leftarrow \text{bone})\frac{\text{Sv}}{\text{Bq}\cdot\text{d}}$$

$$H(\text{skeleton}) = \frac{29.2 \times 10^{-6}\,\text{Bq} \times 6400\,\text{d}}{0.693} \times 5.48 \times 10^{-10}\,\frac{\text{Sv}}{\text{Bq}\cdot\text{d}} = 1.5 \times 10^{-10}\ \text{Sv}$$

Summary of doses in Sv per Bq·s per m^3 exposure

	Lungs	Skeleton
Sr-titinate	3.6×10^{-12}	8×10^{-11}
Sr-chloride	6×10^{-14}	1.5×10^{-10}

13.13 13.13 The following size distribution was obtained on a sample of an aerosol:

Percent by number	Class interval, μm
10	0.5—1.0
15	1.0—1.5
15	1.5—2.0
10	2.0—2.5
10	2.5—3.0
10	3.0—3.5
10	3.5—4.5
10	4.5—6.0
5	6.0—8.0
5	8.0—10.0

(a) Plot the cumulative frequency distributions on linear graph paper, on linear probability paper, and on log probability paper, by number, surface area (assume the particles to be spherical), and by mass (assume the particles to have a density of 2.7 g/cm^3).

Tabulate the cumulative frequency for the diameter, surface area, and mass of the particles below, in order to graph each:

		Less than		
% by number	cumulative %	diameter	surface area, (m)^2	mass, g
10	10	1	3.14	1.41
15	25	1.5	7.07	4.77
15	40	2	12.57	11.31
10	50	2.5	19.63	22.09
10	60	3	28.27	38.17
10	70	3.5	38.48	60.61
10	80	4.5	63.62	128.82
10	90	6	113.09	305.35
5	95	8	201.06	723.80
5	100	10	314.15	1413.68

Linear Graph

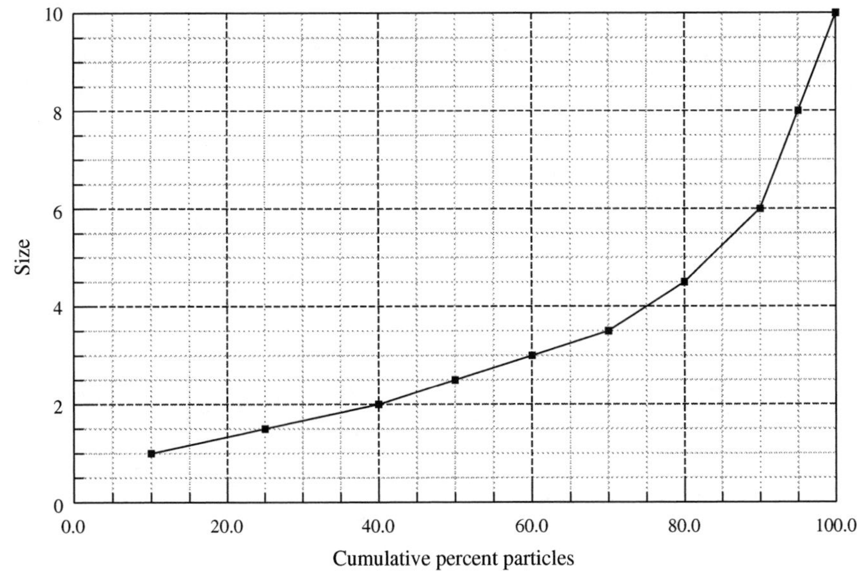

Linear Probability Paper

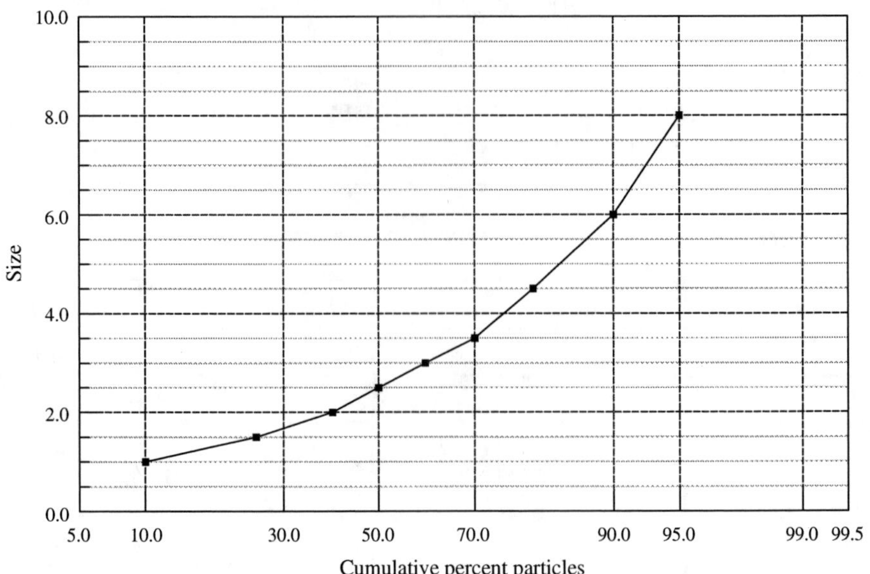

Log Probability Paper

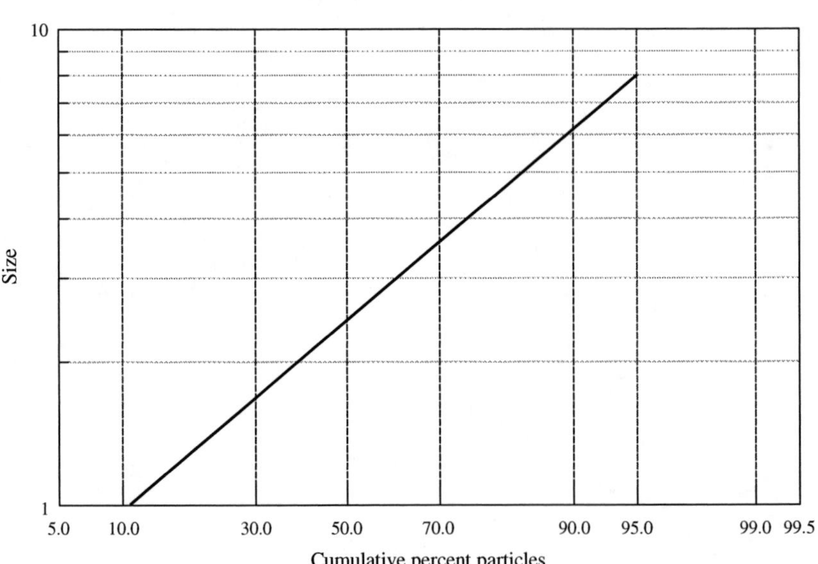

Linear Graph

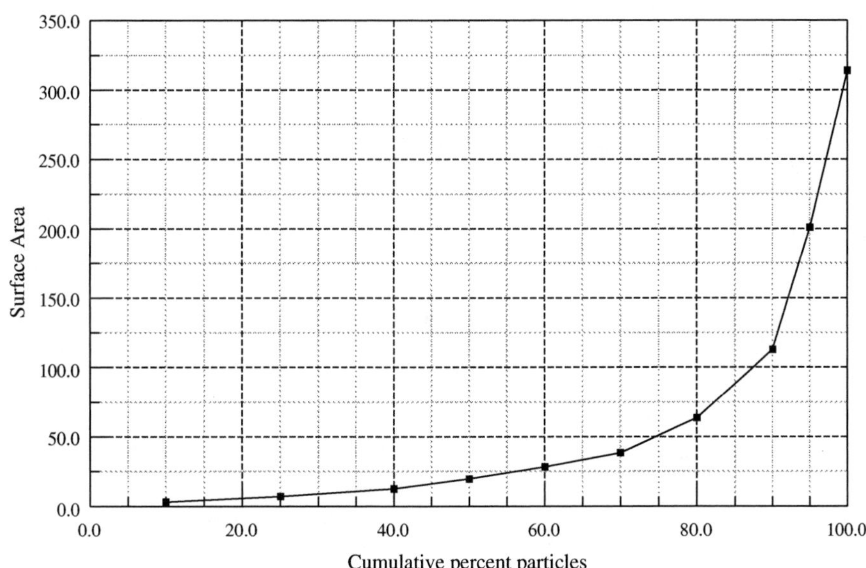

Linear Probability Paper

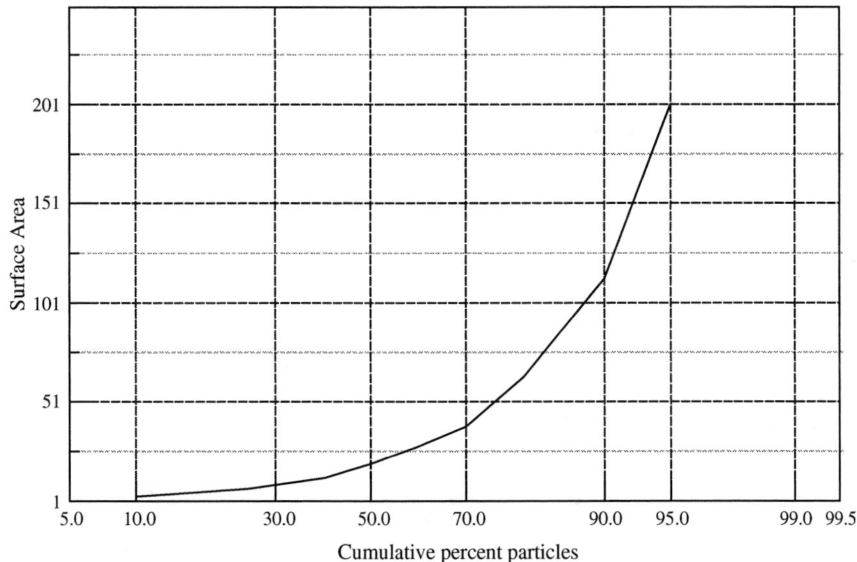

Log Probability Paper

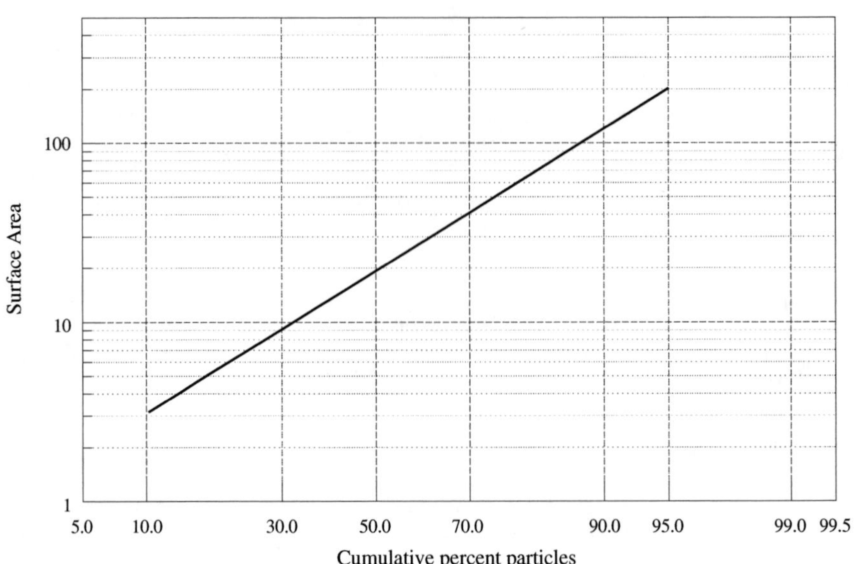

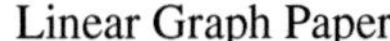

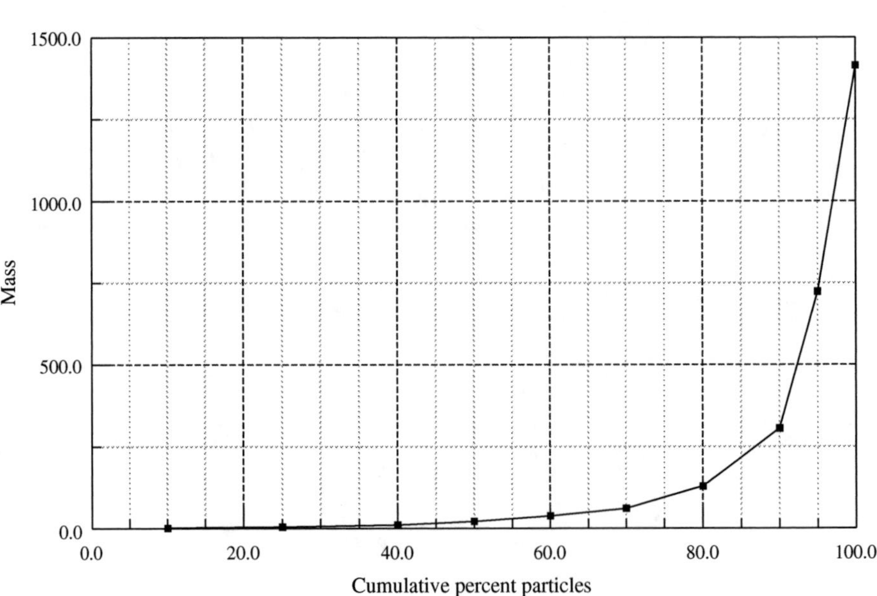

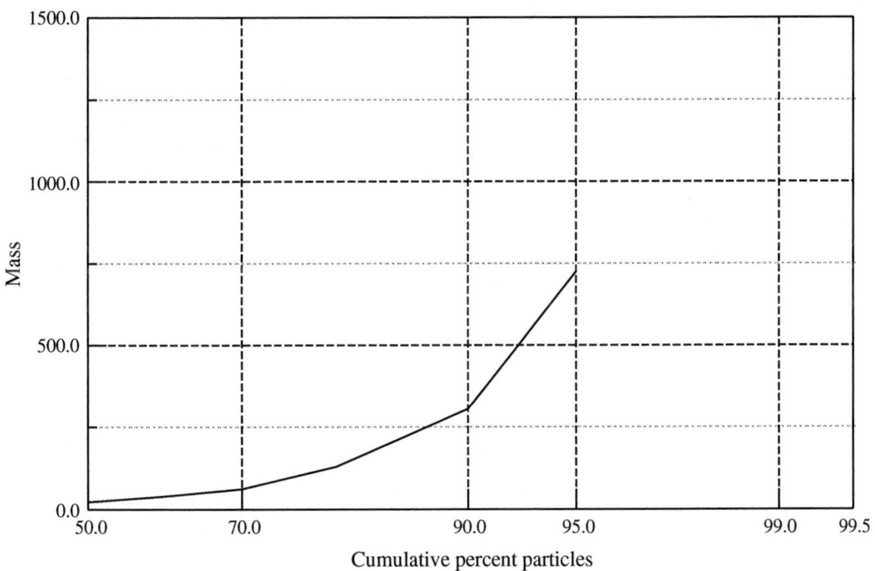
Linear Probability Paper
1500.0
1000.0
500.0
0.0
Mass
50.0
70.0
90.0
95.0
99.0
99.5
Cumulative percent particles

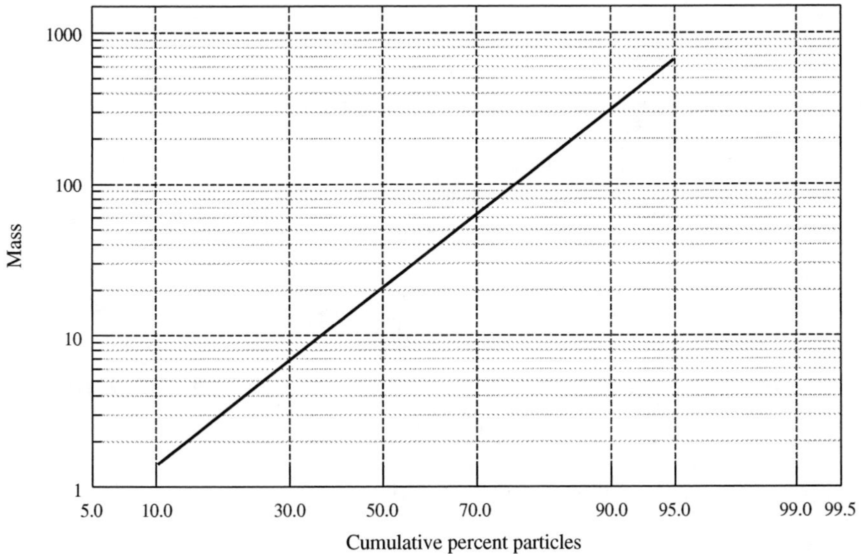
Log Probability Paper
1000
100
10
1
Mass
5.0
10.0
30.0
50.0
70.0
90.0
95.0
99.0
99.5
Cumulative percent particles

(b) Are the size distributions normally or log–normally distributed?

The size distributions are log–normally distributed, as can be seen by the straight line formed when the size, surface area, and mass are plotted on log–probability graphs.

(c) Compute the geometric mean and standard deviations for each of the three types of distributions.
First determining CMD:

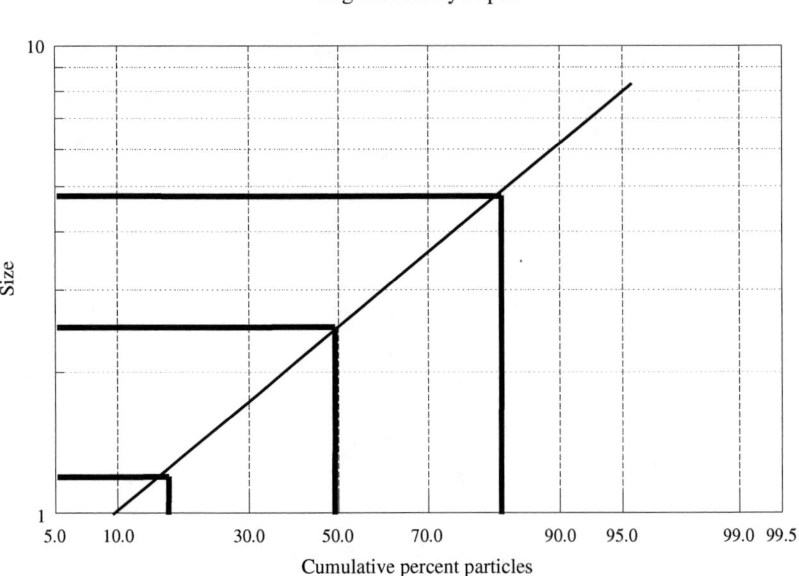

Since we do not know the number of particles in the sample, we must determine the CMD from the graph. On the log-probability plot of cumulative frequency vs. Particle size, we find that the ordinate at the 50% point intersects the plot at 2.5 μ. Next, we determine the size of the particles at one standard deviation above and below the mean to determine the geometric standard deviation.

The geometric standard deviation, σ_g, is given by

$$\sigma_g = \frac{84\% \text{ size}}{50\% \text{ size}}$$

From the graph, we find the 84% size to be 5.1 μ.

$$\sigma_g = \frac{5.1}{2.5} = 2$$

Similarly from the graph, we find the 16% size to be 5 μ.

$$\sigma_g = \frac{2.5}{1.25} = 2$$

Thus, the CMD = 2.5μ $\stackrel{\times}{\div}$ 2

If the number of particles is known,

$$\text{CMD} = \log^{-1} \frac{\sum \log d_i}{N} = \log^{-1} \frac{\sum f_i \log \bar{d}_i}{N}$$

where
N = number of particles
f = number of particles in the ith size interval
$\bar{d}_i$ = average diameter of particles in the ith size interval
d_i = size of the ith particle

The standard deviation can also be calculated as

$$\sigma = \sqrt{\frac{\sum (\log d_i)^2}{N} - (\log \bar{d})^2}$$ where $\log \bar{d}$ is the average logarithm of the particle size.

The mass median diameter, MMD, and the surface median diameter, SMD, can be read from the respective graphs, or they can be calculated if we know the CMD and σ_g.

Log(MMD) = Log(CMD) +6.9 × (Log(σ_{CMD}))^2
Log(MMD) = Log(2.5) +6.908 × (Log(2))^2 = 1.024

MMD = 10.6 μ

The surface median diameter, SMD, is given by:

Log(SMD) = Log(CMD) +5.757 × (Log(σ_{CMD}))^2
Log(SMD) = Log(2.5) +5.757 × (Log(2))^2 = 0.919

SMD = 8.2 μ

13.14

13.14 An instrument repairman suffered an accidental exposure to ^{131}I while working in a customer's laboratory. Two days later his thyroid gland was found to contain 2×10^4Bq (0.54 μCi) ^{131}I. Assuming he is a normal healthy man who weighs 70 kg, calculate
(a) the amount of ^{131}I activity originally deposited in the thyroid,

The activity at any time t after an initial deposit of activity, $A(0)$, is given by the product of the retained fraction and $A(0)$.

$$A(t) = R(t) \times A(0)$$

$$R(t) = 0.7 \exp\left(-\frac{0.693}{0.35}t\right) + 0.3 \exp\left(-\frac{0.693}{100}t\right)$$

$$2 \times 10^4 = 0.7 \times A(0) \times \exp\left(-\frac{0.693}{0.35} \times (2)\right) + 0.3 \times A(0) \times \exp\left(-\frac{0.693}{100} \times (2)\right)$$

$A(0) = 6.5 \times 10^4$ Bq was the activity initially deposited in the thyroid.

(b) the dose commitment to the thyroid as a result of the accident.

Equation 6.97;

$$D(\text{thyroid}) = \tilde{A}(\text{thyroid}) \times S(\text{thyroid} \leftarrow \text{thyroid})$$

Find the cumulated activity, $\tilde{A}$, of the deposited radioactivity using equation 6.91;
Since this particular isotope is in two compartments,

$$\tilde{A} = \frac{A_S(0)}{\lambda} = \frac{0.7 \times (6.5 \times 10^4 \text{ Bq})}{\left(\frac{0.693}{0.35\text{d}}\right)} + \frac{0.3 \times (6.5 \times 10^4 \text{ Bq})}{\left(\frac{0.693}{100 \text{ d}}\right)} = 2.84 \times 10^6 \text{ Bq·d}$$

Next, look in MIRD Pamphlet 11, p. 185, for S(thyroid←thyroid)

$$S(\text{thyroid} \leftarrow \text{thyroid}) = 2.2 \times 10^{-2} \frac{\text{rad}}{\mu\text{Ci} \cdot \text{hr}} \times \frac{0.01 \text{ Gy}}{\text{rad}} \times \frac{1 \text{ }\mu\text{Ci}}{3.7 \times 10^4 \text{ Bq}} \times 24 \frac{\text{h}}{\text{d}}$$

$$S(\text{thyroid} \leftarrow \text{thyroid}) = 1.43 \times 10^{-7} \frac{\text{Gy}}{\text{Bq} \cdot \text{d}}$$

$$S(\text{thyroid} \neg \text{thyroid}) = 1.65 \times 10^{-12} \frac{\text{Gy}}{\text{Bq} \cdot \text{sec}} = 1.43 \times 10^{-7} \frac{\text{Gy}}{\text{Bq} \cdot \text{d}}$$

Replacing values into equation 6.97:

$$D(\text{thyroid}) = \tilde{A}(\text{thyroid}) \times S(\text{thyroid} \neg \text{thyroid})$$

$$D(\text{thyroid}) = 2.84 \times 10^{6}\ \text{Bq·d} \times 1.43 \times 10^{-7} \frac{\text{Gy}}{\text{Bq} \cdot \text{d}} = 0.4\ \text{Gy}$$

13.15 A 20 liter breath sample was collected over 2 minutes. Analysis for ^{222}Rn showed the radon concentration to be 1×10^{-7} Bq per liter. Estimate the body burden of ^{226}Ra from these data. **13.15**

The rate of exhalation of ^{222}Rn is related to the body burden of ^{226}Ra by equation 13.10;

$$A_e = 0.7 \times q\ \text{Bq} \times 1\ \text{min}^{-1}$$

Let:

$C = 1 \times 10^{-7}$ Bq/liter
$V = 20$ liters/2min
$\lambda(^{226}\text{Ra}) = 8.1 \times 10^{-10}\ \text{min}^{-1}$ (chapter 13, p. 550)

The exhalation rate, equation 13.11 is;

$$A_e = \frac{1 \times 10^{-7}\ \text{Bq}}{\text{L}} \times \frac{20\ \text{L}}{2\ \text{min}} = 1 \times 10^{-6} \frac{\text{Bq}}{\text{min}}$$

$$q = \frac{1 \times 10^{-6} \frac{\text{Bq}}{\text{min}}}{0.7 \times 8.1 \times 10^{-10}\ \text{min}^{-1}} = 2 \times 10^{3}\ \text{Bq}$$

13.16

13.16 A lab worker accidentally ingested ^{210}Po by using a contaminated cup for his coffee. Twenty four hour urine samples were taken over a 60 day period and analyzed. The following data were obtained:

Days after ingestion	1	5	10	15	20	25	30	40	50	60
Bq per sample	25	23	21	19	18	16	15	12	11	9

(a) plot the data on semi–log paper and fit an equation to the elimination data.

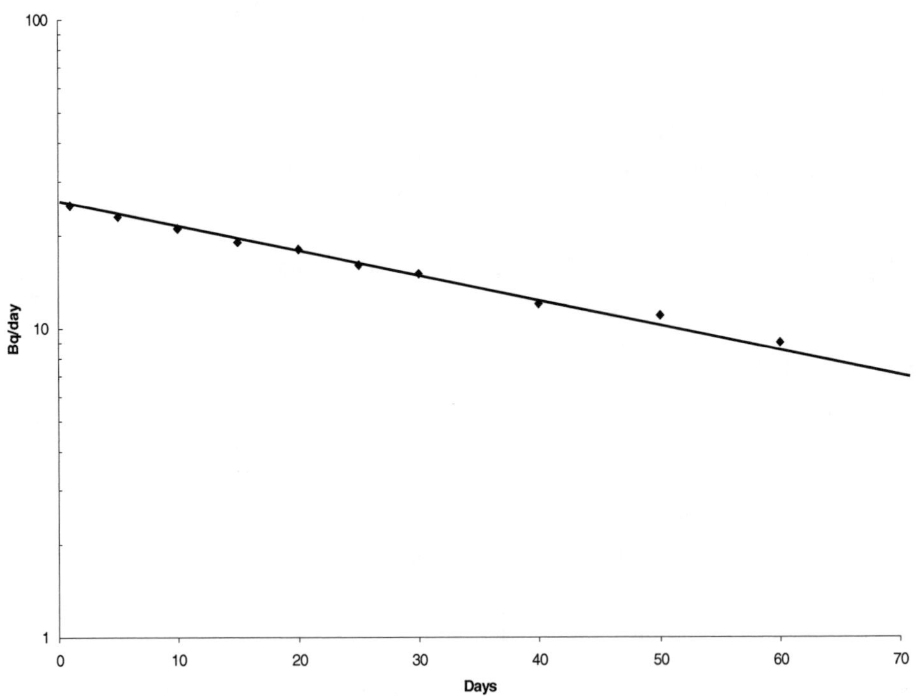

The data, when plotted on semi-log paper, fall on a straight line. Extrapolation of the line intercepts the time axis at 25.4 Bq/d. The graph shows that this value falls by 50% after a time interval of 40 days. The slope of the line, therefore, is $\lambda_E = 0.693/40\text{ d} = 0.0173$ per day. The equation for the urinary clearance data, therefore, is

$U(t) = 25.4 \times e^{-0.017 \times t}$

(b) If 10% of ingested Po is known to be eliminated in the urine, and 90% is eliminated in the feces, how much ^{210}Po was ingested?

The given data represent the effective clearance data, and the slope of the urinary clearance rate. Since the radiological half life of ^{210}Po is 138 days, the biological half life can be calculated. The effective half life, from the data, is 40 days. (Equation 6.54)

$$T_E = \frac{T_R \times T_B}{T_R + T_B}$$

$$40 \text{ d} = \frac{138 \text{ d} \times T_B}{138 \text{ d} + T_B}$$

$T_B = 56.3$ days

$$\lambda_B = \frac{0.693}{56.3 \text{ d}} = 0.0123 \text{ d}^{-1}$$

Since the slope of the biological clearance curve is slightly less than that for the effective clearance curve, the intercept will be different. Since T (^{210}Po) = 138 d, it is reasonable to assume that the 1 day datum is not significantly affected by the 1 day's decay. The new intercept can thus be calculated

$U(1) = U_0 \, e^{-0.0123t}$

$25 = U_0 \, e^{-0.0123 \times 1}$

$U_0 = 25.3$ Bq

The biological urinary clearance curve is

$U(t) = 25.3 \times e^{-0.0123 \times t}$

Since only 10% of the ingested ^{210}Po is eliminated in the urine, the quantity originally deposited = 10 × total activity eliminated in the urine.

$$A(0) = 10\int_0^\infty U(t)dt = 10\frac{A(0)}{\lambda_B} = 10 \times \frac{25.3 \text{ Bq/d}}{0.0123 \text{ d}^{-1}} = 2.06 \times 10^4 \text{ Bq}$$

(c) If 13% of the ^{210}Po was deposited in the kidneys, what was the committed dose equivalent to the kidneys from this accidental ingestion?

Since we have a simple compartment clearance, $\lambda(\text{kid}) = \lambda_E$, and the dose commitment to the kidneys is

$$D = \frac{\dot{D}(0)}{\lambda_E}$$

The activity deposited in the kidney is:

$$A_S(0)_K = 0.13 \times 2.06 \times 10^4 \text{ Bq} = 2.67 \times 10^3 \text{ Bq}$$

The dose rate from this activity is

$$\dot{D}_0 = \frac{q \text{ Bq} \times 1 \text{ tps/Bq} \times E \dfrac{\text{MeV}}{\text{t}} \times 1.6 \times 10^{-13} \dfrac{\text{J}}{\text{MeV}} \times 8.64 \times 10^4 \dfrac{\text{sec}}{\text{d}}}{m \text{ kg} \times 1 \dfrac{\text{J}}{\text{kg}} / \text{Gy}}$$

E (^{210}Po) alpha = 5.4 MeV (including the KE of the recoil nucleus)
w of kidneys = 0.31 kg
Substituting these values into the equation for dose rate, we have:

$$\dot{D}_0 = \frac{2.67 \times 10^3 \text{ Bq} \times 1 \text{ tps/Bq} \times 5.4 \dfrac{\text{MeV}}{\text{t}} \times 1.6 \times 10^{-13} \dfrac{\text{J}}{\text{MeV}} \times 8.64 \times 10^4 \dfrac{\text{sec}}{\text{d}}}{0.31 \text{ kg} \times 1 \dfrac{\text{J}}{\text{kg}} / \text{Gy}}$$

$$\dot{D}_0 = 6.4 \times 10^{-4} \text{ Gy/d}$$

$$D = \frac{\dot{D}_0}{\lambda} = \frac{6.4 \times 10^{-4} \dfrac{\text{Gy}}{\text{d}}}{0.017 \text{ d}^{-1}} = 0.038 \text{ Gy}$$

13.17

13.17 What is the dose commitment to the skeleton due to the ingestion of 100 Bq/day, for 1 year, of ^{90}Sr dissolved in drinking water?

^{90}Sr, a pure beta emitter, rapidly reaches secular equilibrium with its short lived (64.1 h) ^{90}Y daughter. Both isotopes are pure beta emitters. The average energy per ^{90}Sr transformation is the sum of the average beta energies:

$$E_e = 0.1958 \text{ MeV} + 0.9348 \text{ MeV} = 1.13 \text{ MeV/transformation}$$

The dose commitment includes the dose during intake of the ^{90}Sr-^{90}Y, and the dose during the washout from the body following the end of the intake. The dose during the 1 year intake period is given by equation 11.17

$$H(t) = \dot{H}(SS)\left[t_i + \frac{1}{\lambda_E}\left(e^{-\lambda_E t_i} - 1\right)\right]$$

Where $\dot{H}(SS)$ is the steady state dose rate, at which time the daily intake and daily elimination of ^{90}Sr-^{90}Y are equal. This steady state body burden is given by an analog of equation 4.38

$$q(SS) = \frac{K}{\lambda}$$

where

K = the rate of deposition of the activity = intake rate × fraction deposited

λ = the effective turnover rate of the activity. The effective half life of ^{90}Sr in the skeleton is listed by the ICRP, and the ICRP indicates 9% of the ingested ^{90}Sr is deposited in the bone.

T_E (^{90}Sr) = 6400 d in the skeleton (ICRP)

$$\lambda_E = \frac{0.693}{T_E} = \frac{0.693}{6400\text{ d}} = 1.08 \times 10^{-4}\text{ d}^{-1}$$

$$q(SS) = \frac{100\,\frac{\text{Bq}}{\text{d}} \times 0.09}{1.08 \times 10^{-4}\text{ d}^{-1}} = 8.33 \times 10^{4}\text{ Bq}$$

The dose rate to the skeleton, whose weight is 7 kg, is given by:

$$\dot{H} = \frac{q\text{ Bq} \times \frac{1\text{ tps}}{\text{Bq}} \times E_e\,\frac{\text{MeV}}{\text{t}} \times 1.6 \times 10^{-13}\,\frac{\text{J}}{\text{MeV}} \times 8.64 \times 10^{4}\,\frac{\text{sec}}{\text{day}} \times 1\,\frac{\text{Sv}}{\text{Gy}}}{m\text{ kg} \times 1\,\frac{\text{J/kg}}{\text{Gy}}}$$

$$\dot{H}(SS) = \frac{8.33 \times 10^{4}\text{ Bq} \times \frac{1\text{ tps}}{\text{Bq}} \times 1.13\,\frac{\text{MeV}}{\text{t}} \times 1.6 \times 10^{-13}\,\frac{\text{J}}{\text{MeV}} \times 8.64 \times 10^{4}\,\frac{\text{sec}}{\text{day}} \times 1\,\frac{\text{Sv}}{\text{Gy}}}{7\text{ kg} \times 1\,\frac{\text{J/kg}}{\text{Gy}}}$$

$$\dot{H}(SS) = 1.86 \times 10^{-4}\text{ Sv/d}$$

Substituting this value into the dose equation gives:

$$H(365\text{ d}) = 1.86 \times 10^{-4}\ \frac{\text{Sv}}{\text{d}}\left[365\text{ d} + \frac{1}{1.08 \times 10^{-4}\text{ d}^{-1}}\left(e^{-1.08\times10^{-4}\text{ d}^{-1}\,365\text{ d}} - 1\right)\right]$$

$H(365\text{ d}) = 1.3 \times 10^{-3}\text{ Sv}$

The dose during the washout is given by

$$H(\text{washout}) = \frac{\dot{H}(0)}{\lambda_E}$$

where $\dot{H}(0)$ is the dose rate at the beginning of the washout period. Since the steady state has not yet been reached at the end of 1 year (The effective half life = 6400 d = 17.5 years), the dose rate after 1 year is given by a variant of equation 4.40.

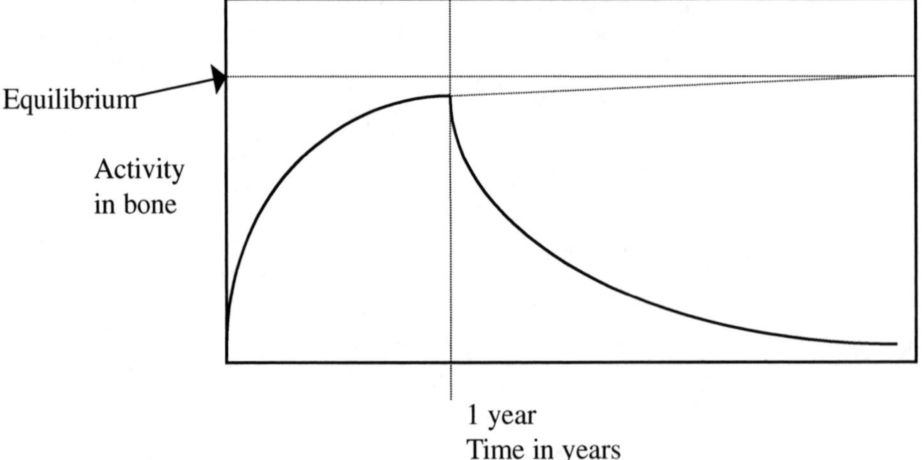

$$\dot{H}(0) = \dot{H}(SS)\left(1 - e^{-\lambda_E t}\right)$$

$$\dot{H}(0) = 1.86 \times 10^{-4}\ \frac{\text{Sv}}{\text{d}}\left(1 - e^{-1.08\times10^{-4}\times365}\right) = 7.19 \times 10^{-6}\ \frac{\text{Sv}}{\text{d}}$$

$$H(\text{washout}) = \frac{7.19 \times 10^{-6}\ \frac{\text{Sv}}{\text{d}}}{1.08 \times 10^{-4}\text{ d}^{-1}} = 66.57 \times 10^{-3}\text{ Sv}$$

Dose commitment = 1.32×10^{-3} Sv + 66.57×10^{-3} Sv = 68×10^{-3} Sv

13.18 An accidental release of $^{210}PoO_2$ from a glove box leads to an atmospheric concentration of 1500 Bq/m^3 (4.05 × 10^{-8} μCi/cm^3). From a recording air monitor whose alarm had failed it was later learned that a worker had been exposed to the airborne $^{210}PoO_2$ for 1 hour. Measurements made with a cascade impactor showed the mass median aerodynamic particle size (MMAD) to be 0.5 μm. Using the data for the reference person, calculate **13.18**
(a) the amount of activity deposited in the lung,

Since 10 CFR 20 is based upon ICRP 30, the ICRP three compartment model is utilized.

The quantity inhaled is based on approximately 10 m^3 air inhaled per 8 hour day (Appendix C).

$$1500\frac{\text{Bq}}{\text{m}^3}\times 1\text{ hr}\times\frac{10\text{ m}^3}{8\text{ hr}} = 1875\text{ Bq is the quantity of activity inhaled.}$$

For a MMAD of 0.5 mm particle, the following deposition occurs (Figure 8.4);

C	Fraction inhaled ^{210}Po deposited in region	Total Activity in Bq inhaled	Deposited activity in regions, Bq
N-P	0.18	1875	Not in lung
T-B	0.08	1875	150
P	0.34	1875	637.5
		Sum	787.5

The total activity deposited in the lung is 787.5 Bq.

(b) the dose commitment to the lung from this accidental exposure.

The dose to the lung is calculated from equation 6.97

$$H(\text{lung}) = \tilde{A}(\text{lung})\text{Bq}\cdot\text{d}\times S(\text{lung}\leftarrow\text{lung})\frac{\text{Sv}}{\text{Bq}\cdot\text{d}}$$

Clearance rates of particles in the lung are given in Fig. 8.3. For $^{210}PoO_2$, which is class W (moderately soluble), the effective clearance half times = the biological half times given in Fig. 8.3 for clearance from the T-B region (since T_R = 138 days). From the P region, 40% of the deposit is cleared with a half time of 1 day. However, 60% of the particles are cleared from the P region with a biological half time of 50 days. The effective half time, therefore, is given by equation 6.54.

$$T_E = \frac{T_R \times T_B}{T_R + T_B} = \frac{138 \text{ d} \times 50 \text{ d}}{138 \text{ d} + 50 \text{ d}} = 37 \text{ d}$$

The activity deposited in each region, and for each clearance pathway. The fraction of the deposit, its retention half time, and its clearance rate λ (= 0.693/ T_E) are listed in the table below.

Region	Bq	f	T_E, d	λ, d^{-1}
N-P	337.5	Not in lung		
T-B	150	0.5 0.5	0.01 0.2	69.3 3.47
P	637.5	0.4 0.6	1 37	0.693 0.0187

The cumulated activity, $\tilde{A}$, for several compartments is given by a variant of equation 6.91,

$$\tilde{A} = \sum \frac{A_i(0)}{\lambda_i}$$

If we substitute the values from the table above, we have

$$\tilde{A} = \frac{0.5 \times 150 \text{ Bq}}{69.3 \text{ d}^{-1}} + \frac{0.5 \times 150 \text{ Bq}}{3.47 \text{ d}^{-1}} + \frac{0.4 \times 637.5 \text{ Bq}}{0.693 \text{ d}^{-1}} + \frac{0.6 \times 637.5 \text{ Bq}}{0.0139 \text{ d}^{-1}}$$

$$\tilde{A} = 2.1 \times 10^4 \text{ Bq·d}$$

The dose rate to the lung, S(lung←lung), Sv/Bq·d is calculated

$$S(\text{lung} \leftarrow \text{lung}) =$$

$$\frac{1 \text{ Bq} \times 1 \frac{\text{tps}}{\text{Bq}} \times \overline{E} \frac{\text{MeV}}{\text{t}} \times 1.6 \times 10^{-13} \frac{\text{J}}{\text{MeV}} \times 8.64 \times 10^4 \frac{\text{sec}}{\text{day}} \times Q \frac{\text{Sv}}{\text{Gy}}}{m \text{ kg} \times 1 \frac{\text{J}}{\text{kg}} / \text{Gy}}$$

The lung has a mass of 1 kg, a ^{210}Po alpha decay releases 5.4 MeV, and the quality factor Q for alpha particles is 20. Substituting these values into the equation above gives

$$S(\text{lung} \leftarrow \text{lung}) = 1.49 \times 10^{-6} \frac{\text{Sv}}{\text{Bq} \cdot \text{d}}$$

The lung dose is

$$H = 2.1 \times 10^4 \text{ Bq} \cdot \text{d} \times 1.49 \times 10^{-6} \frac{\text{Sv}}{\text{Bq} \cdot \text{d}} = 0.031 \text{ Sv}$$

13.19 A demineralizer 20 cm in diameter × 20 cm high processes 200 liters per 13.19
minute contaminated water, and removes the following long lived isotopes:

Isotope	Bq/liter	μCi/L
^{60}Co	1.48 × 104	0.4
^{137}Cs	1.11 × 105	3.0
^{144}Ce	1.85 × 106	50.0

The demineralizer operates for 180 days. Thirty days later,
(a) What is the activity of each of these isotopes in the demineralizer?

The activity buildup in the demineralizer follows the same kinetics as serial transformation. The activity at any time t_b, $A(t)$ after the start of operation is given by a variant of equation 4.38:

$$A = \frac{K}{\lambda}\left(1 - e^{-\lambda t_b}\right),$$

and after a decay time of t_d after the end of buildup, the activity on the resins is reduced to

$$A = \left(\frac{K}{\lambda}\left(1 - e^{-\lambda \times t_b}\right)\right)e^{-\lambda \times t_d}$$

where

$$K = C\frac{\mu\text{Ci}}{\text{L}} \times 200\frac{\text{L}}{\text{min}} \times 1440\frac{\text{min}}{\text{d}} = 2.88 \times 10^5 C\frac{\text{L}}{\text{d}}$$

λ = decay rate

For ^{60}Co, $T = 5.3$ y

$$\lambda_{\text{Co-60}} = \frac{0.693}{T_{1/2}} = \frac{0.693}{5.27\ \text{yr}} \times \frac{1\ \text{yr}}{365\ \text{d}} = 3.58 \times 10^{-9}\ \text{d}^{-1}$$

$$A\left({}^{60}\text{Co}\right) = \left(\frac{0.4 \dfrac{\mu\text{Ci}}{\text{L}} \times 2.88 \times 10^{5} \dfrac{\text{L}}{\text{d}}}{3.58 \times 10^{-4}\ \text{d}^{-1}} \times \left(1 - e^{-3.58\times10^{-4} \times 180\ \text{d}}\right) \right) \times e^{-3.58\times10^{-4} \times 30\ \text{d}}$$

$$A\left({}^{60}\text{Co}\right) = 1.99 \times 10^{7}\ \mu\text{Ci} = 19.9\ \text{Ci}$$

For ^{137}Cs, $T = 30$ y, $\lambda = 6.33 \times 10^{5}\ \text{d}^{-1}$

$$A\left({}^{137}\text{Cs}\right) = \left(\frac{3 \dfrac{\mu\text{Ci}}{\text{L}} \times 2.88 \times 10^{5} \dfrac{\text{L}}{\text{d}}}{3.58 \times 10^{-4}\ \text{d}^{-1}} \times \left(1 - e^{-6.33\times10^{-5} \times 180\ \text{d}}\right) \right) \times e^{-6.33\times10^{-5} \times 30\ \text{d}}$$

$$A\left({}^{137}\text{Cs}\right) = 1.55 \times 10^{8}\ \mu\text{Ci} = 155\ \text{Ci}$$

For ^{144}Ce, $T = 285$ d, $\lambda = 2.43 \times 10^{-3}\ \text{d}^{-1}$

$$A\left({}^{144}\text{Ce}\right) = \left(\frac{50 \dfrac{\mu\text{Ci}}{\text{L}} \times 2.88 \times 10^{5} \dfrac{\text{L}}{\text{d}}}{3.58 \times 10^{-4}\ \text{d}^{-1}} \times \left(1 - e^{-2.43\times10^{-3} \times 180\ \text{d}}\right) \right) \times e^{-2.43\times10^{-3} \times 30\ \text{d}}$$

$$A\left({}^{144}\text{Ce}\right) = 1.95 \times 10^{9}\ \mu\text{Ci} = 1950\ \text{Ci}$$

(b) If the demineralizer approximates a point source at 4 meters, estimate the gamma ray dose rate there.
Equation 10.1

$$\text{Dose rate} = \frac{\Gamma \dfrac{\text{R} \cdot \text{m}^2}{\text{Ci} \cdot \text{hr}} \times \dfrac{\text{rad}}{\text{R}} \times A\ \text{Ci}}{(d,\ \text{m})^2}$$

For ^{60}Co, $\Gamma_{\text{Co-60}} = 1.32 \dfrac{\text{R} \cdot \text{m}^2}{\text{Ci} \cdot \text{hr}}$ (Table 6.3)

$$\dot{D} = \frac{\left(1.32\frac{\text{R}\cdot\text{m}^2}{\text{Ci}\cdot\text{hr}}\right)\times 0.95\frac{\text{rad}}{\text{R}}\times 19.9\text{ Ci}}{(4\text{ m})^2} = 1.56\frac{\text{rads}}{\text{hr}}.$$

For ^{137}Cs, $\Gamma_{\text{Cs-137}} = 0.33\frac{\text{R}\cdot\text{m}^2}{\text{Ci}\cdot\text{hr}}$ (Table 6.3)

$$\dot{D} = \frac{\left(0.33\frac{\text{R}\cdot\text{m}^2}{\text{Ci}\cdot\text{hr}}\right)\times 0.95\frac{\text{rad}}{\text{R}}\times 155\text{ Ci}}{(4\text{ m})^2} = 3.04\frac{\text{rads}}{\text{hr}}$$

For ^{144}Ce, $\Gamma_{\text{Ce-144}} = 0.04\frac{\text{R}\cdot\text{m}^2}{\text{Ci}\cdot\text{hr}}$ (RHH)

$$\dot{D} = \frac{\left(0.04\frac{\text{R}\cdot\text{m}^2}{\text{Ci}\cdot\text{hr}}\right)\times 0.95\frac{\text{rad}}{\text{R}}\times 1950\text{ Ci}}{(4\text{ m})^2} = 4.63\frac{\text{rads}}{\text{hr}}$$

The total dose rate = 1.56 + 3.04 + 4.63 = 9 rads/h

(c) Estimate the gamma ray dose rate at the surface of the demineralizer.

The surface dose rate is estimated with equation 6.68,

$$D = C\Gamma g$$

where D is the mean dose rate from an isotope of concentration C and g is a geometry factor (Table 6.4). The volume of the ion exchanger is

$$V = \pi r^2 h = \pi\,(20)^2\,20 = 6283\text{ cm}^3$$

^{60}Co

$$\dot{D} = \frac{19.9\text{ Ci}}{6.283\times 10^3\text{ cm}^3}\times 1.32\times 10^4\frac{\text{R}\cdot\text{cm}^2}{\text{Ci}\cdot\text{hr}}\times 0.95\frac{\text{rad}}{\text{R}}\times 68.9\text{ cm}$$

$$\dot{D} = 2.74\times 10^3\text{ rads/hr}$$

^{137}Cs

$$\dot{D} = \frac{155 \text{ Ci}}{6.283 \times 10^3 \text{cm}^3} \times 0.33 \times 10^4 \frac{\text{R} \cdot \text{cm}^2}{\text{Ci} \cdot \text{hr}} \times 0.95 \frac{\text{rad}}{\text{R}} \times 68.9 \text{ cm}$$

$\dot{D} = 5.33 \times 10^3$ rads/hr

^{144}Ce

$$\dot{D} = \frac{1950 \text{ Ci}}{6.283 \times 10^3 \text{cm}^3} \times 0.04 \times 10^4 \frac{\text{R} \cdot \text{cm}^2}{\text{Ci} \cdot \text{hr}} \times 0.95 \frac{\text{rad}}{\text{R}} \times 68.9 \text{ cm}$$

$\dot{D} = 8.13 \times 10^3$ rads/hr

Adding the contributions of the 3 radionuclides we have a total of 16.2×10^3 rads/h

Since this is the mean dose rate, the surface dose rate is
$\dot{D}$(surface) = $0.5 \times 16.2 \times 10^3 = 8.1 \times 10^3$ rads/hr

13.20

13.20 In accidental releases to the air in a fuel reprocessing plant, the following mixture of isotopes is usually found. Using DAC values for the air given in 10CFR20, calculate the atmospheric DAC for the total activity that must be applied during cleanup of the contamination.

Isotope	% of total activity
^{89}Sr	7
^{90}Sr	1
^{91}Y	10
^{95}Zr	15
^{95}Nb	25
^{144}Ce	13
^{147}Pm	2

The DAC of a mixture of contaminants is given by

$$\text{DAC(mixture)} = \frac{1}{\Sigma \frac{p_i}{\text{DAC}_i}}$$

where p_i is the proportion of the ith contaminant, and DAC_i is the DAC of the ith contaminant.

For the radioisotopes in the mixture, we have (10CFR20, Appendix B, Table 2, column 1)

$$DAC = \left[\frac{0.07}{6\times 10^{-8}} + \frac{0.01}{2\times 10^{-9}} + \frac{0.1}{5\times 10^{-8}} + \frac{0.15}{5\times 10^{-8}} + \frac{0.25}{5\times 10^{-7}} + \frac{0.13}{6\times 10^{-9}} + \frac{0.02}{6\times 10^{-8}}\right]^{-1}$$

DAC = 3×10^{-8} μCi/mL

Note that the DAC applies only to occupational radiation workers.

13.21 Tritiated water vapor was unknowingly released in a laboratory. An air sample was taken using a freeze–out technique (100% freeze out) when the leak was discovered. Further investigation revealed that the system had been leaking for 24 hours prior to the discovery. Five hundred liters air were drawn through the cold trap, and the collected moisture was diluted to 50 mL. One mL of the dilution was counted for tritium betas in a liquid scintillation counter whose background was 12 cpm and whose counting efficiency was 30%. The 1 mL sample gave 3200 cpm. **13.21**
(a) What was the tritium concentration in the air?

3200 cpm – 12 cpm (background) = 3188 net cpm

Since the counting technique was 30% efficient:

$$3188\,\frac{\text{counts}}{\text{min}} \times \frac{1\text{ min}}{60\text{ sec}} \times \frac{100\text{ decays}}{30\text{ counts}} \times \frac{1\text{ Bq}}{1\frac{\text{decay}}{\text{sec}}} = 177.1\text{ Bq is the actual activity in}$$

1 mL sample collected from the 50 mL dilution.

Convert this to the activity in each cubic meter of air (50 mL sample represented 500 liters of air);

$$\frac{177.1\text{ Bq}}{1\text{ mL}} \times \frac{50\text{ mL}}{500\text{ L}} \times \frac{10^3\text{ L}}{1\text{ m}^3} = 1.77 \times 10^4\ \frac{\text{Bq}}{\text{m}^3}$$

(b) A technician who had been working in the lab for 8 hours left for a vacation without leaving a urine sample. If the principal route of intake was inhalation, and if all the inhaled tritium was taken up by the technician, estimate her dose commitment. (Use the biological data given for reference person.)

First find how much air the technician takes in during 8 hours. From Appendix C, it is found that 9100 liters (female) are taken during 8 hrs.

$q = \frac{1.77 \times 10^4 \text{ Bq}}{\text{m}^3} \times \frac{\text{m}^3}{1000 \text{ L}} \times 9100 \text{ L} = 1.61 \times 10^5 \text{ Bq}$ is the amount of tritium entering her body.

The dose rate, $\dot{D}$, from this activity entering her body is given by equation 6.47:

$$\dot{D} = \frac{q \text{ Bq} \times 1 \frac{\text{tps}}{\text{Bq}} \times E_e \frac{\text{MeV}}{\text{t}} \times 1.6 \times 10^{-13} \frac{\text{J}}{\text{MeV}} \times 8.64 \times 10^4 \frac{\text{sec}}{\text{day}}}{m \text{ kg} \times 1 \frac{\text{J}}{\text{kg}} / \text{Gy}}$$

where the mass of the reference person is 70 kg (Appendix C) and the average energy of the tritium beta is 0.0057 MeV.

$$\dot{D} = \frac{1.61 \times 10^5 \text{ Bq} \times 1 \frac{\text{tps}}{\text{Bq}} \times 0.0057 \frac{\text{MeV}}{\text{t}} \times 1.6 \times 10^{-13} \frac{\text{J}}{\text{MeV}} \times 8.64 \times 10^4 \frac{\text{s}}{\text{day}}}{70 \text{ kg} \times 1 \frac{\text{J}}{\text{kg}} / \text{Gy}}$$

$$\dot{D} = 1.81 \times 10^{-7} \frac{\text{Gy}}{\text{d}}$$

ICRP 30, part 1, p.66, gives the effective half life of tritium in the body as 10 days. Calculating the effective decay constant using equation 4.21;

$$\lambda_E = \frac{0.693}{T} = \frac{0.693}{10 \text{ d}} = 0.0693 \text{ d}^{-1}$$

The dose commitment can now be calculated using equation 6.58;

$$D = \frac{\dot{D}_0}{\lambda_E} = \frac{1.81 \times 10^{-7}\,\frac{\text{Gy}}{\text{d}}}{0.0693\ \text{d}^{-1}} = 2.61 \times 10^{-6}\ \text{Gy}$$

Since the dose is only due to betas, a quality factor of 1 is used, and thus the dose commitment is 2.61×10^{-6} Sv

(c)The technician submitted a urine sample 21 days later. What concentration of tritium would be expected in the urine?

ICRP 30, part 1, p.65, gives the water content of the body as 42000 g = 42 L. Thus, the activity in the technician is distributed over the 42 liters of water in the body, giving an initial concentration of tritium in the body fluids of:

$C({}^3\text{H}) = \frac{1.61 \times 10^5\ \text{Bq}}{42\ \text{L}} = 3.83 \times 10^3\ \frac{\text{Bq}}{\text{L}}$ is the initial concentration of tritium in the body.

Since the urine is a bodily fluid, it will have the same concentration as the rest of the bodily fluids. ICRP 30, part 1, p.65, shows that the retention of tritium follows the following function, with t in days;

$$R(t) = A(0)e^{\frac{-0.693t}{10}} = 3.83 \times 10^3\ \frac{\text{Bq}}{\text{L}} \times e^{\frac{-0.693\ \times\ 21}{10}} = 894\frac{\text{Bq}}{\text{L}}$$

13.22 A worker accidentally ingested an unknown amount of ^{60}Co activity. His body burden was measured by whole–body counting from day 1 until day 14 after the ingestion with the following results: **13.22**

Day	1	2	3	4	7	14
kBq	75.3	63.4	54.3	49.2	42.0	31.0

The whole body retention function for ingested ^{60}Co is given as

$$Q(t) = 0.5e^{-1.386t} + 0.3e^{-0.1155t} + 0.1e^{-0.01155t} + 0.1\,e^{-8.663\times10^{-4}t}.$$

(a) Estimate the amount of ingested activity.

The intake retention function, $Q(t)$, gives the fraction of the intake remaining at time t days after intake. Therefore, the estimated intake, $A_{si}(0)$, from a whole body measurement is:

$$A_{si}(0) = \frac{\text{measured activity}}{Q(t)} = \frac{A_{si}(t)}{Q(t)}$$

Our best estimate of the intake is the mean of the intakes calculated from the successive body burden measurements and the value of $Q(t)$ at the time of the measurement.

$$A_{si}(0) = \frac{\text{measured activity}}{0.5 \times e^{-1.386 \times t} + 0.3 \times e^{-0.1155 \times t} + 0.1 \times e^{-0.01155 \times t} + 0.1 \times e^{-8.663 \times 10^{-t} \times t}}$$

For 1 day, we have

$$A_{s1}(0) = \frac{75.3 \text{ kBq}}{0.5 \times e^{-1.386 \times 1} + 0.3 \times e^{-0.1155 \times 1} + 0.1 \times e^{-0.01155 \times 1} + 0.1 \times e^{-8.663 \times 10^{-t} \times 1}}$$

$A_{s1}(0) = 127.39$ kBq

Similarly, we can calculate the estimated intake from each of the whole body measurements and then take the mean value as our best estimate of the intake. The results, together with the calculated values for $Q(t)$, are tabulated below:

Day	$Q(t)$	$A_{si}(t)$, kBq	$A_{si}(0)$, kBq
1	0.591	75.3	127.39
2	0.467	63.4	135.78
3	0.416	54.3	130.43
4	0.386	49.2	127.42
7	0.325	42	129.10
14	0.243	31	127.32

Mean = 129.6 kBq

(b) What was the committed dose from the ingested radiocobalt?

The committed dose equation is given by equation 6.97.

$$H = \tilde{A}\ \text{Bq·d} \times S_{\text{Co-60}}(\text{body}\leftarrow\text{body})\ \frac{\text{Sv}}{\text{Bq}\cdot\text{d}}$$

The cumulated activity, $\tilde{A}$, is given by equation 6.91.

$$\tilde{A} = \sum \frac{A_{Si}(0)}{\lambda_{Ei}}$$

$$\tilde{A} = 129.6 \times 10^3\ \text{Bq}\left(\frac{0.5}{1.386\ \text{d}^{-1}} + \frac{0.3}{0.1155\ \text{d}^{-1}} + \frac{0.1}{0.01155\ \text{d}^{-1}} + \frac{0.1}{8.663 \times 10^{-4}\ \text{d}^{-1}}\right)$$

$$\tilde{A} = 1.647 \times 10^7\ \text{Bq}\cdot\text{d}$$

$S_{\text{Co-60}}(\text{body}\leftarrow\text{body}) =$

$$= 2.7 \times 10^{-5} \frac{\text{rad}}{\mu\text{Ci}\cdot\text{hr}} \times \frac{0.01\ \text{Gy}}{\text{rad}} \times \frac{1\ \mu\text{Ci}}{3.7 \times 10^4\ \text{Bq}} \times 24 \frac{\text{h}}{\text{d}} \times 1 \frac{\text{Sv}}{\text{Gy}}$$

$$S_{\text{Co-60}}(\text{body}\leftarrow\text{body}) = 1.75 \times 10^{-10}\ \frac{\text{Sv}}{\text{Bq}\cdot\text{d}}$$

$$\text{Dose} = 1.647 \times 10^7\ \text{Bq}\cdot\text{d} \times 1.75 \times 10^{-10}\ \frac{\text{Sv}}{\text{Bq}\cdot\text{d}} = 2.9 \times 10^{-3}\ \text{Sv} = 2.9\ \text{mSv}$$

13.23 A rotameter is calibrated to read directly at 25°C and 760 mm Hg. It is used at an altitude of 5000 ft (1500 m), where the pressure is 633 mm Hg and the temperature is 15°C. What was the actual flow rate when the rotameter reading was 2.5 L/min? **13.23**

Equation 13.17;

$P_0 = 760$ mm
$P_a = 633$ mm
$T_0 = 25°\text{C} = 273 + 25 = 298$ K
$T_a = 15°\text{C} = 273 + 15 = 288$ K

$$Q_a = Q_0\sqrt{\frac{P_0}{P_a}\frac{T_a}{T_0}} = 2.5\frac{\text{L}}{\text{min}} \times \sqrt{\frac{760\text{ mm}}{633\text{ mm}} \times \frac{288\text{ K}}{298\text{ K}}} = 2.7\frac{\text{L}}{\text{min}}$$

13.24

13.24 A rotameter that was calibrated for air at 25°C and 760 mm was used in a room at a temperature of 25°C and 760 mm to measure helium flowing into a gas chromatograph. The rotameter reading was 28.3 L/min (1 cfm). What was the actual flow rate of the helium?

The density of He, MW = 4, differs greatly from that of air, MW = 29. Equation 13.17 relates flow to molecular weight.

$$Q_{actual} = Q_{calibrated}\sqrt{\frac{\rho_{calibrated}}{\rho_{He}}} = Q_{calibrated}\sqrt{\frac{MW_{calibrated}}{MW_{He}}} = 28.3\frac{\text{L}}{\text{min}} \times \sqrt{\frac{29}{4}} = 76.2\frac{\text{L}}{\text{min}}$$

13.25

13.25 The air in a lab 10 m × 8 m × 5 m high has airborne ^{239}Pu at a concentration of 0.1 DAC (DAC = 7 × 10^{-12} μCi/mL = 3 × 10^{-1} Bq/m^3). If all the airborne activity were to settle out, what would be the areal concentration on the floor, tpm, per 100 cm^2?

5 m × 10 m × 8 m = 400 m^3

The ^{239}Pu activity in a column of air 100 cm^2 in an area 500 cm (5 m) high, when all the Pu settled, gives an areal concentration of

$$C_a = 0.1 \times 7 \times 10^{-12}\,\frac{\mu\text{Ci}}{\text{cm}^3} \times \left(100\text{ cm}^2 \times 500\text{ cm}\right) \times 2.22 \times 10^6\,\frac{\text{tpm}}{\mu\text{Ci}}$$

C_a = 0.078 tpm/ 100 cm^2

13.26

13.26 The continuous air monitor (CAM) of a radiochemical manufacturing laboratory that synthesizes various ^{14}C labeled compounds is set to alarm at 0.1 DAC. Long term data show that the mix of ^{14}C in the air is:

Compound	%	DAC, µCi/mL
^{14}CO	20	7×10^{-4}
$^{14}CO_2$	70	9×10^{-5}
Labeled	10	1×10^{-6}

At what ^{14}C concentration should the alarm be set?

The DAC of the mixture is given by:

$$\mathrm{DAC}_{\mathrm{mixture}} = \frac{1}{\sum \frac{p_i}{\mathrm{DAC}_i}} = \frac{1}{\frac{\text{fraction }^{14}\mathrm{CO}}{\mathrm{DAC}\ ^{14}\mathrm{CO}} + \frac{\text{fraction }^{14}\mathrm{CO}_2}{\mathrm{DAC}\ ^{14}\mathrm{CO}_2} + \frac{\text{fraction labeled}}{\text{DAC labeled}}}$$

$$\mathrm{DAC}_{\mathrm{mixture}} = \frac{1}{\frac{0.2}{7 \times 10^{-4}\ \frac{\mu\mathrm{Ci}}{\mathrm{mL}}} + \frac{0.7}{9 \times 10^{-5}\ \frac{\mu\mathrm{Ci}}{\mathrm{mL}}} + \frac{0.1}{1 \times 10^{-6}\ \frac{\mu\mathrm{Ci}}{\mathrm{mL}}}} = 9.25 \times 10^{-6}\ \frac{\mu\mathrm{Ci}}{\mathrm{mL}}$$

Set the CAM for one tenth the DAC,

$9.25 \times 10^{-6}\ \frac{\mu\mathrm{Ci}}{\mathrm{mL}} \times 0.1 = 9 \times 10^{-7}\ \frac{\mu\mathrm{Ci}}{\mathrm{mL}}$ (since DAC's are normally rounded to the nearest whole number)

Solutions for Chapter 14

NONIONIZING RADIATION

14.1 The lethal absorbed dose of 265 nm ultraviolet light for *E. coli* bacteria is 14 MeV. To how many photons of this UV radiation does the lethal absorbed dose correspond? **14.1**

$$14 \text{ MeV} \times \frac{1.6 \times 10^{-13} \text{ J}}{1 \text{ MeV}} = 2.24 \times 10^{-12} \text{ J} \text{ is the energy required to cause lethality}$$

The photon energy is (equation 2.76);

$$E = \frac{hc}{\lambda} = \frac{6.614 \times 10^{-34} \text{ J} \cdot \text{sec} \times 3 \times 10^{8} \frac{\text{m}}{\text{sec}}}{265 \times 10^{-9} \text{ m}} = 7.5 \times 10^{-19} \frac{\text{J}}{\text{photon}}$$

Calculating the number of photons required;

$$2.24 \times 10^{-12} \text{ J} \times \frac{\text{photon}}{7.5 \times 10^{-19} \text{ J}} = 3 \times 10^{6} \text{ photons}$$

14.2 An yttrium-aluminum-garnet (YAG) laser emits near-infrared radiation 1060 nm in wavelength at a power level of 10 W cw. The exit aperture is 3 mm in diameter, and the beam divergence is 5 mrad. Calculate **14.2**
(a) the $1/e^2$ diameter at the aperture,

The aperture area is

$$A = \frac{\pi}{4} d^2 = \frac{\pi}{4} (3 \text{ mm})^2 = 7.069 \text{ mm}^2$$

The $1/e^2$ diameter is the diameter of a circle that intercepts 0.865 of the energy in the laser beam. The $1/e^2$ diameter, d_e, is calculated from

$$0.865 \times 7.069 \text{ mm}^2 = \frac{\pi}{4} d_e^2$$

$d_e = 2.79$ mm
Note that this is normally measured rather than calculated

(b) the $1/e^2$ diameter at a distance of 10 m.

Since the publication of the textbook, the ANSI standards have changed. Using these updated standards, we have the diameter, D_L, of a laser beam at distance r from the aperture diameter, a, and a beam divergence ϕ radians, is given by equation B13 ANSI Z136.1-1993, Appendix B, p. 83.

$$D_L = \sqrt{a^2 + r^2 \phi^2}$$

In this case, the $1/e^2$ aperture diameter is 0.279 cm (2.79 mm). The $1/e^2$ diameter at 1,000 cm (10 m) is

$$D_L = \sqrt{(0.279 \text{ cm})^2 + (10^3 \text{ cm})^2 \left(5 \times 10^{-3} \text{ rad}\right)^2} = 5.0 \text{ cm}$$

Using the former standards, on which the equations in the textbook are based, we have equation 14.15

$$D_L = a + r\phi = 0.279 \text{ cm} + (1000 \text{ cm} \times 5 \times 10^{-3} \text{ rad}) = 5.3 \text{ cm}$$

(c) the irradiance at a distance of 10 m.

Since the publication of the textbook, the ANSI standards have changed. Using these updated standards, and ignoring atmospheric attenuation a this small distance,

$$\text{Irradiance} = \frac{\text{Power}}{\frac{\pi}{4}(D_L)^2} = \frac{10 \times 10^3 \text{ mW}}{\frac{\pi}{4} \times (5 \text{ cm})^2} = 509 \frac{\text{mW}}{\text{cm}^2}$$

Using the former standards, equation 14.12

$$E = \frac{10 \times 10^3 \text{ mW}}{\pi \times \left(\frac{1}{2} \times 5.3\text{cm}\right)^2} = 453 \frac{\text{mW}}{\text{cm}^2}$$

14.3 A 0.1 ruby laser has an aperture of 7 mm and a beam divergence of 1 mrad. **14.3**

(a) What is the radiant exposure at distances of 5 and 10 m from the aperture?

$$\text{Radiant Exposure} = \frac{\text{Radiant energy}}{\text{Irradiated area}}$$

Since the publication of the textbook, the ANSI standards have changed. Using these updated standards, we have the radiant exposure, $H(r)$, at a distance r from a laser is given by equation B11, Appendix B, p.83,
ANSI Z136.1-1993 as

$$H(r) = \frac{Q}{\pi\left(\frac{1}{2}\left(\sqrt{a^2 + r^2\phi^2}\right)\right)^2}$$

where
Q = radiant energy = 0.1 J
a = aperture diameter = 0.7 cm (7 mm)
r = distance = 500 cm (5 m) and 1000 cm (10 m)
ϕ = beam divergence = 0.001 radian

$$H(5\text{ m}) = \frac{0.1\text{ J}}{\pi \times \left(\frac{1}{2} \times \left(\sqrt{(0.7\text{ cm})^2 + \left[(500\text{ cm})^2 \times (0.001)^2\right]}\right)\right)^2} = 0.172 \frac{\text{J}}{\text{cm}^2}$$

$$H(10\text{ m}) = \frac{0.1\text{ J}}{\pi \times \left(\frac{1}{2} \times \left(\sqrt{(0.7\text{ cm})^2 + \left[(1000\text{ cm})^2 \times (0.001)^2\right]}\right)\right)^2} = 0.085 \frac{\text{J}}{\text{cm}^2}$$

Using the former standards, we have equation 14.12

$$E = \frac{0.1 \text{ J}}{\pi \times \left(\frac{1}{2} \times \left(0.7 \text{ cm} + 500 \text{ cm} \times 1 \times 10^{-3}\right)\right)^2} = 0.088 \frac{\text{J}}{\text{cm}^2}$$

$$E = \frac{0.1 \text{ J}}{\pi \left(\frac{1}{2} \times \left(0.7 \text{ cm} + 1000 \text{ cm} \times 1 \times 10^{-3}\right)\right)^2} = 0.044 \frac{\text{J}}{\text{cm}^2}$$

(b) How far behind the laser aperture is the virtual focal point from where the laser light seems to originate?

The virtual focal point is the point where backward projection of the beam boarders intersect, as shown in the figure below. The figure shows that this distance, d, is given by

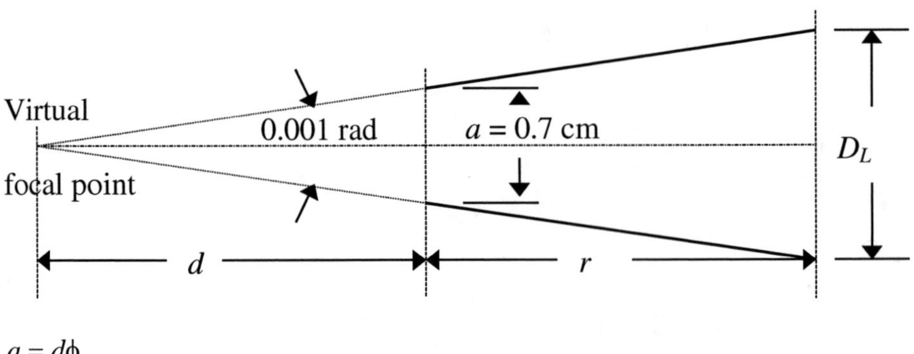

$$a = d\phi$$

$$d = \frac{a}{\phi} = \frac{0.7 \text{ cm}}{0.001 \text{ rad}} = 700 \text{ cm} = 7 \text{ m}$$

(c) Is the inverse square law applicable if distances are measured from the virtual focal point of the laser beam?

Although geometry implies that the inverse square law is applicable, revision of the calculational methods based on better scientific understanding of laser beams which more accurately predict beam shape and intensity, show that the inverse square law is not applicable.

14.4 The output of a cw pumped Nd:YAG laser is Q-switched at a pulse repetition frequency of 10 kHz. If each pulse is 50 nanoseconds wide, and if the mean power output is 10W, calculate **14.4**
(a) the duty cycle,
50 nanoseconds = 50×10^{-9} sec/pulse
10 kHz = 10×10^{3} pulses/sec

$$\text{duty cycle} = \text{fraction of time lasing occurs} = n\frac{\text{pulses}}{\text{sec}} \times \tau\frac{\text{sec}}{\text{pulse}}$$

$$\text{duty cycle} = 10 \times 10^{3}\,\frac{\text{pulses}}{\text{sec}} \times 50 \times 10^{-9}\,\frac{\text{sec}}{\text{pulse}} = 5 \times 10^{-4}$$

(b) the peak power per pulse;

mean power = duty cycle × peak power

$P_{mean} = 10$ W

duty cycle = 5×10^{-4} (part (a))

Equation 14.22;

$$P_{peak} = \frac{P_{mean}}{\text{duty cycle}} = \frac{10\text{ W}}{5 \times 10^{-4}} = 2 \times 10^{4}\text{ W}$$

(c) the energy per pulse.

energy per pulse = peak power × time of pulse

$$E = 2 \times 10^{4}\text{ W} \times \frac{1\,\text{J}/\text{sec}}{1\text{W}} \times 50 \times 10^{-9}\,\frac{\text{sec}}{\text{pulse}} = 0.001\text{ J per pulse}$$

14.5

14.5 What is the recommended MPE value, in mW/cm^2, for direct ocular exposure for 1 sec to a beam from a He-Ne laser operating at a power level of 5 mW cw?

The wavelength for a He-Ne laser is 0.6328 micrometers from Table 14.6.

$MPE(H) = 1.8(t)^{3/4} \times 10^{-3}\ J/cm^2 = 1.8 \times (1)^{3/4} \times 10^{-3}\ J/cm^2 = 1.8 \times 10^{-3}\ J/cm^2$

Equation 14.2 is rearranged;
$t = 1$ sec
$H = Et$

$$MPE\ (E) = \frac{H}{t} = \frac{1.8\times10^{-3}\ \frac{J}{cm^2}}{1\ sec} \times \frac{1\ mW}{10^{-3}\ \frac{J}{sec}} = 1.8\frac{mW}{cm^2}$$

14.6

14.6 What is the protection standard (i.e., the maximum permissible irradiance for a direct intrabeam exposure) to a 0.8 ms wide pulse from a 694.3 nm ruby laser?

$t = 0.8\ msec = 0.8 \times 10^{-3}\ sec$

$MPE(H) = 1.8(t)^{3/4} \times 10^{-3}\ J/cm^2$ (Table 14.6)

$MPE(H) = 1.8 \times (0.8 \times 10^{-3}\ sec)^{3/4} \times 10^{-3}\ J/cm^2 = 8.56 \times 10^{-6}\ J/cm^2$

Equation 14.2 is rearranged;

$H = Et$

$$MPE\ (E) = \frac{H}{t} = \frac{8.56\times10^{-6}\ \frac{J}{cm^2}}{0.8\times10^{-3}\,sec} = 0.0107\frac{W}{cm^2} = 10.7\frac{mW}{cm^2}$$

14.7

14.7 A pulsed ruby laser, $\lambda = 694.3$ nm, is operated in a laboratory at a level of 5×10^{-4} J/pulse, 100 μs pulse width, and a PRF of 60 pulses per second. The beam exit aperture is 1 mm in diameter, and the beam divergence is 0.1 mrad. What optical density is required for protective goggles for
(a) incidental exposure for as long as 2 s?

We will calculate the required OD on the basis of two criteria, and then choose the more conservative OD:
1. MPE for a single pulse
2. MPE for the total exposure

In table 14.6, we find that, for 0.6643 μm wavelength,

$$\text{MPE} = 1.8 \times t^{3/4} \times 10^{-3} \frac{\text{J}}{\text{cm}^2}$$

For a single pulse whose duration is 100 μsec, of 1×10^{-4} sec,

$$\text{MPE} = 1.8\left(1 \times 10^{-4}\right)^{3/4} \times 10^{-3} \frac{\text{J}}{\text{cm}^2} = 1.8 \times 10^{-6} \frac{\text{J}}{\text{cm}^2}$$

Because we have a pulsed beam whose PRF = 60 per sec, we reduce the MPE by a factor C_p (Equation 14.9, Figure 14.9), which depends on the total number of pulses, n, in the exposure:

$$C_p = n^{-1/4} = \left(60 \frac{\text{pulses}}{\text{sec}} \times 2\ \text{sec}\right)^{-1/4} = 0.302$$

Therefore,

$$H(\text{MPE/pulse}) = 0.302 \times 1.8 \times 10^{-6} = 5.44 \times 10^{-7} \frac{\text{J}/\text{cm}^2}{\text{pulse}}$$

In this laser, we have 5×10^{-4} J/pulse

$$H = \frac{5 \times 10^{-4} \dfrac{\text{J}}{\text{pulse}}}{\dfrac{\pi}{4}(0.1\ \text{cm})^2} = 6.37 \times 10^{-2} \frac{\text{J}/\text{cm}^2}{\text{pulse}}$$

$$OD = \log \frac{H}{(H)\text{MPE}} = \log \frac{6.37 \times 10^{-2} \dfrac{\text{J}}{\text{cm}^2}}{5.44 \times 10^{-7} \dfrac{\text{J}}{\text{cm}^2}} = 5.1$$

The MPE for the total exposure of 2 seconds is (Table 14.6)

$$\text{MPE} = 1.8 \times 2^{3/4} \times 10^{-3}\frac{\text{J}}{\text{cm}^2} = 3.03 \times 10^{-3}\ \frac{\text{J}}{\text{cm}^2}$$

$$\text{The total radiant expure} = \frac{5 \times 10^{-4}\ \dfrac{\text{J}}{\text{pulse}} \times 120 \text{ pulses}}{\dfrac{\pi}{4}(0.1\text{ cm})^2} = 7.64\ \frac{\text{J}}{\text{cm}^2}$$

$$OD = \log\frac{H}{(H)\text{MPE}} = \log\frac{7.64\dfrac{\text{J}}{\text{cm}^2}}{3.03 \times 10^{-3}\ \dfrac{\text{J}}{\text{cm}^2}} = 3.4$$

The required OD is 5.1

(b) For “continuous” worst case exposure, we will choose an exposure time of 3 $\times$ 10^4 seconds. Table 14.6 gives the MPE for the exposure as

$\text{MPE(cw)} = 10^{15(1 - 0.550)} \times 10^{-6}\ \text{W/cm}^2$
$\text{MPE(cw)} = 10^{15(0.6943 - 0.550)} \times 10^{-6} = 1.46 \times {}^{10-4}\ \text{W/cm}^2$

The MPE(pulse) is lower than the MPE(cw) by a factor of $n^{-0.25}$. The number of pulses, n, during an exposure time of 3 $\times$ 10^4 seconds:

$$C_P = \left(100\frac{\text{pulses}}{\text{sec}} \times 3 \times 10^4 \text{ sec}\right)^{-0.25} = 0.024$$

$\text{MPE(pulse)} = 0.024 \times 1.46 \times 10^{-4} = 3.51 \times 10^{-6}\ \text{W/cm}^2$

The power density in a single pulse is

$$E = \frac{5 \times 10^{-4}\ \text{J/pulse}}{\dfrac{\pi}{4}(0.1\text{ cm})^2 \times 1 \times 10^{-4}\ \text{sec/pulse}} \times \frac{1\text{ W}}{\text{J/sec}} = 637\frac{\text{W}}{\text{cm}^2}$$

$$\text{OD} = \log \frac{E}{\text{MPE(pulse)}} = \log \frac{637}{3.51 \times 10^{-6}} = 8.3$$

For a continuous exposure

$$E = \frac{60 \dfrac{\text{pulses}}{\text{sec}} \times 5 \times 10^{-4}\ \text{J/pulse}}{\dfrac{\pi}{4}(0.1\ \text{cm})^2} \times \frac{1\ \text{W}}{\text{J/sec}} = 3.82 \frac{\text{W}}{\text{cm}^2}$$

$$\text{OD} = \log \frac{E}{\text{MPE(pulse)}} = \log \frac{3.82}{1.46 \times 10^{-4}} = 4.42$$

Please note that continuous intentional exposure is not intended for any laser system. Typically, an aversion response time of 0.25 seconds is assumed in safety calculations for visible light rather than the maximum time of 3×10^4 seconds.

14.8 A He-Ne laser, $\lambda = 632.8$ nm, is operated at a power level of 3 W cw. The beam aperture is 0.9 mm in diameter, and the beam divergence is 0.9 mrad. If the possibility exists for momentary accidental intrabeam ocular exposure not exceeding 0.25 s, calculate the minimum required optical density of protective goggles for exposure **14.8**
(a) at the laser,

From example 14.7, find the power density at the aperture;

$$E = \frac{\text{power}}{\text{area}} = \frac{3\ \text{W}}{\dfrac{\pi}{4} \times (0.09\ \text{cm})^2} = 472 \frac{\text{W}}{\text{cm}^2}$$

Next find the MPE (Table 14.6);

$\text{MPE}(H) = 1.8(t)^{3/4} \times 10^{-3}\ \text{J/cm}^2 = 1.8 \times (0.25)^{3/4} \times 10^{-3} = 6.36 \times 10^{-4}\ \text{J/cm}^2$

The maximum permissible radiant exposure corresponds to a maximum permissible irradiance of

This MPE(H) corresponds to an irradiance of:

$$\text{MPE }(E) = \frac{636 \times 10^{-4}\ \dfrac{\text{J}}{\text{cm}^2}}{0.25\ \text{sec}} \times \frac{1\ \text{W}}{1\ \text{J}/\text{sec}} = 2.54 \times 10^{-3}\ \frac{\text{W}}{\text{cm}^2}$$

$$OD = \log \frac{E}{\text{MPE}(E)} = \log\left(\frac{472\ \dfrac{\text{W}}{\text{cm}^2}}{2.5 \times 10^{-3}\ \dfrac{\text{W}}{\text{cm}^2}}\right) = 5.3$$

(b) at a distance of 100 m.
Since the publication of the textbook, the ANSI standards have been changed. Using the new standards, we have the downrange irradiance from equation B10, p. 83, ANSI Z136.1-1993,

$$E(r) = \frac{P}{\pi\left(\frac{1}{2}\left(\sqrt{a^2 + r^2\phi^2}\right)\right)^2}$$

$$E(r) = \frac{3\ \text{W}}{\pi \times \left(\frac{1}{2} \times \left(\sqrt{(0.09\ \text{cm})^2 + (10000\ \text{cm})^2 \times \{0.9 \times 10^{-3}\}^2}\right)\right)^2}$$

$$E(r) = 4.72 \times 10^{-2}\ \frac{\text{W}}{\text{cm}^2}$$

$$\text{MPE} = 2.5 \times 10^{-3}\ \frac{\text{W}}{\text{cm}^2} \text{ from part a}$$

Equation 14.21

$$OD = \log\ \frac{E}{\text{MPE}(E)} = \log \frac{4.72 \times 10^{-2}\ \dfrac{\text{W}}{\text{cm}^2}}{2.54 \times 10^{-3}\ \dfrac{\text{W}}{\text{cm}^2}} = 1.3 \text{ is the required OD.}$$

Using the former standards, we have

$$E = \frac{3\text{ W}}{\frac{\pi}{4}\times\left(0.09\text{ cm} + 10000\text{ cm}\times 0.9\times 10^{-3}\right)^2} = 0.0462\frac{\text{W}}{\text{cm}^2}$$

Which will produce the same OD.

(c) what is the minimum required OD for continuous intrabeam viewing for up to 100 s at a distance of 100 m?

The MPE is found in table 14.6. An exposure time of 100 seconds corresponds to T_1 in table 14.6.

$$T_1 = 10\times 10^{[20\times(\lambda - 0.550)]} = 10\times 10^{[20\times(0.6328-0.550)]} = 453\text{ sec}$$

MPE(H) = $1.8 \times (t)^{3/4} \times 10^{-3}$ J/cm^2
MPE(H) = $1.8 \times (100)^{3/4} \times 10^{-3}$ J/cm^2 = 0.057 J/cm^2

which is equivalent to an irradiance of

$$\text{MPE}(E) = \frac{0.057\frac{\text{J}}{\text{cm}^2}}{100\text{ sec}}\times\frac{1\text{ W}}{\text{J}/\text{sec}} = 5.7\times 10^{-4}\ \frac{\text{W}}{\text{cm}^2}$$

$$OD = \log\frac{E}{\text{MPE}(E)} = \log\frac{4.72\times 10^{-2}\ \frac{\text{W}}{\text{cm}^2}}{5.7\times 10^{-3}\ \frac{\text{W}}{\text{cm}^2}} = 1.9 \text{ is the required optical density.}$$

14.9 A scanning He-Ne laser that scans at a rate of 10/s emits 5 mW through an aperture of 0.7 cm. If the beam divergence is 5 mrad, then, for an intrabeam viewing distance of 200 cm, calculate **14.9**
(a) the time during each scan that the pupil of the eye can be exposed,

Since the publication of the textbook, the ANSI standards have changed. Using these updated standards, the beam diameter at 200 cm is estimated with equation B13 from ANSI Z136.1-1993. Note that all scanning lasers are considered pulsed systems per ANSI Z136.1-1993, p. 85.

$$D_L = \sqrt{a^2 + r^2\phi^2} = \sqrt{(0.7\ \text{mm})^2 + (200\ \text{cm})^2 (5 \times 10^{-3}\ \text{rad})^2} = 1.22\ \text{cm}$$

The pupil will be exposed while the entire diameter of the beam sweeps across the pupil. The exposure time for this sweep is given by

$$\text{exposure time} = \frac{\text{diameter}}{\text{velocity}}$$

S = PRF = 10 pulses per second = scanning rate
θ_S = Maximum angular sweep (usually 0.1 radians)

$$t = \frac{D_L}{rS\theta_S}$$

This equation is identical to ANSI Z136.1-1993, p. 85 equation B23 for $D_L > d_e$.

$$t = \frac{1.22\ \text{cm}}{200\ \text{cm} \times 10 \dfrac{\text{pulses}}{\text{sec}} \times 0.1\ \text{rad}}$$

$$t = 6.1 \times 10^{-3}\ \frac{\text{s}}{\text{pulse}}$$

(b) the radiant exposure per scan (pulse),

The radiant exposure must take into account not only the diameter of the beam, but also the scanning area of the beam when performing safety calculations. Each individual scan is considered a pulse. Therefore, the radiant energy is

$$H = \frac{\text{energy}}{\text{scanned area of beam}}$$

$$H = \frac{P\ \text{watts}}{\frac{\pi}{4} D_L\ \text{cm} \times (r\ \text{cm} \times \theta_S\ \text{radians})} \times \frac{1}{S\dfrac{\text{pulse}}{\text{sec}}} \times \frac{1\ \text{J/sec}}{\text{W}}$$

This equation is identical to ANSI Z136.1-1993, p.85 equation B21.

$$H = \frac{5 \times 10^{-3}\,\text{W}}{\frac{\pi}{4} \times 1.22\ \text{cm}(200\ \text{cm} \times 0.1\ \text{radians})} \times \frac{1}{10\frac{\text{pulses}}{\text{sec}}} \times \frac{1\ \text{J/sec}}{\text{W}}$$

$$H = 2.6 \times 10^{-5} \frac{\text{J}}{\text{cm}^2 \cdot \text{pulse}}$$

To determine the total radiant exposure, find the number of pulses which occur during 0.25 sec (aversion response for 400 to 700 nm laser light), then find the energy deposited during that time.

$n = t_{\text{exposure}} \times \text{PRF} = 0.25\ \text{sec} \times 10\ \text{pulses/s} = 2.5\ \text{pulses}$

$$H_{\text{total}} = n \times \frac{H}{\text{pulse}} = 2.5\ \text{pulses} \times 2.6 \times 10^{-5} \frac{\text{J}}{\text{cm}^2 \cdot \text{pulse}} = 6.5 \times 10^{-5} \frac{\text{J}}{\text{cm}^2}$$

(c) the average irradiance at the cornea,

$$E = 6.5 \times 10^{-5} \frac{\text{J}}{\text{cm}^2} \times \frac{1}{0.25\ \text{sec}} \times \frac{\text{W}}{1\,\text{J}/\text{sec}} = 2.6 \times 10^{-4} \frac{\text{W}}{\text{cm}^2}$$

or one could also calculate average irradiance using the radiant energy;

$$E = 2.6 \times 10^{-5} \frac{\text{J}}{\text{cm}^2 \cdot \text{pulse}} \times 10\frac{\text{pulses}}{\text{sec}} \times \frac{\text{W}}{1\,\text{J}/\text{sec}} = 2.6 \times 10^{-4} \frac{\text{W}}{\text{cm}^2}$$

(d) what hazard class should be assigned to this laser?

$5 \times 10^{-3}\ \text{W} = 5 \times 10^{-3}\ \text{J/s}$

Recall that aversion response time is 0.25 seconds.

$J_0 = P_0 \times t_{\text{exposure}} = 5 \times 10^{-3}\ \text{J/s} \times 0.25\ \text{s} = 1.25 \times 10^{-3}\ \text{J} = 1.25\ \text{mJ}$

This is a Class III b laser, according to Table 2 of ANSI Z136.1-1993, p. 38, since the accessible emission levels are greater than 0.25 mJ, but no more than 30 mJ in 0.25 sec. Also, since 5 mW is 5 mJ/sec, this laser emits 1.25 mJ in 0.25 second. Using the former standard and table 14.10 of the text, this laser falls into the Class III category.

14.10

14.10 A microwave beam is pulsed 100 times per second, the pulse width is 1 μsec, and the peak power is 1 MW.
(a) What is the duty cycle?

$1\ \mu\text{sec} = 1 \times 10^{-6}$ sec

From example 14.9,

duty cycle = pulse width × pulse repetition frequency

$$\text{duty cycle} = 1 \times 10^{-6}\ \text{sec} \times 100\ \frac{\text{pulses}}{\text{sec}} = 10^{-4}$$

(b) What is the average power?

Equation 14.22;

$$P_{peak} = \frac{P_{average}}{\text{duty cycle}}$$

$$P_{average} = P_{peak} \times \text{duty cycle} = (1 \times 10^{6}\ \text{W}) \times 1 \times 10^{-4} = 100\ \text{W}$$

14.11

14.11 A radar operates at an average power level of 20 W; its pulse width is 1 μsec, and the PRF is 1000 per second. Calculate
(a) the duty cycle,

duty cycle = pulse width × pulse repetition frequency

$$\text{duty cycle} = 1 \times 10^{-6}\ \text{sec} \times 1000\ \frac{\text{pulses}}{\text{sec}} = 1 \times 10^{-3}$$

(b) the peak power.

Equation 14.18A;

$$P_{peak} = \frac{P_{average}}{\text{duty cycle}} = \frac{20\ \text{W}}{1 \times 10^{-3}} = 20{,}000\ \text{W}$$

14.12 Calculate the gain of a 30 cm diameter parabolic antenna used to transmit at a frequency of 3000 MHz. Express the answer as **14.12**
(a) power ratio,

$$\text{power rato} = \frac{P_{out}}{P_{in}} = \text{Antenna gain}$$

Antenna gain is given by equation 14.26

$$G = \frac{4\pi A}{\lambda^2}$$

A = antenna area = $\pi r^2 = \pi\,(0.15)^2 = 0.07\ \text{m}^2$

Equation 2.57

$$\lambda = \frac{c}{f} = \frac{3\times 10^8\ \frac{\text{m}}{\text{sec}}}{3000\times 10^6\ \text{sec}^{-1}} = 0.1\ \text{m}$$

$$G = \frac{4\pi A}{\lambda^2} = \frac{4\times\pi\times(0.07)}{0.1^2} = 88.8$$

(b) dB.

The power gain in dB is given by equation 14.27

$$G\ (\text{dB}) = (10)\log\left(\frac{P_2}{P_1}\right) = (10)\times\log(88.8) = 19.5\ \text{dB}$$

14.13 A far field measurement shows the power density in a 1000 MHz radiation field to be 4 mW/cm^2. Calculate **14.13**
(a) the electric field strength, in V/m, and the square of the electric field strength,

The electric field, E V/m, and the magnetic field, H A/m, are related to the far field power density, S mW/cm^2, by equation 14.44

$$S = \frac{E^2}{3770} = 37.7H^2$$

$$E^2 = 4 \times 3770 = 15{,}080\ (\text{V/m})^2$$

$$E = \sqrt{15{,}080 \frac{\text{V}^2}{\text{m}^2}} = 122.8 \frac{\text{V}}{\text{m}}$$

(b) the magnetic field strength, in A/m, and the square of the magnetic field strength,

$$H^2 = \frac{4}{37.7} = 0.106 \frac{\text{A}^2}{\text{m}^2}$$

$$H = \sqrt{0.106 \frac{\text{A}^2}{\text{m}^2}} = 0.325 \frac{\text{A}}{\text{m}}$$

(c) energy density, in pJ/cm^3

$$4 \frac{\text{mW}}{\text{cm}^2} = 4 \times 10^{-3} \frac{\text{J}}{\text{cm}^2 \cdot \text{sec}}$$

$$\text{Energy Density} = \frac{\text{Energy flux}}{\text{Energy velocity}} = \frac{4 \times 10^{-3} \dfrac{\text{J}}{\text{cm}^2 \cdot \text{sec}}}{3 \times 10^{10} \dfrac{\text{cm}}{\text{sec}}} = 1.33 \times 10^{-13} \frac{\text{J}}{\text{cm}^3}$$

$$1.33 \times 10^{-13} \frac{\text{J}}{\text{cm}^3} = 0.133 \frac{\text{pJ}}{\text{cm}^3}$$

14.14

14.14 How many dB attenuation of power density are required to reduce a 1 W/cm^2 field to 1 mW/cm^2?

$$P_i = 1 \frac{\text{W}}{\text{cm}^2}$$

$$P_0 = \frac{1\ \text{mW}}{\text{cm}^2} = 1 \times 10^{-3} \frac{\text{W}}{\text{cm}^2}$$

From equation 14.27,

$$\text{dB} = (10)\log\left(\frac{P_i}{P_0}\right) = 10 \times \log\frac{1\dfrac{\text{W}}{\text{m}^2}}{1\times 10^{-3}\dfrac{\text{W}}{\text{m}^2}} = 30\text{ dB}$$

14.15 What is the maximum magnetic intensity in a plane electromagnetic wave whose maximum electric intensity is 100 V/m? **14.15**

The relationship between the E field and the H field is given by equation 2.68

$$H = \frac{E}{Z} = \frac{100\dfrac{\text{V}}{\text{m}}}{377\text{ ohms}} = 0.27\frac{\text{A}}{\text{m}}$$

14.16 A dipole antenna with a 50 cm parabolic dish radiates 100 W of power at a frequency of 2400 MHz. Calculate the **14.16**
(a) mean power density at the aperture,

Equation 14.29 gives the mean power density at the aperture

$$W_0 = \frac{P}{A}$$

where

$P = 100$ W

$$A = \text{dish area} = \pi r^2 = \pi \times \left(\frac{0.5\text{ m}}{2}\right)^2 = 0.196\text{ m}^2$$

$$W_0 = \frac{P}{A} = \frac{100\text{ W}}{0.196\text{ m}^2} = 509.3\frac{\text{W}}{\text{m}^2} = 51\frac{\text{mW}}{\text{cm}^2}$$

(b) maximum power density in the near field,

Equation 14.30 is used with the value from part (a)

$$W = 4W_0 = 4 \times \left(51 \frac{\text{mW}}{\text{cm}^2}\right) = 204 \frac{\text{mW}}{\text{cm}^2}$$

(c) distance to far field,

Distance to the far field is given by equation 14.28

$$R_{ff} = \frac{D^2}{2.83\lambda}$$

where

D = dish diameter = 0.5 m

$$\lambda = \text{wavelength} = \frac{c}{f} = \frac{3 \times 10^8 \dfrac{\text{m}}{\text{sec}}}{2400 \times 10^6 \dfrac{1}{\text{sec}}} = 0.125 \text{ m}$$

$$R_{ff} = \frac{D^2}{2.83\lambda} = \frac{(0.5 \text{ m})^2}{(2.83) \times 0.125 \text{ m}} = 0.707 \text{ m} = 71 \text{ cm}$$

(d) power density at 1 meter,

First, find the distance to the far field using equation 14.34. The power density in the far field is given by equation 14.74;

$$W_{ff} = 2W_0 \left(\frac{R_{ff}}{R}\right)^2$$

where

W_0 = mean power density at the aperture = $51 \dfrac{\text{mW}}{\text{cm}^2}$

R_{ff} = distance to far field = 71 cm

R = downrange distance of interest = 100 cm

$$W_{ff} = 2W_0\left(\frac{R_{ff}}{R}\right)^2 = 2 \times 51\frac{\text{mW}}{\text{cm}^2} \times \left(\frac{70.7\text{ cm}}{100\text{ cm}}\right)^2 = 51\frac{\text{mW}}{\text{cm}^2}$$

(e) distance at which the power density is down to 1 mW/cm^2.

Use equation 14.34 to find the downrange distance R;

$$W = 2W_0\left(\frac{R_{ff}}{R}\right)^2$$

$W_{ff} = 1$ mW/cm^2
$W_0 = 51$ mW/cm^2
$R_{ff} = 0.71$ m (from part (c))

$$1\frac{\text{mW}}{\text{cm}^2} = 2 \times 51\frac{\text{mW}}{\text{cm}^2} \times \left(\frac{0.71\text{ m}}{R}\right)^2$$

$R = 7.14$ m

14.17 A rectangular horn antenna, 17 × 24 cm, and operating at a frequency of 2400 MHz has an effective area of 200 cm^2. If the radiated power is 100 W, calculate the **14.17**
(a) mean power density,

$P = 100$ W $= 100 \times 10^3$ mW
$A = 200$ cm^2

Putting values into equation 14.29;

$$W_0 = \frac{P}{A} = \frac{100 \times 10^3\text{ mW}}{200\text{ cm}^2} = 500\frac{\text{mW}}{\text{cm}^2}$$

(b) the maximum power density in the near field,

using equation 14.30,

$$W_{nf} = 4\ W_0 = 4 \times \left(500 \frac{\text{mW}}{\text{cm}^2}\right) = 2000 \frac{\text{mW}}{\text{cm}^2}$$

(c) the distance to the start of the far field,

To find the distance to the far field, the equation for a rectangular antenna should be used. Note that equation 14.28 applies for circular antennas. ANSI C95.5-1981, "Recommended Practice for Measurement of Hazardous Electromagnetic Fields - RF and Microwaves" provides the following equation for the distance to the far field from a rectangular antenna:

$$R_{ff} = \frac{2a^2}{\lambda}$$

where

a = greatest linear dimension of the antenna = $\sqrt{17^2 + 24^2} = 29.4$ cm

$$\lambda = \frac{c}{f} = \frac{3 \times 10^8 \frac{\text{m}}{\text{sec}}}{2400 \times 10^6 \frac{1}{\text{sec}}} = 0.125 \text{ m} = 12.5 \text{ cm}$$

$$R_{ff} = \frac{2a^2}{\lambda} = \frac{2 \times (29.4 \text{ cm})^2}{12.5 \text{ cm}} = 138 \text{ cm}$$ is the far field for the rectangular horn antenna

(d) the power density in the far field, at a distance of 5 meters,

Since the antenna is a rectangular horn type, the following formula from ANSI C95.5-1981, "Recommended Practice for Measurement of Hazardous Electromagnetic Fields - RF and Microwaves" is used to calculate power density in the far field:

$$W_{ff} = \frac{A_e P_T}{\lambda^2 r^2}$$

where
A_e = effective area of the antenna = 200 cm^2
P_T = radiated power = 1×10^5 mW
λ = wavelength = 12.5 cm
r = downrange distance = 500 cm

$$W_{ff} = \frac{A_e P_T}{\lambda^2 r^2} = \frac{200\text{ cm}^2 \times 1 \times 10^5\text{ mW}}{(12.5\text{ cm})^2 \times (500\text{ cm})^2} = 0.5\frac{\text{mW}}{\text{cm}^2}$$

(e) distance at which the power density is down to 1 mW/cm^2.

According to the ANSI expression for power density in the far field:

A_e = 200 cm^2 (effective antenna area)
P_T = 1×10^5 mW
λ = 12.5 cm
r = ?
W_{ff} = 1 mW

$$W_{ff} = \frac{A_e P_T}{\lambda^2 r^2}$$

$$1\frac{\text{mW}}{\text{cm}^2} = \frac{200\text{ cm}^2 \times 1 \times 10^5\text{ mW}}{(12.5\text{ cm})^2 (r)^2}$$

$$r = \sqrt{\frac{200\text{ cm}^2 \times 1 \times 10^5\text{ mW}}{(12.5\text{ cm})^2 \times 1\frac{\text{mW}}{\text{cm}^2}}} = 358\text{ cm}$$

14.18 A radar installation, using a parabolic dish antenna 1.2 m in diameter, has a peak power output of 2 MW of 10 GHz radiation. If the pulse repetition frequency is 200 per second and the pulse width is 5 μsec, calculate the **14.18**
(a) duty cycle,

duty cycle = pulse width × PRF

duty cycle = 5×10^{-6} sec $\times$ 2×10^{2} sec^{-1} = 1×10^{-3}

(b) average power output,
According to equation 14.22

$$P_{average} = P_{peak} \times \text{duty cycle} = 2 \times 10^{6}\ \text{W} \times 1 \times 10^{-3} = 2000\ \text{W}$$

(c) antenna gain as a power ratio is given by equation 14.26:

$$G = \frac{4\pi A}{\lambda^2}$$

where

$$A = \text{antenna area} = \pi r^2 = \pi \times (0.6)^2 = 1.131\ \text{m}^2$$

$$\lambda = \frac{c}{f} = \frac{3 \times 10^{8}\ \frac{\text{m}}{\text{sec}}}{10 \times 10^{9}\ \frac{1}{\text{sec}}} = 0.03\ \text{m}$$

$$G = \frac{P_{out}}{P_{in}} = \frac{4 \times \pi \times 1.131\ \text{m}}{(0.03\ \text{m})^2} = 15791$$

The gain, expressed as a power ratio, can be converted to gain expressed in dB with equation 14.27

$$G = 10\ \log\left(\frac{P_2}{P_1}\right) = 10 \times \log(15791.37) = 42\ \text{db}$$

(d) downrange distance to an average power density of 1 mW/cm^2.

The distance is calculated with equation 14.34

$$W_{ff} = 2W_0\left(\frac{R_{ff}}{R}\right)^2$$

where

W_0 = average power density at the aperture

$$W_0 = \frac{P}{A} = \frac{2 \times 10^6\ \text{W}}{1.131\ \text{m}^2} = 1.768 \times 10^6\ \frac{\text{W}}{\text{m}^2} = 176.8\,\frac{\text{mW}}{\text{cm}^2}$$

$$R_{ff} = \text{distance to far field} = \frac{D^2}{2.83\lambda} = \frac{1.2^2}{2.83 \times (0.03)} = 17\ \text{m}$$

Substituting into equation 14.24:

$$W_{ff} = 2W_0\left(\frac{R_{ff}}{R}\right)^2$$

$$\frac{1\ \text{mW}}{\text{cm}^2} = 2 \times \left(1.768 \times 10^2\ \frac{\text{mW}}{\text{cm}^2}\right) \times \left(\frac{17\ \text{m}}{R}\right)^2$$

$R = 320$ m

14.19 A radar that rotates 3 rpm operates at a frequency of 10 GHz and peak power of 2 MW. The PRF = 400/s, the pulse width is 3 μs, the beam width is 4½°, and the parabolic dish is 0.5 m in diameter. Calculate the **14.19**

(a) duty cycle,

duty cycle = pulse width × PRF

$$\text{duty cycle} = 3 \times 10^{-6}\ \frac{\text{sec}}{\text{pulse}} \times 400\,\frac{\text{pulses}}{\text{sec}} = 1.2 \times 10^{-3}$$

(b) What is the average power density at the aperture?

Equation 14.22;

$$P_{average} = P_{peak} \times \text{duty cycle} = 2 \times 10^6\ \text{W} \times 1.2 \times 10^{-3} = 2.4 \times 10^3\ \text{W}$$

Divide power by the area of the aperture to find the power density;

$$\frac{2.4 \times 10^3\,\text{W}}{\frac{\pi}{4} \times (0.5\ \text{m})^2} = 1.2 \times 10^4\ \frac{\text{W}}{\text{m}^2} = 1.2 \times 10^3\ \frac{\text{mW}}{\text{cm}^2}$$

(c) What is the power density at 50 m?

The power density, W_{ff}, in the far field, is given by equation 14.34

$$W_{ff} = 2W_0\left(\frac{R_{ff}}{R}\right)^2$$

W_0 = average power density at the aperture = 1.2×10^3 mW/cm^2

$$R_{ff} = \text{distance to far field} = \frac{D^2}{2.83\lambda} = \frac{D^2}{2.83\frac{c}{f}} = \frac{(0.5\ \text{m})^2}{2.83 \times \frac{3 \times 10^8\ \frac{\text{m}}{\text{sec}}}{10 \times 10^9\ \text{sec}^{-1}}} = 2.95\ \text{m}$$

R = downrange distance = 50 m

Substituting these vales into equation 14.34, we have

$$W_{ff} = 2 \times 1.2 \times 10^3\ \frac{\text{mW}}{\text{cm}^2}\left(\frac{2.95\ \text{m}}{50\ \text{m}}\right)^2 = 8.4\frac{\text{mW}}{\text{cm}^2}$$

(d) A person spends 1 hour at this distance. According to OSHA standards, is his exposure within acceptable limits?

The OSHA standard is 10 mW/cm^2 averaged over a 6 minute exposure time. Therefore the permissible exposure is given by

$$10\frac{\text{mW}}{\text{cm}^2} \times 6\ \text{min} = 60\frac{\text{mW} \cdot \text{min}}{\text{cm}^2}$$

Since the antenna is rotating at 3 RPM, during 6 minutes, the antenna rotates 18 times during this time period. Three RPM translates into 20 seconds per revolution. With a beam width of 4.5°, the actual exposure time is

$$\frac{4.5^\circ}{360^\circ} \times 20\frac{\text{sec}}{\text{revolution}} \times 18 \text{ revolutions} = 4.5 \text{ sec}$$

During 6 minutes, a person would actually only be in the beam for 4.5 seconds and the exposure is

$$8.4\frac{\text{mW}}{\text{cm}^2} \times 4.5 \text{ sec} \times \frac{1 \text{ min}}{60 \text{ sec}} = 0.63\frac{\text{mW}\cdot\text{hr}}{\text{cm}^2}$$

which is less than the maximum listed in the OSHA regulations, 29 CFR.1910.97.
Yes, the exposure is within acceptable limits.

14.20 Show by dimensional analysis that the unit for α in equation (14.36) is per meter. **14.20**

We will consider the two parts of the right hand side separately. First, we'll consider the expression to the left of the $\{\ \}^{1/2}$, and substitute the units for each of the respective symbols.

$$\omega\sqrt{\frac{\mu\varepsilon}{2}} = \frac{1}{\text{sec}}\left(\frac{\text{N}}{\text{A}^2} \times \frac{\text{C}^2}{\text{N}\cdot\text{m}^2}\right)^{\frac{1}{2}} = \frac{1}{\text{sec}} \times \frac{\text{C}}{\text{A}\cdot\text{m}} = \frac{1}{\text{sec}} \times \frac{\text{C}}{\frac{\text{C}}{\text{sec}} \times \text{m}} = \frac{1}{\text{m}}$$

Next, we will consider the expression inside the radical inside the $\{\ \}^{1/2}$

$$\frac{\sigma}{\omega\varepsilon} = \frac{1}{\text{ohm}\cdot\text{m}} \times \frac{1}{\frac{1}{\text{s}} \times \frac{\text{C}^2}{\text{N}\cdot\text{m}^2}}$$

$$\text{ohm} = \frac{\text{volt}}{\text{A}} = \frac{\text{V}}{\frac{\text{C}}{\text{sec}}} = \text{V} \times \frac{\text{sec}}{\text{C}}$$

$$\text{Since volt} = \frac{\text{J}}{\text{C}} = \frac{\text{N}\cdot\text{m}}{\text{C}}$$

$$\text{ohm} = \frac{\text{N}\cdot\text{m}}{\text{C}} \times \frac{\text{sec}}{\text{C}}$$

Substituting for $\dfrac{1}{\text{ohm}\cdot\text{m}}$

$$\frac{\sigma}{\omega\varepsilon}=\frac{1}{\dfrac{\text{N}\cdot\text{m}}{\text{C}}\cdot\dfrac{\text{s}}{\text{C}}\cdot\text{m}}\times\frac{1}{\dfrac{1}{\text{s}}\times\dfrac{\text{C}^2}{\text{N}\cdot\text{m}^2}}=\text{dimensionless}$$

$\alpha=\dfrac{1}{\text{m}}$, or "per meter

14.21 Calculate the wavelength of 100 MHz microwaves in muscle and in fat.

The wavelength, λ, of an electromagnetic wave that passes through a medium (which includes all biologic tissues) which absorbs energy from the EM wave, is given by equation 2.61. Numerical values for the parameters are given in table 14.17.

$$\lambda=\frac{\lambda_0}{\sqrt{K_e}}\left(\frac{1}{2}+\frac{1}{2}\sqrt{1+\left(\frac{\sigma}{\omega\varepsilon}\right)^2}\right)^{-\frac{1}{2}}$$

where

$$\lambda_0=\text{wavelength in free space}=\frac{c}{f}=\frac{3\times10^8\,\dfrac{\text{m}}{\text{sec}}}{100\times10^6\,\dfrac{1}{\text{sec}}}=3\text{ m}$$

K_e =dielectric coefficient = 71.7 (muscle); 7.45 (fat)
σ = conductivity = 0.889 $(\text{ohm}\cdot\text{m})^{-1}$ (muscle); 0.025 $(\text{ohm}\cdot\text{m})^{-1}$(fat)
ω = angular velocity = $2\pi f = 2\pi\times100\times10^6\text{ sec}^{-1}$

$$\varepsilon=\text{permittivity}=K_e\times\varepsilon_0=K_e\times8.85\times10^{-12}\,\frac{\text{C}^2}{\text{N}\cdot\text{m}^2}$$

Substituting the values for muscle, we have

$$\lambda = \frac{3\text{ m}}{\sqrt{71.7}} \times \left(\frac{1}{2} + \frac{1}{2}\sqrt{1 + \left(\frac{0.889}{\left(2 \times \pi \times 100 \times 10^{6}\right) \times \left(71.7 \times 8.85 \times 10^{-12}\ \frac{\text{C}^2}{\text{N} \cdot \text{m}^2}\right)} \right)^2} \right)^{\frac{1}{2}}$$

$\lambda = 0.27$ cm

Similarly, when the numerical values for fat are used, we find that

λ (fat, 100 MHz) = 106 cm

14.22 Calculate the penetration depth of 100 MHz radiation in fat and muscle. **14.22**

The penetration depth, δ, is given by equation 14.37

$$\delta = \frac{1}{\alpha}$$

where alpha, the linear absorption coefficient, is given by equation 14.36

$$\alpha = \omega\sqrt{\frac{\mu\varepsilon}{2}}\left\{\sqrt{\left[1 + \left(\frac{\sigma}{\omega\varepsilon}\right)^2\right]} - 1\right\}^{-\frac{1}{2}}$$

where

ω =angular frequency = $2\pi f = 2\pi \times 100 \times 10^{6}\ \text{sec}^{-1}$

μ_0 = permeability $= 4\pi \times 10^{-7}\,\frac{\text{N}}{\text{A}^2}$

ε = permittivity = $K_e \times \varepsilon_0 = K_e \times 8.85 \times 10^{-12}\,\frac{\text{C}^2}{\text{N} \cdot \text{m}^2}$;

K_e = 71.7 (muscle), 7.45 (fat)

σ = conductivity = 0.889 $(\text{ohm}\cdot\text{m})^{-1}$ (muscle); 0.025 $(\text{ohm}\cdot\text{m})^{-1}$(fat)

For fat, alpha is found by substituting the respective values into the equation for the absorptin coefficient:

$\alpha = 1.66\ \text{m}^{-1} = 0.0166\ \text{cm}^{-1}$

Penetration depth is:

$\delta\ (\text{fat}) = \frac{1}{\alpha} = \frac{1}{0.0166\ \text{cm}^{-1}} = 60$ cm is the maximum penetration depth in fat.

Similarly, for muscle

$$\alpha(\text{muscle}) = 15\ \text{m}^{-1} = 0.15\ \text{cm}^{-1}$$

$$\delta(\text{muscle}) = \frac{1}{\alpha} = \frac{1}{0.15\ \text{cm}^{-1}} = 6.7\ \text{cm}$$

14.23

14.23 How many dB attenuation will reduce a field of 800 mW/cm^2 to the power density of 1 mW/cm^2 recommended by ANSI for occupational exposure?

$$P_0 = 1\frac{\text{mW}}{\text{cm}^2}$$

$$P_i = 800\frac{\text{mW}}{\text{cm}^2}$$

Equation 14.27,

$$\text{dB} = 10\log\left(\frac{P_i}{P_0}\right) = 10 \times \log\frac{800\frac{\text{mW}}{\text{m}^2}}{1\frac{\text{mW}}{\text{m}^2}} = 29\ \text{dB}$$

14.24

14.24 (a) How far from a 10 GHz radar transmitter would the far field be expected to begin if the antenna diameter is 0.6 m?

Distance to the far field is estimated using equation 14.28

$$R_{ff} = \frac{D^2}{2.83\lambda} = \frac{D^2}{2.83\frac{c}{f}} = \frac{0.6^2}{2.83 \times \frac{3 \times 10^8 \ \frac{\text{m}}{\text{sec}}}{10 \times 10^9 \ \text{sec}^{-1}}} = 4.24 \text{ m}$$

(b) A power meter whose calibration at 10 GHz gives -10 dB as the power level that corresponds to 1 mW/cm^2, is used to measure the power density at the distance calculated in part (a). The meter reading is + 3.5 dB. What is the power density at this point?

The meter reads 13.5 dB above its 1 mW/cm^2 calibration point. From equation 14.27, we have

$$\text{dB gain} = 10 \log \frac{P_2}{P_1}$$

$$13.5 = 10 \log \frac{P_2}{1 \text{mW/cm}^2}$$

$$P_2 = 22.4 \frac{\text{mW}}{\text{cm}^2}$$

(c) At what distance from the antenna will the power density be down to -7 dB?

A meter reading of -7 dB is 3 dB above the 1 mW/cm^2 calibration point.

$$3 = 10 \log \frac{P_2}{1 \text{mW/cm}^2}$$

$$P_2 = 2 \frac{\text{mW}}{\text{cm}^2}$$

$P_1 = 22.4$ mW/cm^2 (from part (b))
$P_2 = 2$ mW/cm^2
$d_1 = 4.24$ m (from part (a))

The inverse square law is valid in the far field

$$\frac{P_1}{P_2} = \frac{d_2^2}{d_1^2}$$

$$\frac{22.4\,\dfrac{\text{mW}}{\text{cm}^2}}{2\,\dfrac{\text{mW}}{\text{cm}^2}} = \frac{d_2^2}{(4.24\text{ m})^2}$$

$d_2 = 14.19$ m

14.25

14.25 A microwave survey meter that reads in dB is calibrated to read -8 dB in a field whose power density is 0.01 mW/cm^2. It is then used in a radiation survey, and gives a reading of +2.5 dB at a certain point in a microwave field. What is the power density at that point?

The meter reads 10.5 dB above its 0.01 mW/cm^2 calibration point. The dB gain given by equation 14.27.

$$\text{dB gain} = 10 \log \frac{P_2}{P_1}$$

$$10.5 = 10 \log \frac{P_2}{0.01\,\text{mW/cm}^2}$$

$$P_2 = 0.11 \frac{\text{mW}}{\text{cm}^2}$$

14.26

14.26 A power meter reads 5 mW in a 10 GHz microwave field. If the standard gain horn has a gain of 16 dB at this frequency, and if a 30 dB attenuator was used, what is the power density in the microwave field?

The power density is given by equation 14.43

$$W = \frac{4\pi\alpha P}{\lambda^2 G_a}$$

where

α = attenuation factor, $\frac{P_0}{P_i}$, not the attenuation in dB

G = antenna gain, absolute power level, dB

P = absorbed power

$$\lambda = \text{wavelength} = \frac{c}{f} = \frac{3\times 10^8 \frac{\text{m}}{\text{sec}}}{10\times 10^9 \frac{1}{\text{sec}}} = 0.03\text{ m} = 3\text{ cm}$$

Attenuation factor, α:

$$\text{dB} = 10\log\frac{P_0}{P_i} = 10\log a$$

$$30 = 10\log a$$

$$\alpha = \text{anti-log}\frac{30}{10} = 1000$$

Antenna gain, G:

$$\text{dB} = 10\log\frac{P_o}{P_i} = 10\log G$$

$16\text{ dB} = 10\log G$
$G = \text{anti-log } 1.6 = 40$

Substituting these values into equation 14.43 gives:

$$W = \frac{4\times\pi\times 1000\times 5\text{ mW}}{(3\text{ cm})^2\times 40} = 175\frac{\text{mW}}{\text{cm}^2}$$

14.27

14.27 A radar whose beam width is 12° rotates at 3 rpm. What is the irradiation time for a person who remains in the scanning field for 0.1 hr?

The beam only irradiates the person for $\frac{12^\circ}{360^\circ} = 0.033$ part of the total time it is energized. Since 0.1 hr = 360 sec,

0.033 × 360 sec = 12 sec is the total irradiation time.

14.28

14.28 A radar has the following characteristics:

f = 10GHz
Peak Power = 2 MW
PRF = 200 pps
Pulse width = 5 μs
Beam width = 2.5°
Rotational frequency = 4 rpm
Dish diameter = 1.22 m

(a) What is the duty cycle?

duty cycle = pulse width × PRF

$$\text{duty cycle} = \frac{5\times10^{-6}\ \mu\,\text{sec}}{\text{pulse}} \times \frac{200\ \text{pulses}}{\text{sec}} = 1\times10^{-3}$$

(b) What is the average power?

Equation 14.22;

$$P_{avg} = P_{peak} \times \text{duty cycle} = 2\times10^{6}\ \text{W} \times (1\times10^{-3}) = 2000\ \text{W}$$

(c) What is the power density at 100 m?

The power density at 100 m may be estimated with equation 14.34

$$W_{ff} = 2W_0\left(\frac{R_{ff}}{R}\right)^2$$

where

W_0 = average power density at the aperture = $\dfrac{P}{A} = \dfrac{2000\text{ W}}{\dfrac{\pi}{4}(1.22\text{ m})^2}$

$W_0 = 1.71 \times 10^3\text{ W/m}^2 = 171\text{ mW/cm}^2$

R_{ff} = estimated distance to far field, given be equation 14.32 = $\dfrac{D^2}{2.83\lambda}$

$$R_{ff} = \frac{D^2}{2.83\dfrac{c}{f}} = \frac{(1.22\text{ m})^2}{2.83 \times \dfrac{3\times 10^8\ \dfrac{\text{m}}{\text{sec}}}{10\times 10^9\ \text{sec}^{-1}}} = 18\text{ m}$$

$$W(100\text{ m}) = 2 \times 171\frac{\text{mW}}{\text{cm}^2}\left(\frac{18\text{ m}}{100\text{ m}}\right)^2 = 11\frac{\text{mW}}{\text{cm}^2}$$

(d) A person spends 1 hour at this distance. According to OSHA standards, is his exposure within acceptable limits?

OSHA standards allow 10 mW/cm^2 averaged over a six minute period (29 CFR 1910.97)

$$\text{PEL} = 10\frac{\text{mW}}{\text{cm}^2}\times 6\text{ min} = 60\frac{\text{mW}\cdot\text{min}}{\text{cm}^2},$$

or a total radiant exposure of $600\dfrac{\text{mW}\cdot\text{min}}{\text{cm}^2}$ during a 1 hour exposure.

Here, the estimated radiant exposure during the 1 hour time interval at a distance of 100 meters is

$$H = \frac{2.5}{360}\times 60\text{ min}\times 11\frac{\text{mW}}{\text{cm}^2} = 4.6\frac{\text{mW}\cdot\text{min}}{\text{cm}^2}$$

Since estimated radiant exposure is less than $600\dfrac{\text{mW}\cdot\text{min}}{\text{cm}^2}$, the person did not exceed the OSHA standard.

14.29

14.29 A worker is simultaneously exposed to four different radiation sources. Measurements of the electric and magnetic fields produced by each source alone are listed below. Does this work area meet the ACGIH safety requirements listed in Table 14.20?

Radiation		Measured			MPE	
Source	f, MHz	E, V/m	H, A/m	E/H	E, V/m	H, A/m
1	7.5	140	0.2	700	245.6	2.17
2	30	24	0.07	342	61.4	0.54
3	950	13	0.18	73	109.3	0.29
4	2450	54	0.2	270	175.5	0.47

In the far field, $E/H = 377$ ohms. The E/H ratios for the measured values which are listed in the table above, show that none of the measurement locations is in the far field. Therefore, E fields and H fields must be separately considered. For 7.5 MHZ, the MPE's are listed in table 14.20 as

$$\text{MPE}(E) = \frac{1842}{f} = \frac{1842}{7.5} = 245.6\,\frac{\text{V}}{\text{m}}$$

$$\text{MPE}(H) = \frac{16.3}{f} = \frac{16.3}{7.5} = 2.17\,\frac{\text{A}}{\text{m}}$$

The E and H field MPE's for 30 MHz were also found directly in Table 14.20. For 950 and 2450 MHz, only the power density, S, is listed as $f/300$ mW/cm^2. For 950 MHz,

$$S = \frac{f}{300} = \frac{950}{300} = 3.17\,\frac{\text{mW}}{\text{cm}^2} = 31.7\,\frac{\text{W}}{\text{m}^2}$$

We can calculate the far field E and H fields corresponding to this MPE power density, and use these for the MPE's for the E and H fields. According to equation 14.44, the power density is related to the E and H fields by

$$S = \frac{E^2}{3770} = 37.7\,H^2$$

where
$S = \text{mW/cm}^2$
$E = \text{V/m}$
$H = \text{A/m}$

For the 950 MHz E field:

$$3.17 = \frac{E^2}{3770}$$

$E = 109.3$ V/m

and for the H field:

$3.17 = 37.7H^2$

$H = 0.29$ A/m

The values for the 2450 MHz E and H fields that are listed in the table above were calculated in a similar manner.

Equation 14.45 gives the safety criterion for exposure to multiple sources

$$\sum_i \frac{F_i}{L_i} \leq 1$$

where
$F_i = \text{i}^{\text{th}}$ field measurement
$L_i =$ MPE value for the ith radiation

For the E fields:

$$\frac{140}{245.6} + \frac{24}{61.4} + \frac{13}{109.3} + \frac{54}{175.5} = 1.39$$

For the H fields:

$$\frac{0.2}{2.17} + \frac{0.07}{0.54} + \frac{0.18}{0.29} + \frac{0.20}{0.47} = 1.23$$

The safety criteria for both E and H fields are exceeded and the work area does not meet the ACGIH safety standards.

14.30

14.30 An experimental setup employing a 2450 MHz magnetron produces a leakage radiation field of 100 mW/cm^2. It is proposed to use a chicken wire screen, 4 × 4/in., wire diameter = 0.025 in., as a shield. What will the power density be outside the proposed shield?

Equation 14.49 gives the attenuation factor for a wire mesh shield.

$$\frac{I_0}{I} = \frac{1}{4}\left\{\frac{\lambda}{a}\frac{1}{\ln\left[\dfrac{0.83e^{2\pi r/a}}{\left(e^{2\pi r/a}\right)-1}\right]}\right\}^2$$

Where

$$r = \frac{0.025''}{2} = 0.0125'' = 0.032 \text{ cm}$$

$$\lambda = \frac{c}{f} = \frac{3\times10^{10}\ \frac{\text{cm}}{\text{sec}}}{2450\times10^{6}\ \text{Hz}} = 12.24 \text{ cm}$$

Since 4 × 4 mesh is 1/4" between wires;

$$a = \left(\frac{1}{4}\right) \text{in.} = 0.635 \text{ cm}$$

$$\frac{\lambda}{a} = \frac{12.24 \text{ cm}}{0.635 \text{ cm}} = 19.276$$

$$\frac{r}{a} = \frac{0.032 \text{ cm}}{0.635 \text{ cm}} = 0.05$$

$$I_0 = 100\frac{\text{mW}}{\text{cm}^2}$$

Putting the above values into equation 14.49 and solving for I:

$$I = \frac{I_0}{\left\{\frac{1}{4}\left\{\frac{\lambda}{a}\frac{1}{\ln\left[\frac{0.83e^{2\pi r/a}}{\left(e^{2\pi r/a}\right)-1}\right]}\right\}\right\}^2} = \frac{100\frac{\text{mW}}{\text{cm}^2}}{\left\{\frac{1}{4}\times\left\{19.276\times\frac{1}{\ln\left[\frac{0.83\times e^{2\times\pi\times 0.05}}{\left(e^{2\times\pi\times 0.05}\right)-1}\right]}\right\}\right\}^2} = 1.4\frac{\text{mW}}{\text{cm}^2}$$

Index

D

E

F

G

H

I

K

Q

R

S